The new ShopIngenix... redesigned by an expert in the industry...

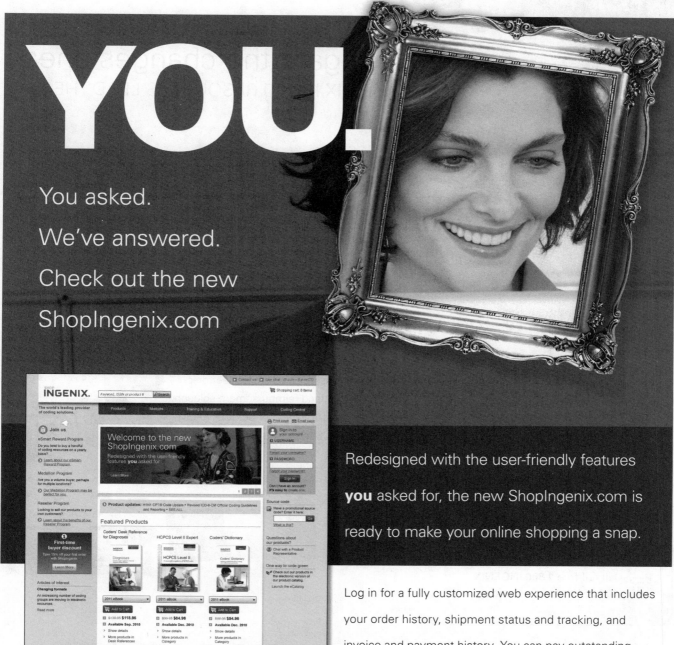

YOU.

You asked.

We've answered.

Check out the new

ShopIngenix.com

Redesigned with the user-friendly features **you** asked for, the new ShopIngenix.com is ready to make your online shopping a snap.

Log in for a fully customized web experience that includes your order history, shipment status and tracking, and invoice and payment history. You can pay outstanding invoices online, manage your address book, and get product recommendations based on your order history. But that's just the beginning. **Use source code FB11M to get 20% off your next ShopIngenix.com order.**

SHOP INGENIX.

www.shopingenix.com

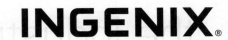
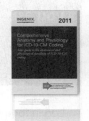 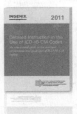 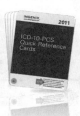 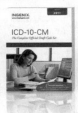 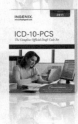

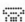

INGENIX®
*e*solutions

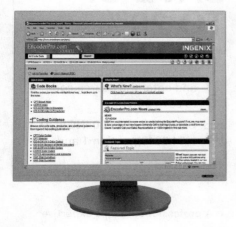

Electronic coding, billing and reimbursement products.

Ingenix provides a robust suite of eSolutions to solve a wide variety of coding, billing and reimbursement issues. As the industry moves to electronic products, you can rely on Ingenix to help support you through the transition.

← **Web-based applications for all markets**

← **Dedicated support**

← **Environmentally responsible**

Key Features and Benefits

Using eSolutions is a step in the right direction when it comes to streamlining your coding, billing and reimbursement practices. Ingenix eSolutions can help you save time and increase your efficiency with accurate and on-time content.

- **Simplify ICD-10 transition.** ICD-10 mapping tools provide crosswalks between ICD-9-CM and ICD-10 codes quickly and easily

- **Save time and money.** Ingenix eSolutions combine the content of over 37 code books and data files

- **Increase accuracy.** Electronic solutions are updated regularly so you know you're always working with the most current content available

- **Get the training and support you need.** Convenient, monthly webinars and customized training programs are available to meet your specific needs

- **Rely on a leader in health care.** Ingenix has been producing quality coding products for over 26 years. All of the expert content that goes into our books goes into our electronic resources

- **Get Started.** Visit **shopingenix.com/ eSolutions** for product listing

SAVE UP TO 20%

with source code FB11B

 Visit **www.shopingenix.com** and enter the source code to save 20%.

 Call toll-free **1.800.INGENIX** (464.3649), option 1 and save 15%.

Ingenix | Information is the Lifeblood of Health Care | Call toll-free 1.800.INGENIX (464.3649), option 1.

100% Money Back Guarantee If our merchandise ever fails to meet your expectations, please contact our Customer Service Department toll-free at 1.800.INGENIX (464.3649), option 1, for an immediate response. Software: Credit will be granted for unopened packages only.

Also available from your medical bookstore or distributor.

INGENIX®

2011 Essential Coding Resources

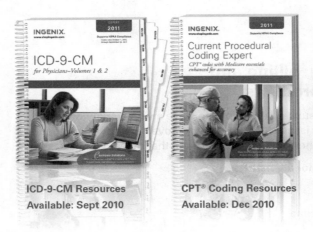

ICD-9-CM Resources
Available: Sept 2010

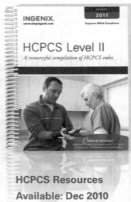

CPT® Coding Resources
Available: Dec 2010

HCPCS Resources
Available: Dec 2010

2011 Essential Coding Resources

Looks can be deceiving. Competitors attempt to imitate Ingenix code books because interpreting coding and reimbursement rules correctly and understanding the professional workflow is what we've helped coding professionals do successfully for over 25 years. Count on Ingenix to deliver accurate information, familiar features, industry-leading content, and innovative additions that help you improve coding practices, comply with HIPAA code set regulations, and realize proper reimbursement.

← A professional team's expertise

← Trusted and proven ICD-9-CM, CPT® and HCPCS coding resources

← Industry-leading content

← More value, competitive prices

Key Features and Benefits

Select from a range of formats for your ICD-9-CM, CPT,® and HCPCS coding resources to fit your individual preferences, skill level, business needs, and budget—you can trust your resource to be accurate and complimentary to your daily work when it's under an Ingenix cover.

2011 ICD-9-CM

Physician, Hospital, Home Health, and Skilled Nursing (with Inpatient Rehabilitation and Hospices) editions available

- New Look! Modified font and more vibrant colors increase readability

- New! Highlighted coding informational notes

- New! Snap-in tab dividers (*Expert* spiral editions only)

- More official coding tips and ICD-10 Spotlight codes

- Hallmark additional digit required symbols, intuitive color-coded symbols and alerts, QuickFlip™ color bleed tabs, dictionary headers, and symbol keys

2011 Current Procedural Coding Expert

- Code "Resequencing" identification

- Interventional radiology guidance section

- Reimbursement and mid-year changes information not found in the American Medical Association's CPT® code books

- Easy-to-navigate design

- Comprehensive and up-to-date listings with an extensive, user-friendly index

- PQRI icons and appendix

2011 HCPCS Level II Expert

- Comprehensive code updates for accurate reporting of supplies and services in physician, hospital outpatient, and ASC settings

- User-friendly format and expanded index to ease code look-up

- Important coding indicators and icons, PQRI icons, detailed illustrations, glossary of terms, and special MUEs

---

Ingenix | Information is the Lifeblood of Health Care | Call toll-free 1.800.INGENIX (464.3649), option 1.

100% Money Back Guarantee If our merchandise ever fails to meet your expectations, please contact our Customer Service Department toll-free at 1.800.INGENIX (464.3649), option 1, for an immediate response. Software: Credit will be granted for unopened packages only.

Also available from your medical bookstore or distributor. CPT is a registered trademark of the American Medical Association.   FB11D

2012

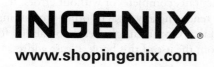

www.shopingenix.com

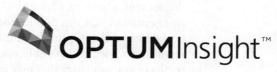

Ingenix is now OptumInsight, part of Optum.
Learn more inside.

Comprehensive Anatomy and Physiology for ICD-10-CM Coding

Publisher's Notice

Comprehensive Anatomy and Physiology for ICD-10-CM Coding is designed to be an accurate and authoritative source of information regarding coding and every reasonable effort has been made to ensure accuracy and completeness of the content. However, OptumInsight makes no guarantee, warranty, or representation that this publication is accurate, complete, or without errors. It is understood that OptumInsight is not rendering any legal or other professional services or advice in this publication and that OptumInsight bears no liability for any results or consequences that may arise from the use of this book. Please address all correspondence to:

OptumInsight
2525 Lake Park Blvd
West Valley City, UT 84120

Our Commitment To Accuracy

OptumInsight is committed to producing accurate and reliable materials.

To report corrections, please visit www.shopingenix.com/accuracy or email accuracy@ingenix.com. You can also reach customer service by calling 1.800.464.3649, option 1.

Copyright

Made in the USA

ISBN 978-1-60151-480-6

Acknowledgments

Michael Grambo, *Product Manager*

Karen Schmidt, BSN, *Technical Director*

Stacy Perry, *Manager, Desktop Publishing*

Lisa Singley, *Project Manager*

Jillian Harrington, MHA, CPC, CPC-P, CPC-I, CCS-P, MHP, *Clinical/Technical Editor*

Kristin Bentley, BS, CPC, *Clinical/Technical Editor*

Kelly Canter, BA, RHIT, CCS, *Clinical/Technical Editor*

Beth Ford, RHIT, CCS, *Clinical/Technical Editor*

Deborah C. Hall, *Clinical/Technical Editor*

Karen Kachur, RN, CPC, *Clinical/Technical Editor*

Temeka Lewis, MBA, CCS, *Clinical/Technical Editor*

Nannette Orme, CCS-P, CPC, CPMA, CEMC, *Clinical/Technical Editor*

Karen Prescott, CMM, CPC, CPC-I, CCS-P, *Clinical/Technical Editor*

Nichole VanHorn, CPC, CCS-P, *Clinical/Technical Editor*

Tracy Betzler, *Desktop Publishing Specialist*

Hope M. Dunn, *Desktop Publishing Specialist*

Kimberli Turner, *Editor*

Kate Holden, *Editor*

Contents

Welcome to Comprehensive Anatomy and Physiology for ICD-10-CM Coding

The transition from ICD-9-CM to ICD-10-CM marks a sea change in coding in the United States. Not only have code choices increased five-fold, but the code descriptions themselves are much more specific. The greater level of detail in ICD-10-CM demands that coders have an in-depth knowledge of anatomy, physiology, and pathophysiology if they are to select the most appropriate code in the new system. OptumInsight's *Comprehensive Anatomy and Physiology for ICD-10-CM Coding* is a great initial step in that education.

Before delving into the details of anatomy and physiology, however, it is important to understand the transition from ICD-9-CM to ICD-10-CM and the differences between the code sets.

ICD-9-CM to ICD-10-CM Transition

The codes within ICD-9-CM fall woefully short of today's medical reporting needs. ICD-9-CM was created more than 25 years ago as a modern and expandable system that was then only partially filled. Thousands of codes have been added to ICD-9-CM over the years to classify new procedures and diseases, and today the remaining space in ICD-9-CM procedure and diagnosis coding systems cannot accommodate new technologies or new understanding of diseases.

In response to ICD-9-CM's shortcomings, new coding systems were developed and soon will be implemented in the United States. The World Health Organization (*WHO*) created and adopted ICD-10 in 1994 and it has been used in much of the world since then. This system is the basis for the new U.S. diagnosis coding system, International Classification of Diseases, version 10, clinical modification (ICD-10-CM).

Concurrent to the clinical modification of ICD-10 by the National Center for Health Statistics (*NCHS*), the Centers for Medicare and Medicaid Services (*CMS*) commissioned 3M Health Information Management to develop a new procedure coding system to replace volume 3 of ICD-9-CM, used for inpatient procedure coding. Now that the coding systems have been designed and written, they need only be implemented, but progress is slow. The government is moving cautiously toward implementation, partly because the scope of change is massive and will profoundly affect all care providers, payers, and government agencies, but also because the change is massive and costly enough to carry considerable political impact.

On January 16, 2009, the Department of Health and Human Services published a final rule in the *Federal Register,* 45 CFR part 162, "HIPAA Administrative Simplification: Modifications to Medical Data Code Set Standards to Adopt ICD-10-CM and ICD-10-PCS" (downloadable at http://edocket.access.gpo.gov/2009/pdf/E9-743.pdf). This final rule adopts modifications to standard medical data code sets for coding diagnoses and inpatient hospital procedures by adopting ICD-10-CM for diagnosis coding, including the Official ICD-10-CM Guidelines for Coding and Reporting, and ICD-10-PCS for inpatient hospital procedure coding, effective October 1,

DEFINITIONS

CMS. Centers for Medicare and Medicaid Services. Federal agency that provides health insurance for more than 74 million Americans through Medicare, Medicaid, and Children's Health Insurance Program. CMS contracted with 3M HIS to develop a new procedure coding system (ICD-10-PCS). Find CMS at http://www.cms.gov/.

NCHS. National Center for Health Statistics. U.S. government agency that, jointly with CMS, refines the diagnostic portion of ICD-9-CM and is responsible for the clinical modification of ICD-10. NCHS holds several hearings a year to consider changes or additions to diagnosis coding. Find NCHS at http://www.cdc.gov/nchs.

WHO. World Health Organization. International agency that maintains an international nomenclature of diseases, causes of death, and public health practices. WHO, with advice from participating countries, developed ICD-9 to track morbidity and mortality statistics worldwide. It recently updated diagnosis coding with ICD-10. Find WHO at http://www.who.int/en.

2013. The most current 2011 draft update release is available for public viewing, and additional updates are expected before implementation. At this time, ICD-10 codes are not valid for any purpose or use other than for reporting mortality data for death certificates. This does not mean it is not time to begin preparing, however. Now is the time to prepare, as the 2013 date is approaching rapidly, and there will be no grace period for using the new codes.

Everyone in facilities will be affected: coders, human resources staff, accountants, information systems staff, physicians—just to name a few. The proposed codes provide tremendous opportunities for disease and procedure tracking but also create enormous challenges. Computer hardware and software, medical documentation, and the revenue cycle are just three elements of medical reimbursement that will be shaken when implementation occurs.

Understanding the changes the World Health Organization made in moving from ICD-9 to ICD-10 is a good basis for learning about the clinical modifications to ICD-10. The first clue to the revisions is in the full title: International Statistical Classification of Diseases and Related Health Problems. WHO felt this change would not only clarify the classification's content and purpose, but show how the scope of the system has moved beyond the classification of disease and injuries to the coding of ambulatory care conditions and risk factors frequently encountered in primary care.

Overall, the 10th revision goes into greater clinical detail than does ICD-9-CM and addresses information about previously classified diseases, as well as those diseases discovered since the last revision. Conditions are grouped with general epidemiological purposes and the evaluation of health care in mind. New features have been added, and conditions have been reorganized, although the format and conventions of the classification remain unchanged for the most part.

Other adaptations of the ICD include:

- International Classification of Diseases for Oncology, third edition (ICD-O-3)
- International Classification of External Causes of Injury (ICECI)
- International Classification of Primary Care, second edition (ICPC-2)
- The ICD-10 for Mental and Behavioral Disorders Diagnostic Criteria for Research
- The ICD-10 for Mental and Behavioral Disorders Clinical Descriptions and Diagnostic Guidelines

In the United States, the clinical modification of ICD-10, ICD-10-CM, will replace the clinical modification of ICD-9, ICD-9-CM. The parent classification system, the International Classification of Disease (ICD), is owned and copyrighted by WHO, which publishes the classification. As with ICD-9-CM, the WHO authorized the development of an adaptation of ICD-10 for use in the United States. This adaptation, the clinical modification (CM), must conform to WHO conventions for the ICD.

If many of the codes considered new in ICD-10 seem familiar to users of ICD-9-CM, it is because ICD-10 is a further evolution of the ICD-9 classification, as ICD-10-CM is a further evolution of ICD-9-CM. The underlying basic structure, conventions, and philosophy remain the same. The clinical modification in use in the United States (ICD-9-CM) has been maintained and updated annually since 1985. The following example using angina pectoris classifications illustrates the evolution from the preclinical modification ICD-9 version to the current 2011 version of ICD-10-CM:

ICD-9

413	Angina pectoris

ICD-9-CM

411.1	Intermediate coronary syndrome (includes unstable angina)
413.0	Angina decubitus
413.1	Prinzmetal angina
413.9	Other and unspecified angina pectoris

ICD-10 and ICD-10-CM

All diseases of the circulatory system appear under the letter "I" in ICD-10.

I20.0	Unstable angina
I20.1	Angina pectoris with documented spasm — (includes Prinzmetal angina)
I20.8	Other forms of angina pectoris — (includes angina of effort and stenocardia)
I20.9	Angina pectoris, unspecified

ICD Structure

The WHO published ICD-10 in three volumes: an index, an instructional manual, and a tabular list. ICD-10-CM will be published in two volumes: an index and a tabular list.

Tabular List

Volume 1 of ICD-9-CM contains the tabular listing of alphanumeric codes. The same hierarchical organization of ICD-9 applies to ICD-10: All codes with the same first three digits have common traits.

Each digit beyond three adds more specificity. In ICD-10, valid codes can contain anywhere from three to five digits. However, ICD-10-CM for use in the United States has been expanded with valid codes containing anywhere from three to seven characters. In some instances, the final character may be an alphabetic character, known as an alpha extension, and not a number. In some cases, the use of a "reserve" subclassification (identified as an "x") has been incorporated into codes that continue with greater specificity beyond the fifth digit to allow for built-in expansion within that established level of specificity. For example:

H83.3 Noise effects on inner ear
    Acoustic trauma of inner ear
    Noise-induced hearing loss of inner ear

H83.3x	**Noise effects on inner ear**	
	H83.3x1	**Noise effects on right inner ear**
	H83.3x2	**Noise effects on left inner ear**
	H83.3x3	**Noise effects on inner ear, bilateral**
	H83.3x9	**Noise effects on inner ear, unspecified ear**

This reserve subclassification, and simply the additional digits themselves, allow for more specific codes. This additional specificity can present a hurdle for some coders who may have not had a great deal of training in anatomy and physiology in the past. New terms are being used in the ICD-10-CM system, and they may be different from what the physician is using in their documentation. For this reason, coders need to be well educated about anatomy and physiology at a deeper level than was previously required for ICD-9-CM coding.

Alphabetic Index

In ICD-9-CM, the alphabetic index is a reference for the tabular list. As in the ICD-9-CM index, terms in the ICD-10 index are arranged alphabetically by diagnosis. This is no different for ICD-10-CM. Therefore, a code for a supernumerary nipple would be accessed by looking under "Supernumerary," then "nipple."

Alphabetical Index to Diseases and Nature of Injury in ICD-10-CM

> **Supernumerary (congenital)**
> aortic cusps Q23.8
> auditory ossicles Q16.3
> bone Q79.8
> breast Q83.1
> carpal bones Q74.0
> cusps, heart valve NEC Q24.8
>   aortic Q23.8
>   mitral Q23.2
>   pulmonary Q22.3
> digit(s) Q69.9
> ear (lobule) Q17.0
> fallopian tube Q50.6
> finger Q69.0
> hymen Q52.4
> kidney Q63.0
> lacrimonasal duct Q10.6
> lobule (ear) Q17.0
> mitral cusps Q23.2
> muscle Q79.8
> nipple(s) Q83.3
> organ or site not listed — *see* Accessory
> ossicles, auditory Q16.3
> ovary Q50.31
> oviduct Q50.6
> pulmonary, pulmonary cusps Q22.3
> rib Q76.6
>   cervical or first (syndrome) Q76.5
> roots (of teeth) K00.2
> spleen Q89.09
> tarsal bones Q74.2
> teeth K00.1
> testis Q55.29
> thumb Q69.1
> toe Q69.2
> uterus Q51.2
> vagina Q52.1
> vertebra Q76.49

Code Structure

All codes in ICD-10 and ICD-10-CM are alphanumeric as opposed to the strictly numeric characters in the main classification of ICD-9-CM. Of the 26 available letters, all but the letter U is used, which is reserved for additions and changes that may need to be incorporated in the future or to resolve classification difficulties that may arise between revisions.

Codes for terrorism were created after September 11, 2001, within the framework of ICD-10 and ICD-9-CM. They have been incorporated into ICD-9-CM since 2002 and proposed for implementation in ICD-10 as U codes for terrorism and have not officially been adopted by WHO. If the codes are adopted, they will be identified as U.S. codes by an asterisk to distinguish them from official ICD codes.

In ICD-10-CM, external causes due to acts of terrorism are classified to code category Y38. This category includes seven-character codes that identify injuries resulting from acts of terrorism, defined as "the unlawful use of force or violence against persons or property to intimidate or coerce a government, the civilian population, or any segment thereof, in furtherance of political or social objective." An additional code from category Y92 should be assigned to specify place of occurrence. The seventh character reports the encounter as A (initial encounter), D (subsequent encounter), or S (sequela).

ICD-9-CM

Diseases of Arteries, Arterioles, and Capillaries (440–449)

440	Atherosclerosis
441	Aortic aneurysm and dissection
442	Other aneurysm
443	Other peripheral vascular disease
444	Arterial embolism and thrombosis
445	Atheroembolism
446	Polyarteritis nodosa and allied conditions
447	Other disorders of arteries and arterioles
448	Disease of capillaries
449	Septic arterial embolism

ICD-10-CM

Diseases of Arteries, Arterioles and Capillaries (I70–I79)

I70	Atherosclerosis
I71	Aortic aneurysm and dissection
I72	Other aneurysm
I73	Other peripheral vascular diseases
I74	Arterial embolism and thrombosis
I75	Atheroembolism
I76	Septic arterial embolism
I77	Other disorders of arteries and arterioles
I78	Diseases of capillaries
I79	Disorders of arteries, arterioles and capillaries in diseases classified elsewhere

The code structures of ICD-9-CM and ICD-10-CM are similar in that each classification system is maintained to be as congruent to the other as possible, pending transition. As ICD-9-CM expands its classification and code structure, ICD-10-CM is similarly expanded and maintained.

Though the use of alphabetic characters I and O may be confused with the numbers 1 and 0, coders should remember that the first character in ICD-10-CM is always a letter. The second character is a numeral, followed by a numeral or alphabetic character in the third character space. Codes may also contain an alphabetic extension in the final character position or a reserve subclassification, denoted as "x."

✓ QUICK TIP

Be careful of alphabetic characters I and O versus numbers 1 and 0. They look similar, but remember that the first character in any ICD-10-CM code is always a letter and the second is always a number. Others could vary, so be cautious with code assignment.

Importance of Anatomy and Physiology to ICD-10-CM

Throughout the many years they have used the ICD-9-CM system, providers have become used to the system's terminology, and many document cases based on that terminology. ICD-9-CM also has many codes that are fairly general; for instance, there are many unspecified or unlisted codes that must be used because more specific codes are not available for the conditions the patient is presenting with. In ICD-10-CM, this lack of specificity is diminished significantly.

ICD-10-CM will require coders to have a greater understanding of human anatomy, physiology, and disease pathology for multiple reasons. First, the code set itself is in many cases much more specific. For example:

Coding for Unspecified Cellulitis and Abscess of Finger

ICD-9-CM		ICD-10-CM	
681.00	Unspecified cellulitis and abscess of finger	L02.511	Cutaneous abscess of right hand
		L02.512	Cutaneous abscess of left hand
		L02.519	Cutaneous abscess of unspecified hand
		L03.011	Cellulitis of right finger
		L03.012	Cellulitis of left finger
		L03.019	Cellulitis of unspecified finger
		L03.021	Acute lymphangitis of right finger
		L03.022	Acute lymphangitis of left finger
		L03.029	Acute lymphangitis of unspecified finger

What was described as an "unspecified" cellulitis or abscess of the finger in ICD-9-CM will now require that the coder review the documentation and determine whether the patient was seen for a cutaneous abscess, cellulitis, or acute lymphangitis. Also, notice that the code set specifies laterality, another level of detail provided by ICD-10-CM.

This greater level of detail will demand that providers beef up their documentation. Previously, a push for a higher level of documentation tended to focus on a few areas—particularly evaluation and management coding in the outpatient realm in addition to various items on the inpatient side. With ICD-10-CM, there will be a big push for documentation improvement across the board for diagnostic information, but much of that push will need to come from the coders. Coders well trained in human anatomy, physiology, and pathophysiology will be able to help providers document accurately what is going on clinically with the patient.

How to Use the *Comprehensive Anatomy and Physiology for ICD-10-CM Coding*

The *Comprehensive Anatomy and Physiology for ICD-10-CM Coding* has been set up to allow coders to study a single body area or organ system at a time if they wish or to review the entire body if that suits their study needs. The body has been broken down into 13 different areas and systems.

- Introduction to the Human Body
- Integumentary System
- Skeletal System and Articulations
- Muscular System
- Nervous System

- Endocrine System
- Cardiovascular System
- Blood and Blood-Forming Organs
- Lymphatic System
- Respiratory System
- Digestive System
- Urinary System
- Reproductive System

Within each chapter is an anatomic overview, providing the coder with a basic knowledge of the anatomy and physiology of the particular body area or organ system. Following the overview is a detailed comparison of the ICD-9-CM and ICD-10-CM codes affecting that section, and how anatomy, physiology, and pathophysiology differ between the two code sets. For example, what is the difference between a cutaneous abscess, cellulitis, and acute lymphangitis? Detailed illustrations are provided for both the basic anatomy and the comparison sections.

Tables are used to illustrate some of the differences between the coding systems. Note that the tables are only examples of the potential mappings between ICD-9-CM and ICD-10-CM and may not show all of the codes for a given situation. These tables demonstrate the anatomic and physiologic terms included in both code sets. For detailed information on ICD-9-CM to ICD-10-CM mapping, see *Ingenix's ICD-10-CM Mappings*. This product provides full mapping tables from the Centers for Medicare and Medicaid Services GEM files for all codes included in those tables.

Also included in the ***Comprehensive Anatomy and Physiology for ICD-10-CM Coding*** are knowledge review questions for each of the chapters to enable the coder to test himself or herself on information in the chapter. Answers as well as rationales are included for the knowledge review questions.

To assist in the overall learning experience, key information has been included in the margins of the book, including interesting anatomy and physiology facts, key points, quick tips, clinical points, definitions, and more. Although much of the medical terminology used in the ICD-10-CM manual is defined within the text itself, there are times when the text doesn't lend itself to this information. In these cases, the terms are placed in bold and italicized font, and the definition can be found in the margin.

Summary

The ***Comprehensive Anatomy and Physiology for ICD-10-CM Coding*** is a great start to learning about ICD-10-CM. Although it is not meant to teach coders how to code under this new code set, it does help them understand the anatomy and physiology differences, as well as provide a ready reference to use side by side with their books when they are learning ICD-10-CM. The new coding system is a much-needed change, and although this is just one part of the training needed before October 2013, it is an important—and essential—first step in coder education.

 KEY POINT

Mapping tables found in the text are simply examples. They will not provide full mapping details. For detailed mapping, see *Ingenix's ICD-10-CM Mappings*.

Chapter 1

Introduction to the Human Body

Anatomy Overview

The human body is a complex organization of body areas and organ systems. Although coders often look at one particular disease process or a group of injuries at a time, it is also important to be aware of certain aspects of the overall function of the human body, as well as the layout of its anatomy. This chapter discusses structural organization of the human body, basic life processes, and anatomical positions and briefly outlines organ systems and body areas.

Structural Organization of the Human Body

Although people tend to think of themselves as simply human beings, the human body really exists on several different levels of organization. From smallest to broadest, these levels include:

- Chemical
- Cellular
- Tissue
- Organ
- System
- Organismal

The most basic level, the **chemical** level, breaks the body down into its most minute parts. Humans are made up of chemicals, atoms, and molecules, which make up the body's cells. Oxygen, carbon, nitrogen, and hydrogen are all important building blocks for genetic material, organs, and everything needed to keep the body functioning on a daily basis.

The cellular level of organization includes cells, the smallest living units in the body and the building blocks for all organs, muscles, blood, and more. Cells serve many roles throughout the body, ranging from helping preserve *homeostasis*, to serving as structural support and helping fight off infections. The principal parts of a cell are the plasma membrane, the cytoplasm, and the nucleus, where *DNA* is housed. A *chromosome*, which is a single molecule of DNA, contains thousands of genes that direct the aspects of cellular structure and function.

The **tissue** level of structural organization is next; it is at this point that items more regularly recognizable in the coding world appear. There are four basic types of tissue found in the human body:

- Epithelial tissue
- Connective tissue
- Muscle tissue
- Nervous tissue

 DEFINITIONS

chromosome. Single thread of genetic material, or DNA, that controls the aspects of cellular function and structure, as well as the inheritance of certain traits.

DNA. Deoxyribonucleic acid. Molecule of genetic information that is found in the nucleus of a cell.

homeostasis. State of relative constancy within the internal environment of the human body.

Figure 1.1: Tissue

Four types of tissue

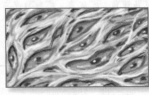

Connective tissue

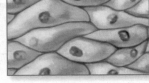

Epithelial tissue

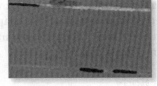

Muscle tissue

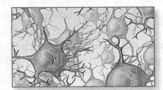

Nervous tissue

Epithelial tissue covers the surfaces of the body and lines body cavities, ducts, and hollow organs, and forms glands in the body. It consists of cells arranged in continuous sheets, in single layers or multiple layers, depending on the thickness of the tissue in that area. Some examples of epithelial tissue are the skin, the lining of the peritoneum, and the thyroid gland.

Connective tissue is found distributed throughout several different areas of the body, making it one of the most abundant tissues found in the human body. Like epithelial tissue, it serves several functions within the body. Connective tissue protects and insulates internal organs, serves as the major transport system throughout the body, supports and strengthens other body tissue, and is the main site of stored energy reserves as well as immune responses. The five main types of connective tissue found in the body are:

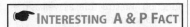

☞ INTERESTING A & P FACT

Connective tissue binds organs together, stores energy reserves as fat, and helps provide immunity.

- **Loose connective tissue:** Fat tissue, subcutaneous layer of the skin
- **Dense connective tissue:** Tendons, ligaments, fascia
- **Cartilage:** Ends of long bones, larynx, trachea
- **Osseous tissue:** Bones
- **Blood:** Within blood vessels and heart

Muscle tissue is made up of elongated cells that are often referred to as muscle fiber. This muscle fiber serves many purposes within the body, such as maintaining posture, generating body heat, and producing the many different movements of the body. There are three types of muscle tissue: skeletal, cardiac, and smooth. Skeletal muscle tissue is found in various places throughout the body and is usually attached to bones. It is commonly referred to as voluntary muscle because its activity, either contraction or relaxation, is under conscious control. Cardiac muscle forms the walls of the heart. It is an involuntary muscle fiber, meaning that its contractions are not consciously controlled. Smooth muscle tissue is also an involuntary type of muscle fiber that is found in the walls of hollow internal structures of the body. For example, smooth muscle can be found in the blood vessels, the intestines, and the urinary bladder. These fibers work involuntarily to move and process food through the gastrointestinal tract, move fluids through the body, and eliminate wastes, among other functions.

Nervous tissue is made up of two main types of cells: neurons and neuroglia. The neurons are the main nerve cells and are sensitive to various stimuli. They take that stimuli and convert it into an electrical impulse, to be sent off to various other parts of the body such as another neuron, muscle tissue, glands, or the brain. Neuroglia cells nourish and protect the neurons, which are very fragile cells.

Organs make up the next level of body structure. Each organ consists of various types of tissue and has a specific function to perform to help the body operate properly. Some examples of organs in the human body include the stomach, the lungs, the skin, and the brain. Proper function of these organs is vital to maintaining good health.

The **system** level of body structure groups related organs together that have some commonality in function. There are 11 commonly accepted systems of the human body, which are described throughout this book in various chapters.

- Integumentary system
- Skeletal system
- Muscular system
- Nervous system
- Endocrine system
- Cardiovascular system
- Lymphatic system
- Respiratory system
- Digestive system
- Urinary system
- Reproductive system

The *integumentary* system includes skin as well as the structures contained in the skin, such as the hair, the nails, and the sweat and oil glands. One of its main purposes is to protect the body. The *skeletal* system consists of the bones and joints. It supports and protects the body and aids in movement. The *muscular* system includes the skeletal muscle tissue throughout the body and produces movement through voluntary muscle control.

The *nervous* system consists of the brain, spinal cord, and nerves, as well as the special sensory organs such as the eyes and the ears. This system plays many important roles for the body, mainly involving monitoring outside activity and communicating that activity to the brain to regulate body activities. The *endocrine* system includes all of the hormone-producing glands throughout the body, such as the hypothalamus and the pituitary gland, as well as any hormone-producing cells that reside in another part of the body. These glands and cells release hormones that help regulate various body activities.

The *cardiovascular* system includes the blood, the heart, and all of the blood vessels. Its main function is to pump the blood throughout the body to carry oxygen and nutrients to the cells and to carry wastes away from the cells. The *lymphatic* system includes lymph nodes and vessels, as well as the lymphatic vessels. It also contains the spleen, the thymus, and the tonsils. One of the lymphatic system's main functions is to return fluid and protein to the

 CLINICAL NOTE

Each organ is made up of several layers of tissue and membrane, each with its own function.

 QUICK TIP

Sometimes organs are part of more than one system, as they may serve several functions. For example, the pancreas is typically included in both the digestive and endocrine systems.

bloodstream. The *respiratory* system consists of the lungs and the air passageways. Its main function is to transfer the oxygen from the inhaled air into something that is usable by the bloodstream, as well as transfer the waste carbon dioxide from the bloodstream into the exhaled air.

The *digestive* system includes all of the organs and accessory structures of the gastrointestinal tract, which include the mouth, the pharynx, the esophagus, the stomach, the small and large intestines, the anus, the salivary glands, the liver, the gallbladder, and the pancreas. The main purpose of the digestive system is to break down food both physically and chemically so that the body can absorb it. The *urinary* system consists of the kidneys, ureters, urinary bladder, and the urethra. Its main function is to produce, store, and eliminate urine. The main function of the *reproductive* system, which contains the reproductive organs, is to produce gametes (oocytes or sperm) in order to reproduce and create a new organism. In males, the testes, epididymis, vas deferens, and penis make up the reproductive organs. In females, the reproductive organs consist of the ovaries, fallopian tubes, uterus, and vagina.

The final and highest level of structural organization of the body is the **organismal** level. The organism is a living, breathing creature. Each of these previous levels rolls up into the organism, a single living person.

Basic Life Processes

Some basic life processes within humans separate us from nonliving things. Problems with these processes are the roots of many of the diseases and disorders that coders deal with each day in their health care organizations. Below is a discussion of six of these basic life processes: metabolism, responsiveness, movement, growth, differentiation, and reproduction.

Metabolism is really an aggregate of all of the various chemical processes that take place within the body. It has two aspects: catabolism and anabolism. Catabolism is the process of breaking down a very complex chemical substance into a simpler one, such as breaking down a protein in food into its component parts such as amino acids. Anabolism is the opposite. It takes those smaller component parts and creates complex chemical substances. In anabolism, the body may take those amino acids it broke down before and build them into new proteins for building muscles and bones throughout the body. The metabolism is a comprehensive bodily function that is necessary for growth, generation of energy, distribution of nutrients, and elimination of wastes throughout the body.

Responsiveness denotes the body's ability to respond to stimuli, be they internal or external. If the body's ability to respond to internal and external environments is diminished, its ability to survive is also diminished. In many instances nerve cells respond to stimuli by telling muscle cells to contract or relax, causing movement, or by raising or lowering body temperature in response to the environment. There are many ways the body can respond to different circumstances, all helping it to survive and maintain health.

Movement is a basic life process that is often associated simply with the external movements of appendages. However, movement also occurs within the body, such as blood moving through the vessels, food moving through the digestive tract, or white blood cells traveling to damaged tissue to speed healing.

Growth is the body's ability to grow from its initial size at birth to its adult size. The body can grow by adding additional cells, by having existing cells grow larger, or by having the material that surrounds the cells expand, such as in the case of bone growth.

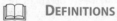

INTERESTING A & P FACT

The body's metabolism tends to slow down as it ages, meaning that these chemical processes are potentially slowing down overall.

📖 **DEFINITIONS**

peristalsis. Symmetrical contraction and relaxation of muscle tissue in a tube-shaped organ that pushes something along it; for example, peristalsis in the digestive tract propels food through its structures

Differentiation is a process whereby unspecialized cells become specialized. Most of the cells in the body are highly specialized in structure and function, with one exception, the *stem cell*. Stem cells, found in the red bone marrow, are considered unspecialized and can undergo differentiation to become one of several types of cells, such as a red blood cell or a white blood cell.

Reproduction is the final basic life process this section examines. This process refers not only to creating a new human being, but also to producing new cells and new tissues for repair. Because cells and tissues constantly die, the body must continually reproduce those cells and tissues. The body also reproduces cells and tissues to repair wounds from traumatic injury.

Body Positions

There are various terms that describe the body in different positions, as well as references that describe imaginary planes that transect the body. These terms are crucial to coders, especially in ICD-10-CM. With the higher level of specificity found in the new coding system, providers often use these terms to describe specific areas of the body affected by a condition. It is important for all coders to be very familiar with these terms and understand their use.

When a body is in the *anatomical position*, the patient is in the forward-facing position, with the head level, and eyes facing forward. His or her feet are flat on the floor, and the palms are turned forward. A patient who is face down in a reclining position is in the *prone* position. In the *supine* position, the patient is face up in a reclining position.

Figure 1.2: Anatomical Position

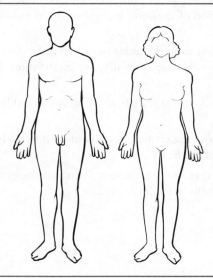

The anatomical position can be divided into imaginary planes and sections and can also be used to demonstrate various directional terms describing parts of the body in relation to one another.

Directional Terms

There are several important directional terms to be aware of, used in various ways. Some describe a body part relative to the anatomical position. Some compare positions of various anatomical structures. It is important to be accurate in descriptions regardless of the type of use.

- **Superior:** Toward the top of the body, or toward the head. The esophagus is superior to the stomach, to which it is attached. (Also referred to as cranial, cephalic)

- **Inferior:** Toward the lower part of the body, or toward the feet. Immediately inferior to the diaphragm lies the abdominal cavity. (Also referred to as caudal)

- **Anterior:** To the front of, or nearer to the front. The nose is on the anterior surface of the head. The anterior surface of the hand is the palm. (Also, ventral)

- **Posterior:** To the back of, or nearer to the back. The heel occupies the posterior part of the foot. (Also, dorsal)

- **Medial:** Toward the middle or toward the medial plane. The external auditory canal extends medially to the tympanic membrane, or eardrum.

- **Lateral:** Farther away from the middle or away from the medial plane. The heart lies in the left lateral compartment of the mediastinum.

- **Intermediate:** Between two structures. The transverse colon is intermediate between the ascending and descending colons.

- **Ipsilateral:** On the same side of the body as another structure. The left lung and the heart are ipsilateral.

- **Contralateral:** On the opposite side of the body from another structure. The ascending colon and the heart are contralateral.

- **Proximal:** Nearest to the point of origin, or nearest to the trunk. The thoracic portion of the aorta is proximal to its passage through the diaphragm.

- **Distal:** Farthest from the point of origin, or farthest from the trunk. The patella, or kneecap, partially overlies the most distal portion of the femur.

- **Superficial:** Closest to the surface. The epidermal layer is superficial to the dermis.

- **Interior:** Nearer the center. Two chambers divided by a septum occupy the interior of the heart.

- **Exterior:** Farther from the center. The muscular exterior of the esophagus works to facilitate swallowing.

Figure 1.3: Body Planes

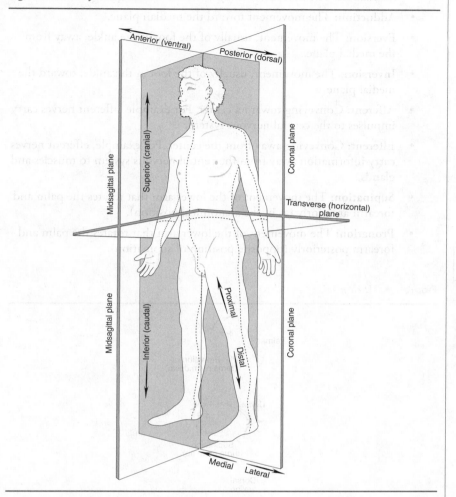

Planes

References to body sites often mention imaginary planes that pass through the body. The median or midsagittal plane runs vertically through the center of the body, dividing it exactly into the right side and the left side. There are any number of sagittal planes that run parallel to the median plane. Frontal or coronal planes run at right angles to the median plane to divide the body into front and back portions. Horizontal planes run at right angles to both the median plane and the coronal planes and may also be called transverse planes or cross-sectional planes. You can see some of these planes denoted in the above illustration.

Types of Movement

Some basic terms describe types of movement, specifically directions of movement usually of the extremities. This information is important for coding purposes, as these terms can often be the difference between one code and another, especially in the more detailed ICD-10-CM code set. Below are definitions of terms used to describe types of movement:

- **Flexion:** The movement causing decreased angle of a joint.

- **Extension:** The movement causing increased angle, or straightening, of a joint.

- **Abduction:** The movement away from the median plane.
- **Adduction:** The movement toward the median plane.
- **Eversion:** The movement, usually of the foot at the ankle, away from the medial plane.
- **Inversion:** The movement, usually of the foot at the ankle, toward the medial plane.
- **Afferent:** Conveying toward a center. For example, afferent nerves carry impulses to the central nervous system.
- **Efferent:** Conveying away from the center. For example, efferent nerves carry information away from the central nervous system to muscles and glands.
- **Supination:** The movement of the lower arm that rotates the palm and forearm anteriorly (as in the anatomical position).
- **Pronation:** The movement of the lower arm that rotates the palm and forearm posteriorly (opposite position of supination).

> ✓ **QUICK TIP**
>
> Internal rotation, also known as medial rotation, is rotation toward the center of the body. External rotation, also known as lateral rotation, is rotation away from the center of the body.

Figure 1.4: Motion

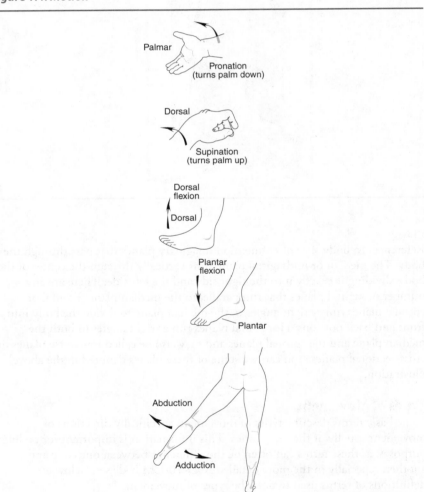

Summary

This chapter has reviewed the basics of the human body and some of the important terminology related to its anatomy and functions. The following chapters go into each of the organ systems and body areas in detail. They also discuss how the transition from ICD-9-CM to ICD-10-CM will require coders to learn more about anatomy and pathophysiology in certain areas.

Chapter 2. **Integumentary System**

Anatomic Overview

The skin is the largest organ system, covering the entire external surface of the body. Known as the integumentary system, the skin serves many purposes. It protects tissue layers from damage and provides waterproofing and cushioning. It also helps the body excrete wastes properly and regulate temperature, and provides the nerves with a surface for originating sensory receptors.

The top layer of the skin is known as the epidermis. This thinner portion of the skin mainly exists to absorb nutrients and to protect deeper tissue layers. The deeper and thicker layer of the skin is the dermis. The dermis is the connective tissue layer and contains the sweat glands, hair roots and follicles, blood vessels, sensory receptors, and other important structures of the integumentary system. Beneath the dermis is the hypodermis, or subcutaneous layer. This layer is not part of the skin itself, but the tie between the integumentary system and the fascia below.

Figure 2.1: Skin

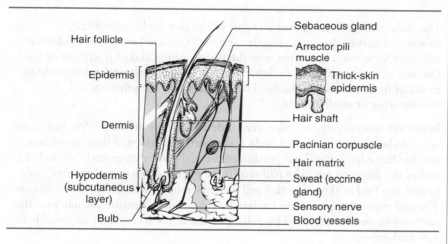

As indicated above, the dermal layer contains many different blood vessels, as well as glands, hair follicles, nerves, and sensory receptors. It is made up mainly of connective tissue, and all of these elements are embedded into that connective tissue.

The sweat glands, also known as sudoriferous glands, are found throughout the body. There are 3 to 4 million of these glands, which release perspiration onto the surface of the skin through small holes known as pores. This process helps regulate body temperature by releasing the perspiration and allowing it to evaporate.

The dermal layer also contains sebaceous glands, which are oil glands. These glands secrete sebum, an oily substance that keeps the skin and hair from drying out. The sebaceous glands are attached to a portion of the hair follicles. The hair and follicles are quite a complex system, allowing for continuous growth and regeneration. Hair, itself, can be thought of as a recycling system, using dead,

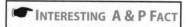

☞ **INTERESTING A & P FACT**

The skin accounts for approximately 16 percent of the body's total weight.

DEFINITIONS

keratin. Tough fibrous protein commonly found in the hair and nails.

keratinized epidermal cells to bond with proteins to create the hair within the follicle. The hair shaft grows out from the follicle, through the epidermis, and out of the skin entirely. The hair's purpose depends on its location—some helps avoid heat loss, while some protects from foreign bodies.

Figure 2.2: Hair and Glands

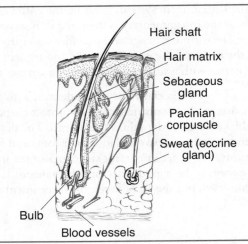

The nails, although not technically part of the skin itself, are typically considered part of the integumentary system. Nails are keratinized epidermal cells that form a solid covering over the surface of the end of the finger or toe. Outside of their aesthetic function, nails provide a protective covering helping to shield from traumatic injuries. They also assist in the gripping and maneuvering of small objects.

While the anatomy of the nail system is detailed, there are only a few important terms to be aware of. The nail body is the portion of the nail that can be seen, and the free edge is the distal portion of the nail body that extends beyond the end of the finger or toe. The nail root is the proximal portion of the nail body buried in a fold of skin. The nail bed is the skin upon which the nail body rests. The nail matrix is a portion of the nail bed found deep beneath the nail root that contains nerves and vessels. This is the portion of the nail system responsible for new nail growth.

Figure 2.3: Nail

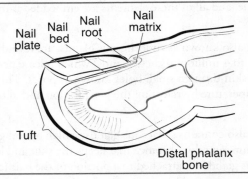

Anatomy and Physiology and the ICD-10-CM Code Set

The integumentary system can be affected by many different disease states. It is also the main site for traumatic injury, such as open wounds and burns. It is important to understand the terminology surrounding many of these disease states and injuries, as the ICD-10-CM code set is intricately detailed.

Skin Infections and Inflammation of Connective Tissue

There are many types of skin infections and inflammations, a few of which are discussed here.

An abscess is an infection in a cavity under the skin that contains pus, surrounded by inflamed tissue. Abscesses can occur nearly anywhere in the body. Those occurring in the integumentary system are known as *cutaneous abscesses*. Often a cutaneous abscess requires incision and drainage to heal appropriately.

A *furuncle*, more commonly known as a boil, is a localized skin infection typically caused by the *Staphylococcus aureus* bacterium. A furuncle is a specific type of abscess that usually begins in a gland or hair follicle, where a core of dead tissue is formed, causing pain, redness, and swelling. The dead tissue may simply reabsorb into the system, which resolves the problem, or it may spontaneously extrude itself. In some instances, surgical removal of the necrotic tissue may be required.

A *carbuncle* is larger than a furuncle and typically consists of several interconnected sites of infection that eventually discharge pus to the skin's surface. Carbuncles are also often caused by the *Staphylococcus aureus* bacterium and can vary greatly in size. Some carbuncles can be small, similar to the size of a pea, but others can grow to be quite large, greater than the size of a golf ball. Much like furuncles, some carbuncles heal on their own by reabsorption into the system or spontaneous extrusion. However, sometimes surgical treatment and antibiotics are required.

Coding for these three types of skin infections is more complex under the ICD-10-CM code set than in ICD-9-CM, and coders need to understand more about the anatomy, physiology, and pathology of the areas in question to code accurately. In ICD-9-CM, carbuncle and furuncle were grouped together under category 680. In ICD-10-CM, carbuncle and furuncle are separate codes, as indicated in the following table.

Coding for Carbuncles and Furuncles

ICD-9-CM		ICD-10-CM	
680.0	Carbuncle and furuncle of face	L02.02	Furuncle of face
		L02.03	Carbuncle of face
680.1	Carbuncle and furuncle of neck	L02.12	Furuncle of neck
		L02.13	Carbuncle of neck

DEFINITIONS

carbuncle. Several interconnected skin infection sites.

cutaneous abscess. Infection in a cavity under the skin that contains pus, surrounded by inflamed tissue.

furuncle. Also known as a boil, a localized skin infection in a gland or hair follicle.

ICD-9-CM		ICD-10-CM	
680.2	Carbuncle and furuncle of trunk	L02.221	Furuncle of abdominal wall
		L02.222	Furuncle of back, any part except buttock
		L02.223	Furuncle of chest wall
		L02.224	Furuncle of groin
		L02.225	Furuncle of perineum
		L02.226	Furuncle of umbilicus
		L02.229	Furuncle of trunk unspecified
		L02.231	Carbuncle of abdominal wall
		L02.232	Carbuncle of back, any part except buttock
		L02.233	Carbuncle of chest wall
		L02.234	Carbuncle of groin
		L02.235	Carbuncle of perineum
		L02.236	Carbuncle of umbilicus
		L02.239	Carbuncle of trunk unspecified
680.3	Carbuncle and furuncle of upper arm and forearm	L02.421	Furuncle of right axilla
		L02.422	Furuncle of left axilla
		L02.423	Furuncle of right upper limb
		L02.424	Furuncle of left upper limb
		L02.429	Furuncle of limb unspecified
		L02.431	Carbuncle of right axilla
		L02.432	Carbuncle of left axilla
		L02.433	Carbuncle of right upper limb
		L02.434	Carbuncle of left upper limb
		L02.439	Carbuncle of limb unspecified
680.4	Carbuncle and furuncle of hand	L02.521	Furuncle of right hand
		L02.522	Furuncle of left hand
		L02.529	Furuncle of unspecified hand
		L02.531	Carbuncle of right hand
		L02.532	Carbuncle of left hand
		L02.539	Carbuncle of unspecified hand

To report skin infections correctly in ICD-10-CM, the type of infection must be known. Did the patient present with a cutaneous abscess, a furuncle, or a carbuncle? Was it *cellulitis* or *lymphangitis*, which is a separate code set within ICD-10-CM. Additionally, the organism causing the infection should be coded, if known.

Once the type of infection has been determined, the location of the skin infection must be identified.

 DEFINITIONS

cellulitis. Sudden, severe, suppurative inflammation and edema in subcutaneous tissue or muscle, most often caused by bacterial infection secondary to a cutaneous lesion.

lymphangitis. Inflammation of the lymph glands.

Coding for Cellulitis and Cutaneous Abscesses

ICD-9-CM		ICD-10-CM	
682.0	Cellulitis and abscess of face	L03.211	Cellulitis of face
682.1	Cellulitis and abscess of neck	L03.221	Cellulitis of neck
682.2	Cellulitis and abscess of trunk	L02.211	Cutaneous abscess of abdominal wall
		L02.212	Cutaneous abscess of back any part except buttock
		L02.213	Cutaneous abscess of chest wall
		L02.214	Cutaneous abscess of groin
		L02.215	Cutaneous abscess of perineum
		L02.216	Cutaneous abscess of umbilicus
		L02.219	Cutaneous abscess of trunk unspecified
		L03.311	Cellulitis of abdominal wall
		L03.312	Cellulitis of back any part except buttock
		L03.313	Cellulitis of chest wall
		L03.314	Cellulitis of groin
		L03.315	Cellulitis of perineum
		L03.316	Cellulitis of umbilicus
		L03.319	Cellulitis of trunk unspecified
		L03.321	Acute lymphangitis of abdominal wall
		L03.322	Acute lymphangitis of back any part except buttock
		L03.323	Acute lymphangitis of chest wall
		L03.324	Acute lymphangitis of groin
		L03.325	Acute lymphangitis of perineum
		L03.326	Acute lymphangitis of umbilicus
		L03.329	Acute lymphangitis of trunk unspecified
682.3	Cellulitis and abscess of upper arm and forearm	L02.411	Cutaneous abscess of right axilla
		L02.412	Cutaneous abscess of left axilla
		L02.413	Cutaneous abscess of right upper limb
		L02.414	Cutaneous abscess of left upper limb
		L02.419	Cutaneous abscess of limb unspecified
		L03.111	Cellulitis of right axilla
		L03.112	Cellulitis of left axilla
		L03.113	Cellulitis of right upper limb
		L03.114	Cellulitis of left upper limb
		L03.119	Cellulitis of unspecified part of limb
		L03.121	Acute lymphangitis of right axilla
		L03.122	Acute lymphangitis of left axilla
		L03.123	Acute lymphangitis of right upper limb
		L03.124	Acute lymphangitis of left upper limb
		L03.129	Acute lymphangitis of unspecified part of limb

In the table above, there are multiple ICD-10-CM codes for cellulitis and cutaneous abscesses. Code selection depends on the type and location of skin infection or inflammation. The detail in these code descriptions is much greater than that provided in ICD-9-CM. For example, take a look at ICD-9-CM code 680.2 Carbuncle and Furuncle of Trunk. In ICD-10-CM, 14 codes are used in its place, seven specific to furuncles and seven specific to carbuncles. The sixth digit indicates the infection site:

1   Abdominal wall

2   Any part of back except buttock

3   Chest wall

4   Groin

5   Perineum

6   Umbilicus

9   Trunk, unspecified

Sixth-digit specifications are added not only to carbuncle and furuncle codes, but also to cutaneous abscess, cellulitis, and acute lymphangitis codes. Similar anatomical breakdowns occur in the other sections as well, such as right side versus left side, upper limbs versus lower limbs, or upper arm versus *axillae*. There is also an unspecified code option in many of these code sets. However, it is not known how payers will handle unspecified codes under the ICD-10-CM code set, so it is important to always code to the highest level of specificity. This may mean querying the provider for additional information. Providers must document any additional information via a query form or an addendum to the medical record.

Dermatitis and Eczema

Simply stated, *dermatitis* is inflammation of the skin. *Eczema* is one form of dermatitis. ICD-10-CM uses these terms interchangeably. Contact dermatitis, a fairly common form of the condition, is inflammation that results from an allergic reaction (allergic contact dermatitis) or exposure to some type of skin irritant (irritant contact dermatitis).

Dermatitis and eczema can be something as simple as redness of the skin or a bumpy rash, to something more serious such as blisters. Generally, the treatment for dermatitis depends on the cause and includes medications such as corticosteroids. In most cases, the use of an antihistamine cream helps control itchiness of the affected area.

Once again, the ICD-10-CM codes for dermatitis and eczema require more detail than their ICD-9-CM counterparts. One of the major differences is the breakdown of allergic- and irritant-related contact dermatitis codes.

Coding for Contact Dermatitis and Eczema

ICD-9-CM		ICD-10-CM	
692.3	Contact dermatitis and other eczema due to drugs and medicines in contact with skin	L23.3	Allergic contact dermatitis due to drugs in contact with skin
		L24.4	Irritant contact dermatitis due to drugs in contact with skin
		L25.1	Unspecified contact dermatitis due to drugs in contact with skin
692.4	Contact dermatitis and other eczema due to other chemical products	L23.1	Allergic contact dermatitis due to adhesives
		L23.5	Allergic contact dermatitis due to other chemical products
		L24.5	Irritant contact dermatitis due to chemical products
		L25.3	Unspecified contact dermatitis due to other chemical products

ICD-10-CM codes differentiate between the various types of skin responses to solar radiation. These more detailed ICD-10-CM codes provide additional granularity in coding but also require that the coder be more knowledgeable about these types of conditions.

A phototoxic response to a drug is different clinically from a photoallergic response, and they are coded differently in ICD-10-CM. A phototoxic response is a rapidly appearing, sunburn-like response generated by exposure to light and a photosensitizing substance. A photoallergic response is a delayed skin reaction of some sort, due to hypersensitivity to light caused by a photosensitizing substance. Photocontact dermatitis is yet another type of dermatitis that involves an interaction between UV radiation and certain substances, fruits, or vegetables. Finally, solar *urticaria* is a condition classified as hives or wheals caused specifically by exposure to the sun or UV radiation. In ICD-9-CM, these services are classified to general acute dermatitis code 692.72, but now all have specific diagnosis codes in ICD-10-CM.

DEFINITIONS

excoriated. Condition resulting from abrading the skin or otherwise scratching off the surface of the skin.

lichenification. Thickening and hardening of the epidermis, which often results in an exaggeration of its normal markings.

urticaria. Well circumscribed areas of redness and edema of the skin, commonly referred to as hives.

Coding for Acute Dermatitis Due to Solar Radiation

ICD-9-CM		ICD-10-CM	
692.72	Acute dermatitis due to solar radiation	L56.0	Drug phototoxic response
		L56.1	Drug photoallergic response
		L56.2	Photocontact dermatitis [berloque dermatitis]
		L56.3	Solar urticaria

ICD-9-CM code 691.8 Other atopic dermatitis and related conditions, includes a list of less common types of dermatitis that can be reported with this code. However, in ICD-10-CM, many of these conditions have their own codes, making it imperative that providers adequately document the different types of dermatitis in medical record documentation.

Besnier's prurigo is a form of atopic dermatitis associated with pregnancy. Also known as prurigo gestationis, it is a dermatological condition of pregnancy typically affecting women between the 20th and 34th week of gestation. It normally consists of an eruption of itchy, red papules that can be *excoriated* as well. There are several treatments that can make the patient more comfortable, although given the pregnancy, not all prescription treatments are an option.

Flexural eczema is a form of atopic dermatitis found in the flexures of the body, such as the elbows, wrists, and knees. This type of dermatitis often affects children, although it isn't exclusive to youth. It typically results in *lichenification,* as well as cracking and weeping of the area.

There are various other conditions that fall within this section. It is important to review documentation and determine whether the information best fits within a detailed diagnosis, or whether the diagnosis is still a more general atopic dermatitis diagnosis. Coders unable to identify the diagnosis based on incomplete documentation should query the provider.

Coding for Other Atopic Dermatitis

ICD-9-CM		ICD-10-CM	
691.8	Other atopic dermatitis and related conditions	L20.0	Besnier's prurigo
		L20.81	Atopic neurodermatitis
		L20.82	Flexural eczema
		L20.84	Intrinsic allergic eczema
		L20.89	Other atopic dermatitis
		L20.9	Atopic dermatitis unspecified

ICD-9-CM code 692.9 Contact dermatitis and other eczema due to an unspecified cause, maps to several ICD-10-CM codes, some unspecified codes, but others more specific.

Nummular dermatitis is typically characterized by itchy, oval lesions. In ICD-9-CM, nummular dermatitis is reported with 692.9. In ICD-10 CM, it has its own code (L30.0).

Cutaneous autosensitization is a secondary dermatitis caused by an inflammatory response somewhere else in the body. This autosensitization dermatitis is also coded to 692.9 in ICD-9-CM but has its own code (L30.2) in ICD-10-CM. Although there are several code options for unspecified dermatitis diagnoses, it is important to note that there is a great deal of uncertainty as to how payers will react to unspecified codes in the ICD-10-CM environment. There are many specific dermatitis codes as well, and it could be a good idea to query the provider for additional detail on the specific type of dermatitis.

Coding for Contact Dermatitis

ICD-9-CM		ICD-10-CM	
692.9	Contact dermatitis and other eczema due to unspecified cause	L23.9	Allergic contact dermatitis, unspecified cause
		L24.9	Irritant contact dermatitis, unspecified cause
		L25.9	Unspecified contact dermatitis, unspecified cause
		L30.0	Nummular dermatitis
		L30.2	Cutaneous autosensitization
		L30.8	Other specified dermatitis
		L30.9	Dermatitis unspecified

ICD-9-CM code 692.73 Actinic reticuloid and actinic granuloma, is separated into two codes in ICD-10-CM: L57.1 Actinic reticuloid, and L57.5 Actinic granuloma. Actinic reticuloid is a form of chronic photosensitivity dermatitis in which the patient's skin becomes inflamed due to sunlight exposure or other artificial light sources, often of the face and neck. Treatment includes a prescription for oral steroids and avoidance of light sources.

Actinic granuloma typically manifests itself as ring-shaped lesions on the skin. It is thought that these are the result of sun damage. Although the lesions tend to generally be asymptomatic, they can cause the patient problems when exposed to the sun. There is some confusion about whether actinic granuloma is related to another skin condition, granuloma annulare. However, there is no proof of a definitive link between the two conditions, although they are similar.

Figure 2.4: Surface and Solid Lesions

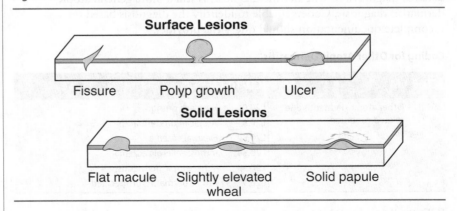

Psoriasis and Other Similar Disorders

In ICD-9-CM, psoriasis and other similar disorders group to category 696 without a great deal of detail. In ICD-10-CM, there are more than 25 codes representing these conditions, providing much more detail in the code description than in ICD-9-CM.

Arthropathic Psoriasis

Arthropathic psoriasis is a form of inflammatory arthritis that affects patients with psoriasis. It causes joint inflammation but can also cause tendinitis, issues with the nails, and swelling of the digits. There are various forms of this condition, described by distinctive names. Many of these forms have been assigned different codes in the ICD-10-CM code set.

Distal interphalangeal psoriatic arthropathy is arthropathic psoriasis characterized by inflammation in the distal portions of the fingers and toes. In this particular type of arthropathy, there are often changes noted in the nails as well, including pitting, discoloration, ridging, and thickening.

Psoriatic arthritis mutilans is a severe, deforming form of arthritis. It gets progressively worse over months or even years, causing resorption of bones and severe joint damage. It is not a common condition, affecting less than 5 percent of patients with arthropathic psoriasis.

Psoriatic spondylitis is a type of arthropathic psoriasis that results in pain and stiffness of the spine and neck. This occurs predominantly in male patients. These patients may show unusual radiological features, such as paravertebral ossification.

Psoriatic juvenile arthropathy is arthropathic psoriasis with an onset in childhood. The average age of onset is 9 to 10 years, and it occurs predominantly in female patients. Luckily, the disease tends to be mild in children. Psoriatic juvenile arthropathy accounts for 8 to 20 percent of all childhood arthritis.

Other Psoriasis and Similar Disorders

Psoriasis vulgaris is the most common form of psoriasis, affecting 80 to 90 percent of all psoriasis diagnoses. Also known as plaque psoriasis, it presents as raised and inflamed red areas covered with silvery/white scaly skin. These areas are known as plaques and can be itchy and painful. Treatment for psoriasis varies based on the severity, but ranges from topical agents to oral pharmaceuticals to various types of phototherapies.

Acrodermatitis continua is a form of pustular psoriasis that results in skin lesions on the ends of the fingers and toes. It is quite rare and is referred to by many different names, such as acropustulosis, acrodermatitis continua of Hallopeau, dermatitis repens, and pustular acrodermatitis. This condition tends to be resistant to common psoriasis treatment, so it can require more aggressive treatment even for what seems like a less serious form of psoriasis.

Pustulosis palmaris et plantaris, or palmoplantar pustulosis (PPP), causes pustules specifically on the hands and feet, hence its name. It is a persistent condition, typically recurring over and over. Interestingly, it is suggested that patients with PPP refrain from smoking, as nicotine has been known to cause flare-ups.

Guttate psoriasis is characterized by small red spots on the skin, as opposed to the large, scaly regions of other types of psoriasis. They are usually found on the upper body, specifically the trunk and upper limbs. It is predominantly found in adolescents and young adults and can be precipitated by many different types of illnesses, such as an upper respiratory infection, strep throat, tonsillitis, or even simply stress or the administration of certain drugs. It is important this condition be treated so it does not become a more serious form of psoriasis in the future.

Parapsoriasis

Pityriasis lichenoides et varioliformis acuta (PLEVA) is a serious disease involving the immune system. It is characterized mainly by rashes and small lesions on the skin, caused by the immune system inappropriately "fighting" the skin cells and causing damage. It is often misdiagnosed as various similar looking conditions, such as chicken pox or rosacea. Common treatment for the condition is a combination of pharmaceuticals and phototherapy. Localized wound care may be required for large ulcerations or infections.

Pityriasis lichenoides chronica is the milder, chronic form of PLEVA. This condition is characterized by the gradual development of symptomless, small, scaling papules that spontaneously flatten and regress over a period of weeks or months. The patient may have lesions at various stages present at any one time. Patients with this condition often have exacerbations and relapses of the condition, which can last for months or years.

Lymphomatoid papulosis is a chronic skin disease with histological features consistent with malignant lymphoma. It is characterized by pruritic papules on the trunk and limbs that heal over time but leave scarring. What is interesting about this condition is that it is histologically malignant, exhibiting the clinical features of a lymphoma. However, its benign clinical course and fairly spontaneous resolution make clinicians reluctant to classify this as a malignancy. Treatment usually includes oral and/or topical medications.

Small plaque parapsoriasis is a mild version of parapsoriasis, resulting in small skin lesions typically on the trunk. This condition often resolves on its own and rarely, if ever, progresses.

Large plaque parapsoriasis is a serious chronic inflammatory disorder that results in large skin lesions. This condition can be concerning, not because of the skin issues themselves, which are quite treatable, but because approximately 10 percent of patients with large plaque parapsoriasis progress to cutaneous T-cell lymphoma or mycosis fungoides, both serious conditions. Treatments include topical pharmaceuticals in conjunction with phototherapy.

Retiform parapsoriasis is a form of large plaque parapsoriasis. It causes large skin lesions that result in a netlike pattern on the body and can also cause the skin to atrophy. As is the case with all large plaque parapsoriasis, treatment is important in avoiding disease progression.

Poikiloderma vasculare atrophicans (PVA) is a condition characterized by hypopigmentation or hyperpigmentation of the skin, atrophy of the skin, and telangiectasia (dilated blood vessels) near the surface of the skin. These issues are often related to another condition, such as mycosis fungoides, other parapsoriasis, and other conditions that might cause the skin issues. Treatment for PVA is typically geared toward the underlying condition.

Other Psoriasis and Similar Disorders, Other

Pityriasis rubra pilaris is a chronic skin condition resulting in reddish orange scaly plaques and keratotic papules of the follicles. It can also cause palmoplantar keratoderma, which is a thickening of the skin on the palms of the

INTERESTING A & P FACT

Many skin conditions, including many of the psoriasis and parapsoriasis conditions, have no identifiable cause. Many researchers hypothesize, but in most cases have not been able to agree on, a solid cause for most of these conditions.

hands and the soles of the feet. Treatment for this condition can include topical and/or oral medications and possibly phototherapy.

Infantile papular acrodermatitis, also known as Gianotti-Crosti syndrome, is a skin condition in children caused by the body's reaction to a viral infection. It is typically characterized by pink to pale flesh-colored papules covering the buttocks, the extremities, and the face. Rarely are other areas of the body involved. Hepatitis B was one of the initial viruses thought to cause this condition, although it is now just one of many seen as the root cause. In general, medications treat the symptoms but do not lessen the course of the condition. Topical agents can be used to soothe the itching, as can oral antihistamines.

Coding for Psoriasis and Other Similar Disorders

ICD-9-CM		ICD-10-CM	
696.0	Psoriatic arthropathy	L40.50	Arthropathic psoriasis unspecified
		L40.51	Distal interphalangeal psoriatic arthropathy
		L40.52	Psoriatic arthritis mutilans
		L40.53	Psoriatic spondylitis
		L40.54	Psoriatic juvenile arthropathy
		L40.59	Other psoriatic arthropathy
696.1	Other psoriasis and similar disorders	L40.0	Psoriasis vulgaris
		L40.1	Generalized pustular psoriasis
		L40.2	Acrodermatitis continua
		L40.3	Pustulosis *palmaris* et *plantaris*
		L40.4	Guttate psoriasis
		L40.8	Other psoriasis
		L40.9	Psoriasis
696.2	Parapsoriasis	L41.0	Pityriasis lichenoides et varioliformis acuta
		L41.1	Pityriasis lichenoides chronica
		L41.2	Lymphomatoid papulosis
		L41.3	Small plaque parapsoriasis
		L41.4	Large plaque parapsoriasis
		L41.5	Retiform parapsoriasis
		L41.8	Other parapsoriasis
		L41.9	Parapsoriasis unspecified
		L94.5	Poikiloderma vasculare atrophicans
696.8	Other psoriasis & similar disorders other	L44.0	Pityriasis rubra pilaris
		L44.8	Other specified papulosquamous disorders
		L45	Papulosquamous disorders in diseases classified elsewhere

Pemphigoid

Pemphigoid is another skin condition in which there is a notable difference between the ICD-9-CM and ICD-10-CM code sets, with the ICD-10-CM code set requiring that the coder have a greater understanding of the different types of pemphigoid to code accurately.

Pemphigoid is an autoimmune disease that results in the body's own immune system attacking the cells of the integumentary system. It is important not to confuse it with pemphigus, which is a somewhat similar condition but is coded differently (L10.9 Pemphigus unspecified).

Bullous pemphigoid presents with blistering at the site of the attack and is accompanied by itching and pain. Treatment includes corticosteroids and/or immunosuppressants, as well as wound care to make sure the site stays clean and uninfected.

DEFINITIONS

infantile. Having to do with infants or children. When this term is used in conjunction with a condition or disease state, it usually indicates onset at a young age.

palmar. Pertaining to the palm. The root term is "palmo-."

plantar. Pertaining to the foot.

Other types of pemphigoid, such as mucous membrane pemphigoid, cicatricial pemphigoid, and gestationis pemphigoid, are reported with L12.8 Other pemphigoid, as more specific codes are not available.

Coding for Pemphigoid

ICD-9-CM		ICD-10-CM	
694.5	Pemphigoid	L12.0	Bullous pemphigoid
		L12.8	Other pemphigoid
		L12.9	Pemphigoid unspecified

Rosacea

Rosacea is a common skin condition coded to a single ICD-9-CM code, 695.3. In ICD-10-CM, however, there are four separate codes with more specific terminology.

Perioral dermatitis is not exclusively related to rosacea but is a condition afflicting many with rosacea. Perioral refers to the area around the mouth. This form of dermatitis typically results in redness, small bumps that can be pus-filled, and peeling of the skin on the chin, the sides of the mouth, and around the nose. There is usually a band of skin around the mouth that is spared. There are various treatments for this condition, but the most common is the use of oral antibiotics, such as tetracycline. Corticosteroid creams are used in some cases but have been known to cause additional flare-ups.

Rhinophyma is the most recognizable condition related to rosacea. Although this condition isn't exclusive to rosacea, in most instances rosacea is involved. Rhinophyma results in the nose taking on a large, bulbous, distorted appearance, typically red in color. This distortion is caused over time by the hypertrophy of the sebaceous glands of the nose. It is often thought to be related to alcoholism, although there is no direct link. Heavy alcohol use, however, can aggravate the condition in patients with existing disease. Treatment for rhinophyma can include dermabrasion, laser resurfacing procedures, or other plastic surgery techniques to remove the damaged skin.

Coding for Rosacea and Related Conditions

ICD-9-CM		ICD-10-CM	
695.3	Rosacea	L71.0	Perioral dermatitis
		L71.1	Rhinophyma
		L71.8	Other rosacea
		L71.9	Rosacea unspecified

Acne

In ICD-9-CM, acne codes are fairly generic, with most types of acne mapping to one of two codes. In ICD-10-CM, there are several codes for acne, all of which require that the coder have extensive knowledge about the specific form.

Acne vulgaris, also known as common acne, is a skin disorder faced by many adolescents who may deal with the disorder into adulthood. It is typically characterized by outbreaks of pimples, cysts, comedones, and inflammation. In youth, acne can have psychological effects as well, such as reduced self-esteem. Treatment for acne vulgaris can be as simple as over-the-counter benzoyl peroxide creams, or as complex as dermabrasion and surgical treatments, depending on severity.

Acne conglobata is a severe but somewhat rare form of acne that causes nodules on the skin, typically the trunk, upper arms, buttocks, thighs, and face. Also called cystic acne, these nodules create abscesses that become interconnected under the skin, creating a network of abscesses. This can cause significant scarring, to the point of disfigurement. It is typically treated with pharmaceuticals, but surgical excision may be required as well.

Acne tropica, or tropical acne, is seen in tropical climates. The warm air and humidity cause this condition, especially when the body is not used to higher temperatures. Acne tropica is caused by a significant build-up of oil, dead skin cells, and bacteria in the pores, which causes a heat rash-like reaction. Perspiration from the hot and humid weather exacerbates the condition, causing a vicious cycle. Treatment for acne tropica is much like that for acne vulgaris. Most patients are advised to use an over-the-counter benzoyl peroxide or salicylic acid treatment.

It is important that medical documentation differentiate between acne vulgaris and acne tropica, as well as between acne tropica and a heat rash, as each is coded differently under the ICD-10-CM system. If needed, the coder should query the provider for additional information.

Infantile acne affects infants, typically starting around 2 to 3 months of age. There is no specific explanation for this form of acne, although there is a hypothesis that it is genetic in nature. It typically affects the nose and cheeks of the infant, but can spread to the chin and forehead. It usually dissipates by 6 months of age, but some cases have lasted up to age 3. Depending on the severity and the age of the patient, treatment may consist of nothing or may be similar to other acne treatments outlined above. In most instances, there is little to no treatment, as this tends to be a fairly mild form of acne.

Acne excoriée des jeunes filles, also known as excoriated acne or picker's acne, is characterized by *comedones* or *pustules* that have been excoriated, or "picked," leaving open wounds or scratch marks. In most instances, much of the acne resolves, but scarring and sores remain. Treatment for this condition varies, based on severity and the root cause of excoriation. In some cases, the excoriation can be caused by an underlying psychological condition, for which the patient may need to seek treatment. The acne itself can be treated with oral pharmaceuticals. In some cases, aggressive treatment to resolve the acne can curtail the patient's habitual picking, thus breaking the cycle.

Acne keloids are a form of *keloid* scarring that typically occurs at the base of the neck. It is associated with the occlusion of hair follicles in that area and is most often encountered in black and Asian men. The skin in the area becomes inflamed and bumpy, and it can be quite painful. Treatment varies, based on the severity of the condition. The use of antibiotics and steroid gels is common and, in more advanced cases, intralesional steroid injections may be required. Larger keloids may require surgical removal.

 DEFINITIONS

comedones. Accumulation of sebum in the opening of a hair follicle. An open comedone is a blackhead, and a closed comedone is a whitehead.

keloid. Progressive overgrowth of cutaneous scar tissue that is raised and irregular in shape, caused by excessive formation of collagen during connective tissue repair.

pustule. Small skin elevation typically containing a purulent fluid,

Coding for Acne

ICD-9-CM		ICD-10-CM	
706.1	Other acne	L70.0	Acne vulgaris
		L70.1	Acne conglobata
		L70.3	Acne tropica
		L70.4	Infantile acne
		L70.5	Acne excoriée des jeunes filles
		L70.8	Other acne
		L70.9	Acne unspecified
		L73.0	Acne keloid

Heat-Related Skin Conditions

Prickly heat, or heat rash, uses significantly different terminology in ICD-9-CM from that used in ICD-10-CM. ICD-9-CM uses a more "layman" approach to the condition, whereas ICD-10-CM has taken a more clinical approach.

Miliaria rubra is the second most serious heat rash condition. It tends to affect adults in hot and humid conditions or neonates aged 1 to 3 weeks. It occurs deep within the epidermis and can cause pruritic papules across the body. The lesions tend to resolve quickly after the patients leave hot and humid climates.

Miliaria profunda is the most serious form of heat rash, caused by repeated episodes of miliaria rubra. This condition causes deep pustules to form at the dermal/epidermal junction. These pustules block the sweat glands and can make it impossible for the body to cool itself properly if widespread. In warm climates, patients with this condition are more likely to be predisposed to heat exhaustion.

Miliaria crystallina is the mildest form of heat rash. It tends to affect adults with other conditions that may be causing a fever or neonates younger than 2 weeks. Some adults who have relocated to a significantly warmer climate may be affected by this condition as well. This form affects the most superficial layer of the skin, causing what almost looks like tiny beads of liquid on the skin. It tends to be asymptomatic and often disappears on its own within a few days.

Coding for Prickly Heat/Heat Rash

ICD-9-CM		ICD-10-CM	
705.1	Prickly heat	L74.0	Miliaria rubra
		L74.1	Miliaria crystallina
		L74.2	Miliaria profunda
		L74.3	Miliaria unspecified

Other Skin Conditions, Cysts

Sebaceous cysts are another type of skin condition difficult to code in ICD-10-CM without extensive knowledge. In ICD-9-CM, sebaceous cysts are grouped to a single code, 706.2. In ICD-10-CM, codes are assigned based on location and depth.

Figure 2.5: Sac Lesions

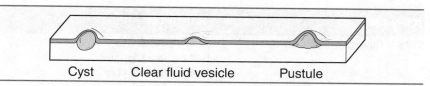

Cyst   Clear fluid vesicle   Pustule

Epidermal cysts, L72.Ø, are benign cysts of the skin resulting from any number of things, including a blocked pore or a traumatic injury. Such a cyst can be filled with pus or other purulent material and most likely needs to be removed surgically.

Trichodermal cysts, L72.1, are benign, fluid-filled cysts found at the hair follicle. They are often found on the scalp, although not exclusively. These cysts can grow together and form groups or channels, which can become problematic. Surgical excision is usually required.

Steatocystoma multiplex, L72.2, is a condition typically described as congenital, causing multiple cysts over the body. These cysts, typically small and fluid filled, are usually found in areas with the highest concentration of sebaceous glands (chest, arms, axillae, and neck). Treatment includes excision of particularly large or disfiguring lesions and pharmaceuticals to help prevent complications.

Nail Conditions

In ICD-9-CM, diseases of the nail are classified to one of three codes, two of which are generic. In ICD-10-CM, more specificity has been added, requiring that the coder be more knowledgeable about the various conditions that affect the nail.

Onychocryptosis, or an ingrown nail, is a painful condition that results in the nail plate growing and penetrating the skin, frequently causing infection. Although similar in appearance, this condition is different from onychia, which is an infection of the nail bed that can result in nail loss, or paronychia, which is an infection of the soft tissue surrounding the nail.

In onycholysis, the nail separates from the nail bed, typically starting at the distal free margin and separating proximally. It can occur for many reasons, including traumatic injuries, systemic diseases, and infections. Patients may be placed on medication to avoid a potential fungal infection related to this nail separation.

Onychogryphosis is a nail condition also known as "ram's horn nails." It is a hypertrophy of the nail that causes the nail to grow in a claw or a horn shape. It can be caused by various disease states or trauma, or it can be caused by neglect of the nail over a long period of time. Treatment often involves surgical avulsion of the nail plate.

Nail dystrophy is a general term relating to malformation of the nail. It can be a congenital malformation, but, in many cases, it is a deformity caused by some other condition or a drug or substance the patient has taken or been exposed to.

Beau's lines are horizontal depressions or lines across the nail bed. These lines grow out as the nail continues to grow. They can be caused by infections or trauma, or potentially even medication use.

Yellow nail syndrome is a rare condition characterized by yellow-tinted nails. The nails lack cuticles and can grow quite slowly. These patients are also typically affected by onycholysis.

Coding for Other Specified Diseases of the Nail

ICD-9-CM	ICD-10-CM	
703.8 Other specified disease of nail	L60.1	Onycholysis
	L60.2	Onychogryphosis
	L60.3	Nail dystrophy
	L60.4	Beau's lines
	L60.5	Yellow nail syndrome
	L60.8	Other nail disorders
	L62	Nail disorders in diseases classified elsewhere

Hair Conditions

Conditions related to the hair are more detailed in ICD-10-CM than in ICD-9-CM, requiring more knowledge to assign codes accurately. Various conditions affecting the hair and hair follicles, grouped to nonspecific codes in ICD-9-CM, have their own code descriptor.

In ICD-9-CM, unspecified alopecia is reported with 704.00. In ICD-10-CM, this condition maps to four codes.

Drug-induced androgenic alopecia, L64.0, is a hair loss condition in males and females caused by the ingestion of or exposure to some drug or substance. In many cases, this hair loss can be stopped by preventing exposure, and there is potential that the patient will have hair regrowth as well.

Androgenic alopecia, L64.8 and L64.9, is a general term for the most common form of hair loss. It is often referred to as male or female pattern baldness. There are various causes of hair loss, including stress, abnormal hormone levels, and disease states. In most instances, people are genetically predisposed to certain types of hair loss. Treatments available for androgenic alopecia include topical pharmaceuticals to attempt to generate hair growth, as well as surgical hair transplant techniques. However, most of these treatments are considered cosmetic in nature.

Alopecia areata (AA) is another type of hair loss affecting a smaller population than androgenic alopecia. Several researchers believe alopecia areata is an autoimmune disorder in which the immune system attacks the hair follicles causing the hair to fall out. In ICD-9-CM, alopecia areata is coded to 704.01. In ICD-10-CM, coding for AA isn't terribly complex, but there is one variant of the condition mentioned separately—ophiasis, L63.2. Patients with ophiasis typically have hair loss on the back of their head in the shape of a wave, near the nape of the neck. Outside of this specific pattern, there is no difference between ophiasis and other types of alopecia areata.

Other alopecia, previously coded as 704.09 in ICD-9-CM, has been separated into several components in ICD-10-CM.

Alopecia capitis totalis is total, typically permanent, hair loss on the scalp. Alopecia universalis is a total hair loss on the body, including eyebrows and eyelashes. Unlike alopecia totalis, however, the hair can grow back in some cases. Interestingly, there is no known cause for these conditions, as is the case for most forms of alopecia. Some researchers consider these conditions to be autoimmune disorders.

Anagen effluvium is hair loss that affects hair follicles specifically in the anagen stage of hair development. This hair loss most commonly occurs in patients undergoing radiation therapy or systemic chemotherapy treatments but can be

☛ **INTERESTING A & P FACT**

The name of the ophiasis pattern of alopecia areata comes from the Greek word for snake, ophis. A patient with the opposite hair loss pattern from the ophiasis pattern (hair loss everywhere except for the wave on the back of the head) is said to have sisaipho (the inverse of ophiasis, slightly altered for the sake of pronunciation).

caused by exposure to other pharmaceuticals or chemicals. Unfortunately, there is no treatment for the hair loss, but hair does typically regrow following conclusion of the therapies.

Alopecia mucinosa is characterized by patches of hair loss, as well as purulent papules and plaques. There is no known cause for this condition. Treatments can include topical medications and phototherapies, although these help with the papules and plaques more than they do hair loss. There is no standard treatment protocol for this condition, and it seems that in many cases the issue resolves on its own.

Pseudopelade is a form of cicatricial alopecia. It is characterized by irregularly shaped, slightly depressed lesions of the scalp. Sometimes there are a few hairs remaining in the lesion; otherwise it is typically hypopigmented in appearance. Once these lesions have occurred, there is unfortunately no medical treatment available. However, the patient may take pharmaceuticals to avoid other lesions from occurring. In serious cases, skin grafts and hair transplants may be used to replace hair loss if the disease has stabilized.

Folliculitis decalvans is another form of scarring alopecia. This condition is characterized by recurrent waves of follicular pustules that cause the hair to fall out. Treatment for this condition is typically a combination of topical corticosteroids and oral tetracycline to control the infection and thus the hair loss.

Coding for Other Types of Alopecia

ICD-9-CM	ICD-10-CM	
704.09 Other alopecia	L63.0	Alopecia capitis totalis
	L63.1	Alopecia universalis
	L64.0	Drug-induced androgenic alopecia
	L64.8	Other androgenic alopecia
	L65.1	Anagen effluvium
	L65.2	Alopecia mucinosa
	L65.8	Other specified nonscarring hair loss
	L66.0	Pseudopelade
	L66.2	Folliculitis decalvans
	L66.8	Other cicatricial alopecia
	L66.9	Cicatricial alopecia unspecified

Skin Ulcers

In ICD-9-CM, pressure and other types of ulcers are reported with multiple codes, although they are not specific to anatomical location. In ICD-10-CM, coders can pinpoint with a single code the ulcer site, type of ulcer, and whether it is related to a disease process. The coding of ulcers will not be reviewed in this publication; however, some anatomy and physiology concepts will be discussed to aid with coding accuracy.

Pressure Ulcer Stages

Pressure ulcer stages play an important role in ICD-9-CM and ICD-10-CM coding. Unfortunately, providers do not always document the specific stage of the ulcer, so wound descriptors may need to be scrutinized.

Figure 2.6: Four Stages of Pressure Ulcers

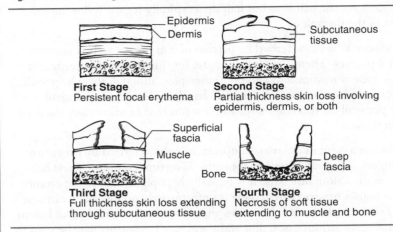

First Stage
Persistent focal erythema

Second Stage
Partial thickness skin loss involving epidermis, dermis, or both

Third Stage
Full thickness skin loss extending through subcutaneous tissue

Fourth Stage
Necrosis of soft tissue extending to muscle and bone

Anatomy

When reporting skin ulcers in ICD-10-CM, the anatomical site must be identified. For example, in ICD-9-CM, pressure ulcer of the lower back is reported with 707.03. In ICD-10-CM, documentation needs to specify whether the ulcer is on the right or left lower back, the sacral region, or the buttock or hip. If the site is not specified, the coder must query the provider.

Conditions Involving the Skin and Subcutaneous Tissue in Other Areas of ICD-10-CM

Diseases involving the skin and subcutaneous tissue are generally found in chapter 12 of ICD-10-CM (LØØ–L99). However, these conditions are not limited to this chapter and can be found throughout the ICD-10-CM manual.

Neoplasms

According to the most widely accepted definition, a neoplasm is an abnormal mass of tissue, the growth of which exceeds and is uncoordinated with that of normal tissues. It persists in the same excessive manner after cessation of the stimulus that evoked the cell changes.

For coding classification purposes, neoplasms are described in the following four ways:

- Behavior
- Functional activity
- Morphology
- Site

The behavior of a neoplasm refers to its biological behavior. The ICD-10-CM coding system recognizes the following behavioral types:

- **Malignant:** Tumors that behave in a life-threatening manner. The behavior that makes certain neoplasms malignant is their ability to invade surrounding tissues, as well as to metastasize. Malignant tumors can be further subdivided as:

  - **malignant primary:** Originating site of the tumor.

  - **malignant secondary:** Site to which a primary tumor has metastasized.

- **carcinoma in situ:** Tumors confined to their point of origin that have not invaded surrounding tissue.

- **Benign:** Tumors in which the dividing cells adhere to each other, with the resulting neoplastic mass remaining as a circumscribed lesion.

- **Uncertain:** Neoplasm whose behavior cannot be determined at the time of discovery and that require continued study to accurately classify the neoplasm by behavior.

- **Unspecified:** Assigned when medical documentation does not specify the neoplasm behavior.

Functional activity refers to the effects certain neoplasms have on tissues that are functionally active and is reported with a secondary code from another chapter of ICD-10-CM.

A *basal cell* carcinoma is a malignant tumor found in the lowest layer of the epidermis, usually in areas exposed to sunlight, such as the head or neck. This is the most common form of carcinoma in the United States. These tumors are slow growing and rarely spread.

A *squamous cell* carcinoma originates in the squamous cells of the epidermis. Like basal cell, these lesions most frequently develop in areas exposed to the sun. However, unlike basal cell carcinoma, squamous cell carcinoma may spread to distant parts of the body and can be fatal.

Malignant *melanoma* begins in the melanocytes, the pigment-producing skin cells. Melanomas vary in size, shape, and color. Melanomas may grow deep into the skin and subcutaneous tissues, with the deepest ones having an increased risk of spreading through the lymphatic and blood system and metastasizing elsewhere in the body. Melanomas that spread are often fatal.

There are also a number of benign neoplasms that affect the skin. Examples include:

- Papilloma
- Acquired keratoderma
- Seborrheic keratosis
- Hemangioma

Site refers to the anatomic location of the neoplasm and is used as a subdivision for the four types of behaviors. ICD-9-CM codes do not differentiate greatly between neoplasm sites. In ICD-10-CM, however, there is greater differentiation in laterality, as well as upper versus lower. The following table illustrates the difference in anatomical terminology used in ICD-9-CM versus ICD-10-CM for neoplasms of the ear.

Coding for Other Malignant Neoplasm of the Skin of the Ear and External Canal

ICD-9-CM		ICD-10-CM	
173.2	Other malignant neoplasm of skin of ear and external auditory canal	C44.20	Malignant neoplasm of skin of unspecified ear and external auricular canal
		C44.21	Malignant neoplasm of skin of right ear and external auricular canal
		C44.22	Malignant neoplasm of skin of left ear and external auricular canal

 DEFINITIONS

basal cell. Malignant epithelial cell tumor that begins as a papule, but enlarges peripherally. They tend to develop a central crater that erodes, crusts, and then bleeds.

melanoma. Highly metastatic malignant neoplasm composed of melanocytes that occur most often on the skin from a preexisting mole or nevus but may also occur in the mouth, esophagus, anal canal, or vagina. Melanoma has four stages. Stage 0: cells are found only in the outer layer of skin cells and have not invaded deeper tissues. Stage I: Tumor is no more than 1 mm thick and the outer layer of skin may appear scraped or ulcerated; or the tumor is between 1 and 2 mm thick with no ulceration and no spread to nearby lymph nodes. Stage II: Tumor is at least 1 mm thick with ulceration or the lesion is more than 2 mm thick without ulceration and no spread to lymph nodes. Stage III: Cells have spread to one or more nearby lymph nodes or to tissues just outside the original lesion. Stage IV: Malignant cells have spread to other organs, lymph nodes, or areas of the skin distant from the original tumor.

squamous cell. Slow-growing malignant tumor of the squamous epithelium, found in the skin as well as the lungs, anus, cervix, larynx, nose, and bladder.

Note that in ICD-9-CM, the term auditory canal describes the external portion of the ear canal. However, in ICD-10-CM that term has been changed to auricular canal.

ICD-10-CM provides a few options for coding benign neoplasms. It is important that the coder have as much detail as possible before selecting the appropriate code.

Coding for Benign Neoplasm of Skin of Other and Unspecified Parts of the Face

ICD-9-CM		ICD-10-CM	
216.3	Benign neoplasm of skin of other and unspecified parts of face	D22.30	Melanocytic nevi of unspecified part of face
		D22.39	Melanocytic nevi of other parts of face
		D23.30	Other benign neoplasm of skin of unspecified part of face
		D23.39	Other benign neoplasm of skin of other parts of face

Melanocytic nevi do not have their own code in ICD-9-CM, although they are included in morphology coding scenarios. These benign neoplasms are made of melanocytes, which are pigment-producing cells, typically giving them a dark color varying from tan to black. These nevi can be surgically removed for cosmetic purposes or if the provider is concerned that they may progress into something more serious.

Symptoms, Signs, and Ill-Defined Conditions Involving the Skin and Subcutaneous Tissue

In ICD-9-CM, chapter 16 is reserved for signs and symptoms that cross over many body and organ systems. ICD-10-CM chapter 18 is similar, and some of the conditions listed involve the integumentary system.

From an anatomy and physiology perspective, most of the signs and symptoms involving the skin and subcutaneous tissues are similar between the two manuals. However, in ICD-10-CM, special attention needs to be paid to anatomical site. For example, in ICD-9-CM, localized superficial swelling, mass, or lump is assigned to a single code, 782.2. In ICD-10-CM, there are 12 distinct codes, differentiated by anatomical site, including:

R22.0	**Localized swelling, mass and lump, head**
R22.1	**Localized swelling, mass and lump, neck**
R22.2	**Localized swelling, mass and lump, trunk**
R22.30	**Localized swelling, mass and lump, upper limb, unspecified side**
R22.31	**Localized swelling, mass and lump, right upper limb**
R22.32	**Localized swelling, mass and lump, left upper limb**
R22.33	**Localized swelling, mass and lump, upper limb, bilateral**
R22.40	**Localized swelling, mass and lump, lower limb, unspecified side**
R22.41	**Localized swelling, mass and lump, right lower limb**
R22.42	**Localized swelling, mass and lump, left lower limb**
R22.43	**Localized swelling, mass and lump, lower limb bilateral**
R22.9	**Localized swelling, mass and lump, unspecified**

There is also some additional specificity added to ICD-10-CM for some skin conditions. For example, in ICD-9-CM, disturbance of skin sensation is reported with a single code, 782.0. In ICD-10-CM, there is a series of codes representing various levels of the disturbance.

Anesthesia of skin is a disturbance of skin sensation resulting in a complete loss of sensation to a particular area of the skin. In most instances, anesthesia refers to induction of an anesthetic for a surgical procedure or pain control; however, this is not the case for this diagnosis.

Hypoesthesia of the skin is a reduced sense of touch or feeling in the skin. It is not a complete anesthesia, but is a noticed decrease in sensation in the affected area. Hyperesthesia is the opposite, an increased sensitivity in the skin.

Paraesthesia is a combination of hypoesthesia with a tingling or prickling feeling in the affected area. It is commonly referred to as "pins and needles" or the area "falling asleep." Patients often complain of paraesthesias in the extremities, which can be secondary to various conditions or pharmaceutical therapies. Treatment depends on the root cause.

Coding for Disturbance of Skin Sensation

ICD-9-CM	ICD-10-CM	
782.0 Disturbance of skin sensation	R20.0	Anesthesia of skin
	R20.1	Hypoesthesia of skin
	R20.2	Paraesthesia of skin
	R20.3	Hyperesthesia
	R20.8	Other disturbances of skin sensation
	R20.9	Unspecified disturbances of skin sensation

Injuries Involving the Skin and Subcutaneous Tissue

In the ICD-10-CM code set, lacerations and open wounds with and without complications are no longer the "norm." Close attention must be paid to the injury site, the mechanism of the injury, the patient encounter, and whether foreign bodies are involved.

Coding for Open Wounds of Scalp

ICD-9-CM	ICD-10-CM	
873.0 Open wound of scalp without mention of complication	S01.00xA	Unspecified open wound of scalp, initial encounter
	S01.01xA	Laceration without foreign body of scalp, initial encounter
	S01.03xA	Puncture wound without foreign body of scalp, initial encounter
	S01.05xA	Open bite of scalp, initial encounter
	S08.0xxA	Avulsion of scalp, initial encounter
873.1 Open wound of scalp, complicated	S01.02xA	Laceration with foreign body of scalp, initial encounter
	S01.04xA	Puncture wound with foreign body of scalp, initial encounter

As illustrated in the table above, what was previously an open wound in ICD-9-CM is now a *laceration,* a *puncture wound,* an *open bite,* or an *avulsion* in ICD-10-CM.

In ICD-9-CM, codes for lacerations and open wounds include descriptors "with or without complications." In ICD-10-CM, this terminology is no longer used,

> **CODING AXIOM**
>
> Examples for injuries involving the skin and subcutaneous tissue include only initial encounters in this publication. However, codes are also differentiated between subsequent encounters and sequelae in ICD-10-CM.

> **DEFINITIONS**
>
> **avulsion.** Traumatic injury caused by the forcible tearing away of a part.
>
> **laceration.** Tearing injury, or a torn, ragged-edged wound.
>
> **open bite.** Traumatic injury caused by an animal or another human.
>
> **puncture wound.** Traumatic injury caused by an object, such as a knife, nail, or fragment of a solid substance like glass or wood.

but code descriptions focus instead on whether the wound includes a foreign body.

Burns

Burns are the result of an injury or destruction to the tissue and can be due to the effects of thermal energy, chemicals, electricity, or radiation. Many complications arise in burn patients, including hypovolemic shock, inhalation injury, inability to regulate temperature, infection, scarring, and contractures.

There are three degrees of burn depending on the level of skin lost:

- **First-degree burns:** Also known as erythema, first degree burns are limited to tissue damage to the outer layer of the epidermis.

- **Second-degree burns:** Extend beyond the epidermis to partial thickness of the dermis.

- **Third-degree burns:** Full-thickness skin loss. Third-degree burns with presence of necrotic tissue is termed deep necrosis and is further specified as with or without loss of body parts.

Figure 2.7: Degrees of Burns

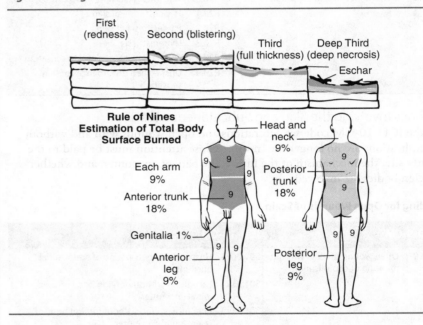

The terminology used for burns varies between ICD-9-CM and ICD-10-CM. Common terminology includes first-, second-, and third-degree burns, as well as the "rule of nines" for calculating the total body surface area (TBSA) burned. However, ICD-10-CM also differentiates between burn types.

There are separate ICD-10-CM codes for burns and corrosions. Burns are traditional thermal burns, and corrosions are chemical burns.

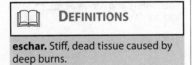

📖 **DEFINITIONS**

eschar. Stiff, dead tissue caused by deep burns.

Coding for Burns of Chin

ICD-9-CM		ICD-10-CM	
941.14	Erythema due to burn of chin	T20.13xA	Burn of first degree of chin, initial encounter
		T20.53xA	Corrosion of first degree of chin, initial encounter

Summary

The integumentary system is truly a diverse system, literally covering the human body from head to toe. In this chapter, the basics of the integumentary system were covered, as well as some of the coding differences between ICD-9-CM and ICD-10-CM. Pay close attention to detail when coding anatomical sites, as a simple left versus right or upper versus lower makes a major difference in ICD-10-CM coding. Also note that because new terminology is used in ICD-10-CM, the coder may have to ask the physician for clarification. Physicians and other providers will be learning about this new code set as well, and most will be happy to help coders learn more about the clinical side of medicine.

Chapter 3.
Skeletal System and Articulations

Anatomic Overview

The skeletal system comprises bones, cartilage, articulations, and ligaments. It is responsible for shaping and supporting the body, providing protection for internal organs, and aiding in and restricting movement. It also plays a role in blood cell production and mineral storage.

Bones

Bones provide the support for and shape of the body. They are the structural foundation for the rest of the body, as well as protection for many vital organs. For instance, the ribs, sternum, scapula, and clavicle protect the heart and lungs, while the bony spine protects the spinal cord and blood vessels within the vertebrae.

A bone consists of two tissue types, the difference between which is seen only microscopically. Compact bone, also known as cortical bone, is tightly packed tissue with minimal gaps and spaces. Spongy or cancellous bone looks disorganized with what appears to be random gaps and holes in the tissue.

The bones also produce and house a highly specialized connective tissue called bone marrow. There are two types of bone marrow: yellow and red. Yellow bone marrow stores fat for the body and is found mainly in the hollow spaces in the long bones of adults. Blood cell formation occurs in red bone marrow, which is primarily stored in spongy bone.

Bones can be classified into five major categories: long, short, flat, irregular, and sesamoid.

Long bones, such as the femur (the thigh bone), are longer than they are wide. They are made up of a shaft, or *diaphysis*, and two bulbous ends, or *epiphyses*. The epiphyses form a joint with another bone and are covered in *articular cartilage* where bones meet to lessen friction during movement. The rest of a long bone is covered in a hard, vascular shell called the periosteum. Within the shaft of a long bone is compact tissue surrounding a space called the medullary cavity; this is where yellow marrow is stored. The epiphyses are covered in an outer layer of compact bone but are mostly composed of spongy bone.

The composition of short, flat, and irregular bones is different from that of a long bone, but similar to each other. They each consist of thin plates of compact bone covering the spongy bone in the middle. Red marrow is found within the spongy tissue of these bones, but there is no actual hollow cavity present. These bone types are classified according to their individual shapes. Short bones are cubelike, such as the bones in the wrist or ankle. Flat bones are platelike; most bones in the skull are flat bones. Irregular bones are those that have complicated shapes, such as the pelvic bones, vertebrae, and some facial bones.

Sesamoid bones are a unique type of bone that forms within *tendons*. They are small and round (some classify these as a type of short bone) and vary in size and number in different individuals. The function of most sesamoid bones is to

 INTERESTING A & P FACT

The skeleton accounts for approximately 30 to 40 percent of the body's total weight.

CLINICAL NOTE

Red marrow is primarily found in the spongy bone of the ribs, skull, sternum, clavicles, vertebrae, and pelvis of adults.

 DEFINITIONS

articular cartilage. Smooth living tissue that covers and protects moving surfaces, resulting in the reduction of friction.

diaphysis. Central shaft of a long bone.

epiphysis. Enlarged proximal and distal ends of a long bone.

tendon. Dense fibrous connective tissue that connects muscle to bone.

direct the pull of a tendon. The kneecap, or patella, is the most commonly recognized bone associated with this classification.

The external surfaces of all bone types have visible bulges, depressions, and holes for various physiological purposes, including providing sites for muscle, ligament, and tendon attachment to passageways for blood vessels and nerves. Some of the more commonly referred to markings for the purposes of coding are:

- **Condyle:** Rounded process that articulates with another bone.
- **Epicondyle:** Raised area on or above a condyle.
- **Facet:** Smooth surface that articulates with another bone.
- **Foramen:** Round opening through a bone.
- **Process:** Prominent projection.
- **Trochanter:** Very large, blunt process (found only on the femurs).
- **Tubercle:** Small rounded process.
- **Tuberosity:** Large rounded process.

The Axial Skeleton

The 206 bones that make up the adult skeleton can be divided into two classifications: the axial skeleton and appendicular skeleton. The axial, or "center," skeleton is formed by the bones and cartilaginous tissue in the skull, vertebral column, and thoracic cage. It supports and protects the organs of the head, neck, and trunk.

The skull consists of eight cranial bones, 14 facial bones, and the hyoid bone. The cranial bones form the cranium, which protects the brain and provides attachments for the muscles of the head and neck. The bones that form the cranium are:

- Two parietal
- Two temporal
- Frontal
- Occipital
- Sphenoid
- Ethmoid

Figure 3.1: Cranium

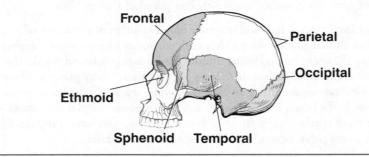

The facial bones provide the facial structure and provide attachments for the muscles that control facial and jaw movement. The face consists of 13 stationary bones and one mobile bone. The mandible (jawbone) is the only facial bone that moves and is also the largest and strongest bone of the face. The remaining bones of the face are:

- Two maxilla
- Two palatine
- Two zygomatic (cheekbones)
- Two lacrimal
- Two nasal
- Two inferior nasal concha (thin, curved bones that form the lateral walls of the nasal cavity)
- Vomer (located along the midline of the nasal cavity forming part of the nasal septum)

Figure 3.2: Facial Bones

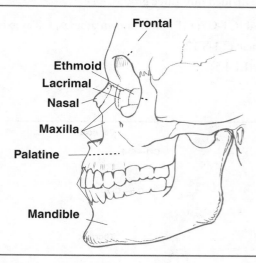

The hyoid bone is not really a part of the skull, as it does not articulate with any bones of the head. It is located in the neck just below the mandible. It supports the tongue and provides attachments for the muscles that move the larynx during speech and swallowing.

Also found in the head but outside of the skull are the bones that make up the middle ear. There are three bones found in each ear: the malleus, incus, and stapes. These bones are the smallest in the human body.

Attaching the skull to the body is the vertebral column, or bony spine. The vertebral column supports the head and trunk of the body and protects the spinal cord. It is composed of 26 individual bones. Of these bones, 24 are vertebrae that are separated by cartilage called intervertebral discs. Vertebrae have a common structure consisting of a body, *pedicles*, and *lamina* that form the vertebral arch. The body and arch come together and form an opening called the vertebral foramen, through which the *spinal cord* passes. Extending laterally off the vertebral arch are three processes: the two on each side are transverse processes, and the one in the middle is the spinous process. There are also processes that extend above and below the vertebral arch, known respectively as the inferior and superior articular processes.

 DEFINITIONS

lamina. Thin plate of membrane or other tissue.

pedicle. Narrow bony spike coming off a larger bone.

spinal cord. Portion of the central nervous system that extends from the brain through the vertebral canal.

Figure 3.3: Figure Vertebrae

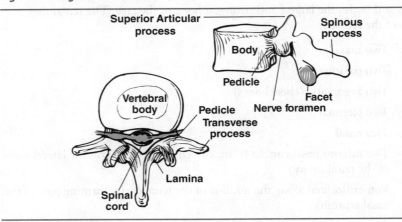

The vertebrae can be divided into three groups:

- Seven cervical (C1-C7; C1 is also known as atlas, C2 as axis)
- Twelve thoracic (T1-T12)
- Five lumbar (L1-L5)

Figure 3.4: Spine

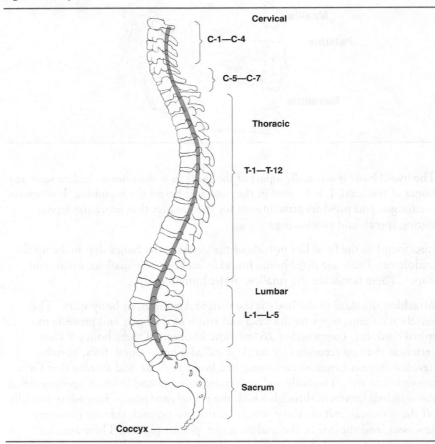

Below the lumbar vertebrae is the sacrum, which articulates with the pelvic bones of the appendicular skeleton. The last bone at the end of the vertebral column is the coccyx, or tail bone.

The spine has naturally occurring curves in it to increase its resilience. These curves allow it to function as a spring, bending and flexing with movement and impact. The names of the curves correspond with the vertebrae associated with it: the cervical, thoracic, and lumbar curvatures.

Articulating with the thoracic vertebrae are 12 pairs of flat bones known as the ribs. The first seven pairs of ribs meet up with the sternum directly via costal cartilage. The cartilage for the next three pairs of ribs joins with the costal cartilage of the seventh rib. The last two rib pairs do not join the sternum at all. The combination of these bones and cartilage form the thoracic cage, or bony thorax. This structure protects the lungs, heart, and great blood vessels. It also supports the shoulders and upper limbs and provides attachments for the muscles of the neck, back, chest, and shoulders.

Figure 3.5: Spine

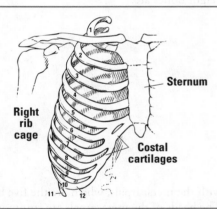

The Appendicular Skeleton

The bones that attach to the axial skeleton are referred to as the appendicular skeleton, which consists of the extremities and their respective girdles. This part of the skeleton enables the body to move.

The shoulder girdle consists of two bones on each side: the clavicle, or collar bone, and the scapula, or shoulder blade. It supports the upper limbs and provides the greatest range of movement found in the human body. The clavicle is found on the anterior side of the shoulder and the scapula on the posterior. The clavicles act as braces for the scapulas and arms by holding them outward.

The upper extremities are formed by 30 bones each and can be distinguished regionally as the upper arm, forearm, wrist, and hand. The bone in the upper arm is the humerus. Its superior epiphysis, or the humeral head, articulates with the glenoid cavity of the scapula to form the shoulder joint. At its inferior end, it articulates with the radius and ulna, the two bones that form the forearm. The radius is the long bone on the thumb side of the arm, and the ulna is located on the side of the little finger.

Figure 3.6: Shoulder/Upper Extremity

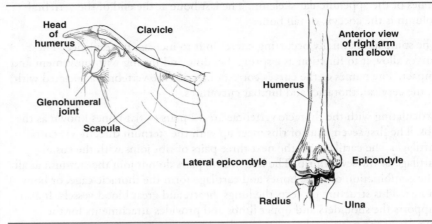

The wrist is composed of eight short bones called carpals that meet with the radius and ulna. These eight bones are:

- Scaphoid
- Capitate
- Trapezium
- Trapezoid
- Hamate
- Pisiform
- Triquetral
- Lunate

The carpals articulate with the metacarpals, which are the five bones that form the palm of the hand. The heads of the metacarpals are commonly referred to as knuckles, where the metacarpals join with the phalanges. Phalanges are the bones that form the fingers. There are three phalanges in all fingers, except for thumbs, which have only two. The phalanges that meet with the metacarpal heads are known as the proximal phalanges, then the middle phalanges, and, last, the distal phalanges.

Figure 3.7: Hand

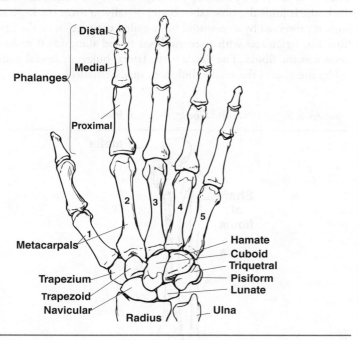

Similar to the upper extremity, the lower extremity follows the same basic structure with the pelvic girdles to attach the lower limbs to the axial skeleton. The pelvic or hip girdle distributes the weight of the body to the legs. It is composed of a coxal bone on each side that joins with the sacrum of the spine at the sacroiliac joint. The coxal bones can be divided into three parts:

- Ilium
- Ischium
- Pubis

Figure 3.8: Right Coxal Bone

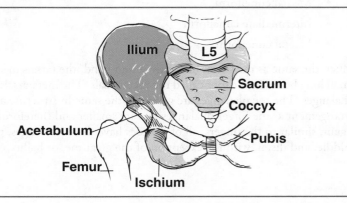

Where the three parts of the pelvic bone fuse is referred to as the acetabulum. It is a deep-seated pocket that accepts the rounded upper epiphysis of the thigh bone, or femoral head, to form the hip joint.

☞ **INTERESTING A & P FACT**

The coxal bones are three separate bones at birth. By adulthood, they are fused together as a single bone. However, the names of the three original bones are retained to identify the different regions of the bone: ilium, ischium, and pubis.

The femur is the only bone in the thigh and is the largest and strongest bone in the body. It joins the tibia (shin bone) distally to form the knee joint. The knee joint is protected by a sesamoid bone called the patella, or the knee cap. The tibia also articulates with a second bone found alongside it within the lower leg known as the fibula. The fibula is the lateral bulge, or lateral malleolus, of the ankle; the tibia is the medial bulge, or medial malleolus.

Figure 3.9: Right Tibia and Fibula, Anterior View

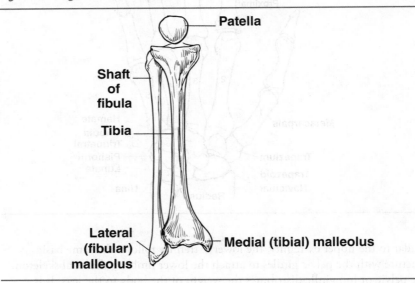

The tibia and fibula meet with the talus, the most superior of the seven tarsal bones, to form the ankle. The talus sits upon the calcaneus, or heel bone. Between the calcaneus and the metatarsals are the remaining five tarsals, known as:

- Cuboid
- Navicular
- Medial cuneiform
- Intermediate cuneiform
- Lateral cuneiform

Much the same as the bones in the wrist and hand, the tarsals meet with five small long bones in the foot called the metatarsals. The metatarsals meet up with phalanges. The toe phalanges are generally the same in structure and arrangement as the finger phalanges but are smaller and therefore less agile. Again, similar to the fingers, all of the toes have three phalanges, proximal, middle, and distal, with the exception of the great toe, or hallux.

Figure 3.10: Right Foot, Dorsal

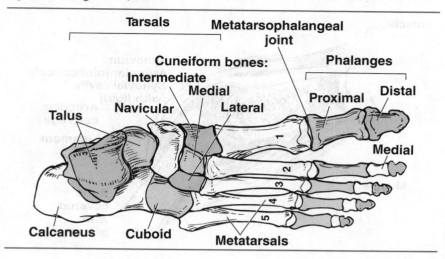

Articulations

Articulations, or joints, join two bones together and allow for movement in response to muscle contractions. There are three classifications of joints based on the structure or type of tissue the joint is composed of, including:

- Fibrous
- Cartilaginous
- Synovial

Fibrous joints are held together by dense tissue and are limited in movement by the length of that tissue. Most of these types of articulations are immovable or slightly moveable at best. There are three types of fibrous joints: sutures, or seams, between bones held together by connective tissue, such as those found in the cranium; gomphosis, a second type of fibrous joint, is found only as a tooth in its socket; and syndesmoses are bones joined by a *ligament*. The articulation between the tibia and fibula is an example of syndesmoses.

Cartilaginous joints are joined by cartilage. The first rib to the sternum is a cartilaginous articulation, as are the intervertebral joints and pubic symphysis. These types of joints do provide for some movement, albeit extremely minimal.

The majority of joints in the human body are synovial. These are free moving and therefore structurally more complex than the preceding two types. Synovial articulations all have a fluid-filled cavity separating the bones it joins. This cavity is called the synovial cavity, and the fluid is synovial fluid. The joint cavity is surrounded by a two-layer capsule called the articular capsule. The external layer of the capsule is a dense connective tissue that is contiguous with the periosteum of the related bones. The internal layer is a synovial membrane that covers all surfaces within the joint cavity except for the opposing bone surfaces. Articular cartilage covers those surfaces. Synovial joints are also unique in that they are reinforced by ligaments.

📖 **DEFINITIONS**

ligament. Fibrous tissue binding joints together connecting bone to bone or bone to cartilage.

Figure 3.11: Synovial Joint Structures

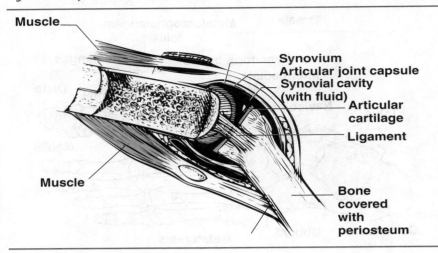

Synovial joints can be further classified by the movements they allow, including:

- **Ball-and-socket:** Head of a long bone ("ball") and depression of another bone ("socket") joint. The shoulder (humeral head and glenoid depression of the scapula) and hip joints (femoral head and acetabulum of a coxa bone) are ball-and-socket articulations.

- **Condyloid:** Protrusion of one bone meets a depression of another to form this type of joint. Examples are the wrist (radius and carpals) and knuckles (metacarpal and proximal phalange).

- **Hinge:** Convex portion of a bone meets with the concave part of another to form a hinge joint. The elbow and knee are large hinge joints.

- **Pivot:** Rounded or pointed protrusion of one bone fits into a ring composed of bone or bone and ligaments of another bone. The articulation between the C1 and C2 vertebrae that allows the head to move back and forth is a pivot joint.

- **Planar:** Flat surfaces of two bones glide against one another. The joints between the short carpals (intercarpal joint) and tarsals (intertarsal joint) are planar.

- **Saddle:** One bone has a depression shaped somewhat like an equestrian saddle; the joint is formed by a second bone straddling that depression. An example of this type of articulation is where the trapezium meets the metacarpal of the thumb. This joint allows the unique *opposition* of the human thumb.

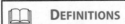

DEFINITIONS

opposition. Act of touching the thumb to the tips of each finger on the same hand.

Anatomy and Physiology and the ICD-10-CM Code Set

It is important to recognize the many differences between ICD-9-CM and ICD-10-CM when it comes to the skeletal system and its articulations. To assign the appropriate ICD-10-CM code, the coder needs advanced knowledge of the anatomy and physiology of the skeletal system and its articulations, as well as the ability to identify what additional information is needed.

Injuries

Injuries to the skeletal system are quite common as it is a rigid structure. The joints are also fairly susceptible to injury because part of their purpose is to maintain alignment, regardless of extraneous external forces.

Fractures, or breaks in the bone, are a common injury. There are roughly 6.8 million fractures reported in the United States annually.

In ICD-9-CM, the appropriate fracture code depends on the bone fractured, whether the fracture was *pathological* or traumatic, and whether it was considered open or closed. ICD-10-CM requires much more information than does ICD-9-CM.

For discussion purposes, ICD-9-CM and ICD-10-CM coding of a closed fracture of the greater tuberosity of the humerus will be compared. A difference in coding can be spotted immediately just by looking at the ICD-10-CM and ICD-9-CM alphabetic index. In ICD-10-CM, the fracture must be identified as traumatic or pathological before proceeding any further in code selection. In ICD-9-CM, the site of the fracture may be selected first, followed by whether it is pathological in nature. In ICD-9-CM, an injury is assumed to be traumatic unless further clarified. With the information provided, code 812.03 Fracture of humerus, upper end, closed, greater tuberosity, may be assigned in ICD-9-CM.

In ICD-10-CM, the above information is not sufficient for code assignment—there are two more considerations. First, is the fracture traumatic or pathological? Second, does the patient also have a diagnosis of *osteoporosis*? If the patient does have osteoporosis, according to ICD-10-CM coding guidelines, the fracture should automatically be reported as a pathological fracture of the humerus, regardless of whether it is specified as such. For demonstration purposes, assume the fracture is specified as traumatic, which leads us to category S42.25 Fracture of greater tuberosity of humerus.

Traumatic fractures must be further clarified with the following information:

- Is the bone *displaced*? If this is unspecified, ICD-10-CM Coding Guidelines direct the coder to assume the fracture is displaced.

- On which side of the body did the injury occur?

These two answers determine the sixth digit of the ICD-10-CM code. However, since fracture codes require a seventh character, even more information is needed. This alphabetic character is based on multiple factors as listed below:

- Is this the initial encounter for the fracture? If yes, is the fracture:
  - *open*
  - *closed*

DEFINITIONS

malunion. Fractured bone that has healed or is healing in an incorrect position.

nonunion. Fractured bone that has failed to heal.

- Is this a subsequent encounter? If yes:
  - Is the healing of the fracture routine or delayed?
  - Is there a *nonunion* or *malunion*?
  - Is there a sequela or late effects of the fracture?

Due to the extensive nature of code selection for a fracture in ICD-10-CM, there is a "one-to-many" match between the two coding classification systems as demonstrated in the table below.

Coding for Closed Fracture of Greater Tuberosity of the Humerus

ICD-9-CM		ICD-10-CM	
812.Ø3	Fracture of greater tuberosity of humerus, closed	S42.251A	Displaced fracture of greater tuberosity of right humerus, initial encounter for closed fracture
		S42.252A	Displaced fracture of greater tuberosity of left humerus, initial encounter for closed fracture
		S42.253A	Displaced fracture of greater tuberosity of unspecified humerus, initial encounter for closed fracture
		S42.254A	Nondisplaced fracture of greater tuberosity of right humerus, initial encounter for closed fracture
		S42.255A	Nondisplaced fracture of greater tuberosity of left humerus, initial encounter for closed fracture
		S42.256A	Nondisplaced fracture of greater tuberosity of unspecified humerus, initial encounter for closed fracture

Note that in ICD-9-CM, if a fracture is specified as complicated by a malunion or nonunion, the fracture site is irrelevant as there are only two applicable codes: 733.81 Malunion of fracture, and 733.82 Nonunion of fracture. However, documentation of the site, laterality, and type of complication is imperative in ICD-10-CM, as the same traumatic fracture codes are used but with a seventh character identifying malunion or nonunion.

Additionally, to appropriately assign a seventh digit for malunion or nonunion of an open fracture, a coder must be aware of the differences between the types of open fractures as described below:

- Type I: The wound is less than 1 cm in length and clean.
- Type II: The wound is greater than 1 cm in length, clean, and there is minimal to no soft tissue injury.
- Type III: The wound is greater than 1 cm in length, and there is significant soft tissue injury. Type III fractures can be further classified as:
  - IIIA: There is enough local soft tissue to cover the wound and bone without the need for skin grafting.
  - IIIB: The injury to the soft tissue is significant enough that skin grafting is necessary to cover the bone.
  - IIIC: The injury is associated with an arterial injury that requires repair.

The differences in coding for malunion and nonunion are captured in the following table. Please note that due to extensive mapping, the table is a sample of the ICD-10-CM codes that represent the various concepts.

Coding for Malunion and Nonunion of Traumatic Fractures

ICD-9-CM		ICD-10-CM	
733.81	Malunion of fracture	S42.021P	Displaced fracture of shaft of right clavicle, subsequent encounter with malunion
		S42.022P	Displaced fracture of shaft of left clavicle, subsequent encounter with malunion
		S42.023P	Displaced fracture of shaft of unspecified clavicle, subsequent encounter with malunion
		S42.024P	Nondisplaced fracture of shaft of right clavicle, subsequent encounter with malunion
		S42.025P	Nondisplaced fracture of shaft of left clavicle, subsequent encounter with malunion
		S42.026P	Nondisplaced fracture of shaft of unspecified clavicle, subsequent encounter with malunion
		S52.011P	*Torus fracture* of upper end of right ulna, subsequent encounter for closed fracture with malunion
		S52.011Q	Torus fracture of upper end of right ulna, subsequent encounter for open fracture type I or II with malunion
		S52.011R	Torus fracture of upper end of right ulna, subsequent encounter for open fracture type IIIA, IIIB or IIIC with malunion
733.82	Nonunion of fracture	S42.021K	Displaced fracture of shaft of right clavicle, subsequent encounter with nonunion
		S42.022K	Displaced fracture of shaft of left clavicle, subsequent encounter with nonunion
		S42.023K	Displaced fracture of shaft of unspecified clavicle, subsequent encounter with nonunion
		S42.024K	Nondisplaced fracture of shaft of right clavicle, subsequent encounter with nonunion
		S42.025K	Nondisplaced fracture of shaft of left clavicle, subsequent encounter with nonunion
		S42.026K	Nondisplaced fracture of shaft of unspecified clavicle, subsequent encounter with nonunion
		S52.011K	Torus fracture of upper end of right ulna, subsequent encounter for closed fracture with malunion
		S52.011M	Torus fracture of upper end of right ulna, subsequent encounter for open fracture type I or II with nonunion
		S52.011N	Torus fracture of upper end of right ulna, subsequent encounter for open fracture type IIIA, IIIB or IIIC with nonunion

 DEFINITIONS

torus fracture. Buckling or bowing of the bone with little or no displacement at the end and no breakage, usually occurring in children due to softer bone tissue.

In addition to expanding the traumatic fracture categories to include malunion and nonunion, ICD-10-CM expands the same traumatic fracture codes to capture sequelae or the late effects of fractures. In ICD-9-CM, codes 905.0 through 905.5 report any abnormal condition arising as a reaction to a fracture. In ICD-10-CM, the same codes for the initial fracture are reported but with a seventh character of S as demonstrated in the following table. Please note that due to extensive mapping, the table is a sample of the ICD-10-CM codes that represent the various concepts.

apophyseal fracture. Avulsion fracture in which a bony prominence, such as a process or tuberosity, is removed from its bone.

comminuted fracture. Any type of fracture in which the bone is splintered or crushed, resulting in multiple bone fragments.

greenstick fracture. Incomplete fracture in which the bone is bent but fractured only on the outer arc of the bend.

Monteggia's fracture. Break in the proximal half of the ulnar shaft accompanied by a dislocation of the radial head.

neoplastic. Relating to any abnormal growth of new tissue, benign or malignant; in this case, usually a malignancy.

osteomyelitis. Inflammation of bone that may remain localized or spread to the marrow, cortex, or periosteum, in response to an infecting organism.

Salter-Harris fracture. Fractures through a growth plate.

spiral fracture. Bone break in which the disruption of the bone is spiral to the shaft of the bone.

Coding Late Effects of Traumatic Fractures

ICD-9-CM		ICD-10-CM	
905.0	Late effect of fracture of skull and face bones	S02.110	Type I occipital condyle fracture, sequela
905.1	Late effect of fracture of spine and trunk without mention of spinal cord lesion	S12.030S	Displaced posterior arch fracture of first cervical vertebra, sequela
		S12.031S	Nondisplaced posterior arch fracture of first cervical vertebra, sequela
905.2	Late effect of fracture of upper extremities	S042.011S	Anterior displaced fracture of sternal end of right clavicle, sequela
		S042.15S	Posterior displaced fracture of sternal end of left clavicle, sequela
		S52.271S	*Monteggia's fracture* of right ulna, sequela
		S52.311S	*Greenstick fracture* of shaft of right radius, sequela
905.3	Late effect of fracture of neck of femur	S72.111S	Displaced fracture of greater trochanter of right femur, sequela
		S72.134S	Nondisplaced *apophyseal fracture* of right femur, sequela
905.4	Late effect of fracture of lower extremities	S72.341S	Displaced *spiral fracture* of shaft of right femur, sequela
		S72.354S	Nondisplaced *comminuted fracture* of the shaft of the right femur, sequela
		S79.011S	*Salter-Harris* Type I physeal fracture of upper end of right femur, sequela
		S82.035S	Nondisplaced transverse fracture of left patella, sequela
905.5	Late effect of fracture of multiple or unspecified bones	Coded to the sites of the fractures with seventh character of S; if the bone is unspecified, a code cannot be determined.	

Just as with traumatic fractures, the coding of pathological fractures is also extremely different in ICD-10-CM. In ICD-9-CM, the only documentation needed to assign a code from category 733.1 Pathological fracture, is the location of the fracture and confirmation that it is pathological in nature. However, in ICD-10-CM, much more information is needed.

The most obvious difference is the division of the pathological codes by the disease process responsible for the fracture. Because these types of fractures are caused by underlying disease processes, ICD-10-CM has split the code sets to reflect the most common causes of pathological fractures. There are categories for fractures due to *neoplastic* disease, age-related and other osteoporosis, and other specified diseases to capture the not-so-common contributing factors, such as *osteomyelitis*.

After identifying the disease process, the coder must also specify site and laterality, whether the encounter is initial or subsequent, and any healing issues.

Coding for Initial Visit for Pathological Fracture of Neck of Femur

ICD-9-CM		ICD-10-CM	
733.14	Pathologic fracture of neck of femur	M80.051A	Age related osteoporosis with current pathological fracture, right femur, initial encounter
		M80.052A	Age related osteoporosis with current pathological fracture, left femur, initial encounter
		M80.059A	Age related osteoporosis with current pathological fracture, unspecified femur, initial encounter
		M80.851A	Other osteoporosis with current pathological fracture, right femur, initial encounter
		M80.852A	Other osteoporosis with current pathological fracture, left femur, initial encounter
		M80.859A	Other osteoporosis with current pathological fracture, unspecified femur, initial encounter
		M84.451A	Pathological fracture, right femur, initial encounter
		M84.452A	Pathological fracture, left femur, initial encounter
		M84.459A	Pathological fracture, unspecified femur, initial encounter
		M84.551A	Pathologic fracture in neoplastic disease, right femur, initial encounter
		M84.552A	Pathologic fracture in neoplastic disease, left femur, initial encounter
		M84.593A	Pathologic fracture in neoplastic disease, unspecified femur, initial encounter
		M84.559A	Pathologic fracture in neoplastic disease, hip, unspecified, initial encounter
		M84.651A	Pathologic fracture in other disease, right femur, initial encounter
		M84.652A	Pathologic fracture in other disease, left femur, initial encounter
		M84.653A	Pathologic fracture in other disease, unspecified femur, initial encounter
		M84.659A	Pathologic fracture in other disease, hip, unspecified, initial encounter

Note that in ICD-9-CM, the verbiage "collapsed vertebra" is synonymous with a pathological fracture and, therefore, 733.13 is reported for this condition. ICD-10-CM, however, differentiates between a vertebral collapse and pathological fracture. There is an entire category for collapsed vertebrae that are not specified as being due to a pathological fracture.

DEFINITIONS

acromioclavicular joint. Joint between the acromion of the scapula and the clavicle.

dislocation. Displacement of a bone from its normal position within an articulation.

subluxation. Incomplete dislocation.

Coding for Collapsed Vertebra

ICD-9-CM		ICD-10-CM	
733.13	Pathological fracture of vertebrae	M48.50xA	Collapsed vertebra, not elsewhere classified, site unspecified, initial encounter
		M48.51xA	Collapsed vertebra, not elsewhere classified, occipito-atlanto-axial region, initial encounter
		M48.52xA	Collapsed vertebra, not elsewhere classified, cervical region, initial encounter
		M48.53xA	Collapsed vertebra, not elsewhere classified, cervicothoracic region, initial encounter
		M48.54xA	Collapsed vertebra, not elsewhere classified, thoracic region, initial encounter
		M48.55xA	Collapsed vertebra, not elsewhere classified, thoracolumbar region, initial encounter
		M48.56xA	Collapsed vertebra, not elsewhere classified, lumbar region, initial encounter
		M48.57xA	Collapsed vertebra, not elsewhere classified, lumbosacral region, initial encounter
		M48.58xA	Collapsed vertebra, not elsewhere classified, sacral and sacrococcygeal region, initial encounter

Another fairly common acute injury affecting the skeletal system is dislocation of a joint. ICD-9-CM coding for this condition is straightforward; the code system classifies *subluxation* and *dislocation* together, and the code is based on the articulation that has been disrupted and whether that disruption is open or closed. For most body sites in ICD-10-CM, code selection is also basic, being determined by site and laterality, but it is further divided by whether the injury is a subluxation or true dislocation. For certain sites of dislocation or subluxation, code selection is further divided by degree or direction of separation. Please note that due to extensive mapping, the table below is a sample of the ICD-10-CM codes that represent the various concepts discussed.

Coding for Dislocation and Subluxation

ICD-9-CM		ICD-10-CM	
831.04	Closed dislocation of the *acromioclavicular (joint)*	S43.101A	Unspecified dislocation of right acromioclavicular joint, initial encounter
		S43.102A	Unspecified dislocation of left acromioclavicular joint, initial encounter
		S43.109A	Unspecified dislocation of unspecified acromioclavicular joint, initial encounter
		S43.111A	Subluxation of right acromioclavicular joint, initial encounter
		S43.121A	Dislocation of right acromioclavicular joint, 100%-200% displacement, initial encounter
		S43.131A	Dislocation of right acromioclavicular joint, greater than 200% displacement, initial encounter
		S43.141A	Inferior dislocation of right acromioclavicular joint, initial encounter
		S43.151A	Posterior dislocation of right acromioclavicular joint, initial encounter

ICD-9-CM		ICD-10-CM	
839.61	Closed dislocation of sternum (*sternoclavicular joint*)	S43.201A	Unspecified subluxation of right sternoclavicular joint, initial encounter
		S43.202A	Unspecified subluxation of left sternoclavicular joint, initial encounter
		S43.203A	Unspecified subluxation of unspecified sternoclavicular joint, initial encounter
		S43.204A	Unspecified dislocation of right sternoclavicular joint, initial encounter
		S43.205A	Unspecified dislocation of left sternoclavicular joint, initial encounter
		S43.206A	Unspecified dislocation of unspecified sternoclavicular joint, initial encounter
		S43.211A	Anterior subluxation of right sternoclavicular joint, initial encounter
		S43.221A	Posterior subluxation of right sternoclavicular joint, initial encounter

> **DEFINITIONS**
>
> **sternoclavicular joint.** Joint between the sternum and the clavicle.

Another common affliction impacting certain joints of the skeletal system is a torn meniscus. This is most commonly seen in the knee joint where two C shaped, cartilage-based cushions are found. They are sandwiched between the lateral and medial condyles of each femur where they articulate with the condyles of the tibia; one on the inside of the knee (the medial meniscus) and one on the outside (lateral meniscus). There are two usual causes of a meniscus tear: trauma and degeneration. A traumatic tear is usually acute and repairable; a tear caused by degeneration is usually chronic or old and irreparable. Only a physician can determine the acuity of the injury. ICD-10-CM guidelines help coders distinguish between acute versus old or chronic by stating that recurrent conditions or conditions that are the result of a healed injury are considered old.

Coding old, chronic, or recurrent meniscus tears is relatively the same in both classification systems, with the exception that ICD-10-CM differentiates laterality of the injury. On the other hand, acute meniscus tears are different. In ICD-9-CM, the site of the tear, lateral or medial meniscus, is the only consideration. The newer classification, however, expands that information to also include the laterality and type of tear. The different types of meniscus tears included in ICD-10-CM code selection are:

- **Bucket handle:** Tear in which the inner portion of the meniscus displaces into the joint causing the meniscus to resemble a bucket and its handle. These are always traumatic injuries.

- **Complex:** Describes more than one type of tear or a tear that goes in more than one direction.

- **Peripheral:** Indicates tears located in the peripheral or outer third of the meniscus. This area is susceptible to healing as it has access to a rich blood supply.

Figure 3.12: Tears of Meniscus

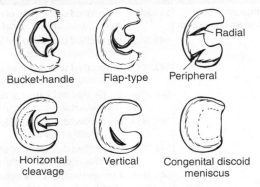

It is important to note, that like fractures and dislocations, acute meniscus tears also require a seventh character distinguishing the encounter as initial (A), subsequent (D), or a sequela of the injury (S). For discussion purposes, only the initial encounter is highlighted below.

Coding for Meniscus Tears

ICD-9-CM		ICD-10-CM	
836.0	Tear medial cartilage or meniscus of knee, current	S83.211A	Bucket handle tear of medial meniscus, current injury, right knee, initial encounter
		S83.212A	Bucket handle tear of medial meniscus, current injury, left knee, initial encounter
		S83.219A	Bucket handle tear of medial meniscus, current injury, unspecified knee, initial encounter
		S83.221A	Peripheral tear of medial meniscus, current injury, right knee, initial encounter
		S83.222A	Peripheral tear of medial meniscus, current injury, left knee, initial encounter
		S83.229A	Peripheral tear of medial meniscus, current injury, unspecified knee, initial encounter
		S83.231A	Complex tear of medial meniscus, current injury, right knee, initial encounter
		S83.232A	Complex tear of medial meniscus, current injury, left knee, initial encounter
		S83.239A	Complex tear of medial meniscus, current injury, unspecified knee, initial encounter
		S83.241A	Other tear of medial meniscus, current injury, right knee, initial encounter
		S83.242A	Other tear of medial meniscus, current injury, left knee, initial encounter
		S83.249A	Other tear of medial meniscus, current injury, unspecified knee, initial encounter

ICD-9-CM		ICD-10-CM	
836.1	Tear lateral cartilage or meniscus of knee, current	S83.251A	Bucket handle tear of lateral meniscus, current injury, right knee, initial encounter
		S83.252A	Bucket handle tear of lateral meniscus, current injury, left knee, initial encounter
		S83.259A	Bucket handle tear of lateral meniscus, current injury, unspecified knee, initial encounter
		S83.261A	Peripheral tear of lateral meniscus, current injury, right knee, initial encounter
		S83.262A	Peripheral tear of lateral meniscus, current injury, left knee, initial encounter
		S83.269A	Peripheral tear of lateral meniscus, current injury, unspecified knee, initial encounter
		S83.271A	Complex tear of lateral meniscus, current injury, right knee, initial encounter
		S83.272A	Complex tear of lateral meniscus, current injury, left knee, initial encounter
		S83.279A	Complex tear of lateral meniscus, current injury, unspecified knee, initial encounter
		S83.281A	Other tear of lateral meniscus, current injury, right knee, initial encounter
		S83.282A	Other tear of lateral meniscus, current injury, left knee, initial encounter
		S83.289A	Other tear of lateral meniscus, current injury, unspecified knee, initial encounter

Infections

Like any other system in the body, the skeletal system and its joints are susceptible to infection. An infection of the bone is known as osteomyelitis. Bacteria, most commonly *Staphylococcal aureus,* are usually the infecting agent, but occasionally fungi are responsible. Infection can be caused by direct exposure to the organism via open fracture or bone surgery and can occur at the site of internal orthopedic devices or adjacent soft tissue infections. Osteomyelitis can be acute or chronic in nature. Chronic osteomyelitis persists over time and can cause many complications, such as bone deformity and pathological fractures. ICD-9-CM categorizes osteomyelitis by acuity and site, as does ICD-10-CM. However, that is just the beginning of code selection for ICD-10-CM. In addition to distinguishing laterality, the coder must also determine whether the osteomyelitis is:

- Acute:
  - Is the infection *hematogenous*?
  - Is the infection actually acute or is it *subacute*?
- Chronic
  - Is there a draining *sinus*?
  - Is the infection hematogenous?
  - Is the infection *multifocal*?

 CLINICAL NOTE

Chronic osteomyelitis occurs in 5 to 25 percent of patients that have had acute osteomyelitis.

DEFINITIONS

hematogenous. Originating or transported in blood.

multifocal. Having many points of origin.

sinus. Cavity or channel leading to a pocket of purulent material.

subacute. Being present as a disease or other abnormal condition in a person who appears to be clinically well.

Coding for Osteomyelitis of the Sternum

ICD-9-CM		ICD-10-CM	
730.08	Acute osteomyelitis, other specified site	M86.08	Acute hematogenous osteomyelitis, other sites
		M86.18	Other acute osteomyelitis, other sites
		M86.28	Subacute osteomyelitis, other sites
730.18	Chronic osteomyelitis, other specified site	M86.38	Chronic multifocal osteomyelitis, other sites
		M86.48	Chronic osteomyelitis with draining sinus, other sites
		M86.58	Other chronic hematogenous osteomyelitis, other sites
		M86.68	Other chronic osteomyelitis, other sites
		M86.8x8	Other osteomyelitis, other sites

An infection of the fluid and tissues of a joint is referred to as septic or pyogenic arthritis. These infections are also caused mainly by bacteria but can also be caused by fungi. ICD-10-CM has divided the classification for septic arthritis by bacterial organism in addition to the site and side affected.

Coding for Septic Arthritis of the Hip

ICD-9-CM		ICD-10-CM	
711.05	Pyogenic arthritis pelvic region and thigh	M00.051	Staphylococcal arthritis, right hip
		M00.052	Staphylococcal arthritis, left hip
		M00.059	Staphylococcal arthritis, unspecified hip
		M00.151	Pneumococcal arthritis, right hip
		M00.152	Pneumococcal arthritis, left hip
		M00.159	Pneumococcal arthritis, unspecified hip
		M00.251	Other streptococcal arthritis, right hip
		M00.252	Other streptococcal arthritis, left hip
		M00.259	Other streptococcal arthritis, unspecified hip
		M00.351	Arthritis due to other bacteria, right hip
		M00.352	Arthritis due to other bacteria, left hip
		M00.359	Arthritis due to other bacteria, unspecified hip

Occasionally, a joint is affected by an infection elsewhere. Inflammation of a joint as a reaction to another disease is referred to as reactive arthropathy. A secondary infection can also arise within a joint, referred to as direct infection. Although the two conditions are very different, ICD-9-CM classifies both under the same categories, 711.4 to 711.6, distinguished by site of the affliction and type of organism: bacterial, viral, or fungal (mycosis). On the other hand, ICD-10-CM has distinguished between reactive arthropathy and a direct infection, giving each its own category, but it has lost some of the detail of ICD-9-CM by not distinguishing the type of organism afflicting the joint. Both code sets require a code be assigned first for the underlying disease, such as leprosy, mycoses, or paratyphoid fever.

Coding for Arthropathy of the Right Shoulder Associated with Other Infectious Diseases

ICD-9-CM		ICD-10-CM	
711.41	Arthropathy associated with other bacterial disease, shoulder region	M01.x11	Direct infection of right shoulder in infectious and parasitic diseases classified elsewhere
		M02.811	Other reactive arthropathies, right shoulder
711.51	Arthropathy associated with other viral diseases, shoulder region	M01.x11	Direct infection of right shoulder in infectious and parasitic diseases classified elsewhere
		M02.811	Other reactive arthropathies, right shoulder
711.61	Arthropathy associated with mycoses, shoulder region	M01.x11	Direct infection of right shoulder in infectious and parasitic diseases classified elsewhere
		M02.811	Other reactive arthropathies, right shoulder

Inflammatory and Degenerative Conditions

As the human body ages, the cartilage of the joints begins to degenerate and lose its elasticity from wear and tear and the natural aging process. This degeneration is referred to as primary osteoarthritis. The same type of disorder can also be caused by other disease processes, such as trauma, obesity, and some metabolic disorders. Osteoarthritis caused by something other than aging is called secondary osteoarthritis.

ICD-9-CM and ICD-10-CM osteoarthritis codes are similar in that there are categories for generalized, primary, secondary, localized, and unspecified osteoarthritis, further divided by site. In fact, localized and unspecified osteoarthritis codes are direct, one-to-one matches between the two classification systems. However, in many instances ICD-10-CM requires more detail, including laterality and cause in the case of secondary osteoarthritis. When the osteoarthritis site is the hand, ICD-10-CM also distinguishes between the first carpometacarpal joint and all other joints. The following table is not a complete mapping of all of the types of osteoarthritis that may occur, but gives the coder an idea of what may be seen in ICD-10-CM. For detailed information on ICD-9-CM to ICD-10-CM mapping, see *Ingenix's ICD-10-CM Mappings*.

Coding for Secondary Osteoarthritis

ICD-9-CM		ICD-10-CM	
715.21	Secondary localized osteoarthrosis, shoulder region	M19.111	Post-traumatic osteoarthritis, right shoulder
		M19.112	Post-traumatic osteoarthritis, left shoulder
		M19.119	Post-traumatic osteoarthritis, unspecified shoulder
		M19.211	Secondary osteoarthritis, right shoulder
		M19.212	Secondary osteoarthritis, left shoulder
		M19.219	Secondary osteoarthritis, unspecified shoulder
715.22	Secondary localized osteoarthrosis, upper arm	M19.121	Post-traumatic osteoarthritis, right elbow
		M19.122	Post-traumatic osteoarthritis, left elbow
		M19.129	Post-traumatic osteoarthritis, unspecified elbow
		M19.221	Secondary osteoarthritis, right elbow
		M19.222	Secondary osteoarthritis, left elbow
		M19.229	Secondary osteoarthritis, unspecified elbow

ICD-9-CM		ICD-10-CM	
715.23	Secondary localized osteoarthrosis, forearm	M19.131	Post-traumatic osteoarthritis, right wrist
		M19.132	Post-traumatic osteoarthritis, left wrist
		M19.139	Post-traumatic osteoarthritis, unspecified wrist
		M19.231	Secondary osteoarthritis, right wrist
		M19.232	Secondary osteoarthritis, left wrist
		M19.239	Secondary osteoarthritis, unspecified wrist
715.25	Secondary localized osteoarthritis, pelvic region and thigh	M16.2	Bilateral osteoarthritis resulting from hip dysplasia
		M16.3Ø	Unilateral osteoarthritis resulting from hip dysplasia, unspecified hip
		M16.31	Unilateral osteoarthritis resulting from hip dysplasia, right hip
		M16.32	Unilateral osteoarthritis resulting from hip dysplasia, left hip
		M16.4	Bilateral post-traumatic osteoarthritis
		M16.5Ø	Unilateral post-traumatic osteoarthritis, unspecified hip
		M16.51	Unilateral post-traumatic osteoarthritis, right hip
		M16.52	Unilateral post-traumatic osteoarthritis, left hip
		M16.6	Other bilateral secondary osteoarthritis of hip
		M16.7	Other unilateral secondary osteoarthritis of hip
715.26	Secondary localized osteoarthritis, lower leg	M17.2	Bilateral post-traumatic osteoarthritis of knee
		M17.3Ø	Unilateral post-traumatic osteoarthritis, unspecified knee
		M17.31	Unilateral post-traumatic osteoarthritis, right knee
		M17.32	Unilateral post-traumatic osteoarthritis, left knee
		M17.4	Other bilateral secondary osteoarthritis of knee
		M17.5	Other unilateral secondary osteoarthritis of knee

📖 **DEFINITIONS**

paresthesia. Sensation of tingling, pricking, or numbness of skin.

spastic paresis. Condition in which the muscles are affected by persistent spasms and exaggerated tendon reflexes.

Degenerative osteoarthritis occurring in the spine is called spondylosis. Spondylosis can cause compression on nerves and blood vessels that are affiliated with or near the spine. Compression that disturbs spinal cord function is referred to as myelopathy. Myelopathy manifests itself in various ways, including *paresthesia* and *spastic paresis*. Another manifestation, radiculopathy, also known as a pinched nerve, can occur, causing pain, weakness, and numbness. In severe cases of spondylosis, the anterior spinal artery and/or the vertebral artery may be compressed, called compression syndrome.

ICD-9-CM divides the spondylosis codes by spinal region and whether myelopathy was present. ICD-10-CM also uses these distinct identifiers to assign codes but increases detail by further specifying the spinal region and differentiating between myelopathy and radiculopathy. New codes identify when the spondylosis has progressed to include blood vessel compression.

Coding for Spondylosis

ICD-9-CM		ICD-10-CM	
721.0	Cervical spondylosis without myelopathy	M47.21	Other spondylosis with radiculopathy, occipito-atlanto-axial region
		M47.22	Other spondylosis with radiculopathy, cervical region
		M47.23	Other spondylosis with radiculopathy, cervicothoracic region
		M47.811	Spondylosis without myelopathy or radiculopathy, occipito-atlanto-axial region
		M47.812	Spondylosis without myelopathy or radiculopathy, cervical region
		M47.813	Spondylosis without myelopathy or radiculopathy, cervicothoracic region
		M47.891	Other spondylosis, occipito-atlanto-axial region
		M47.892	Other spondylosis, cervical region
		M47.893	Other spondylosis, cervicothoracic region
721.1	Cervical spondylosis with myelopathy	M47.011	Anterior spinal artery compression syndromes, occipito-atlanto-axial region
		M47.012	Anterior spinal artery compression syndromes, cervical region
		M47.013	Anterior spinal artery compression syndromes, cervicothoracic region
		M47.021	Vertebral artery compression syndromes, occipito-atlanto-axial region
		M47.022	Vertebral artery compression syndromes, cervical region
		M47.029	Vertebral artery compression syndromes, site unspecified
		M47.11	Other spondylosis with myelopathy, occipito-atlanto-axial region
		M47.12	Other spondylosis with myelopathy, cervical region
		M47.13	Other spondylosis with myelopathy, cervicothoracic region
721.2	Thoracic spondylosis without myelopathy	M47.24	Other spondylosis with radiculopathy, thoracic region
		M47.25	Other spondylosis with radiculopathy, thoracolumbar region
		M47.814	Spondylosis without myelopathy or radiculopathy, thoracic region
		M47.815	Spondylosis without myelopathy or radiculopathy, thoracolumbar region
		M47.894	Other spondylosis, thoracic region
		M47.895	Other spondylosis, thoracolumbar region

ICD-9-CM		ICD-10-CM	
721.3	Lumbosacral spondylosis without myelopathy	M47.26	Other spondylosis with radiculopathy, lumbar region
		M47.27	Other spondylosis with radiculopathy, lumbosacral region
		M47.28	Other spondylosis with radiculopathy, sacral and sacrococcygeal region
		M47.816	Spondylosis without myelopathy or radiculopathy, lumbar region
		M47.817	Spondylosis without myelopathy or radiculopathy, lumbosacral region
		M47.818	Spondylosis without myelopathy or radiculopathy, sacral and sacrococcygeal region
		M47.896	Other spondylosis, lumbar region
		M47.897	Other spondylosis, lumbosacral region
		M47.898	Other spondylosis, sacral and sacrococcygeal region
721.41	Spondylosis with myelopathy, thoracic region	M47.14	Other spondylosis with myelopathy, thoracic region
		M47.15	Other spondylosis with myelopathy, thoracolumbar region
721.42	Spondylosis with myelopathy, lumbar region	M47.16	Other spondylosis with myelopathy, lumbar region
		M47.17	Other spondylosis with myelopathy, lumbosacral region
		M47.18	Other spondylosis with myelopathy, sacral and sacrococcygeal region

As mentioned earlier, secondary arthritis can also be caused by certain disorders, such as *gout*. In gout, uric acid crystals can collect around the joint structures, causing inflammation. ICD-9-CM and ICD-10-CM give gouty arthropathy its own categories arranged first by acute versus chronic diagnosis. ICD-10-CM further clarifies acute gouty arthropathy by anatomical site and laterality (where applicable), as well as whether the gout is *idiopathic* or drug-induced.

📖 **DEFINITIONS**

gout. Metabolic condition causing painful and inflamed joints.

idiopathic. Having no known cause.

Coding for Acute and Unspecified Gouty Arthropathy

ICD-9-CM	ICD-10-CM	
274.00 Gouty arthropathy, unspecified	M10.00	Idiopathic gout, unspecified site
	M10.01[1,2,9]	Idiopathic gout, shoulder
	M10.02[1,2,9]	Idiopathic gout, elbow
	M10.03[1,2,9]	Idiopathic gout, wrist
	M10.04[1,2,9]	Idiopathic gout, hand
	M10.05[1,2,9]	Idiopathic gout, hip
	M10.06[1,2,9]	Idiopathic gout, knee
	M10.07[1,2,9]	Idiopathic gout, ankle and foot
	M10.08	Idiopathic gout, vertebrae
	M10.09	Idiopathic gout, multiple sites
	M10.20	Drug-induced gout, unspecified site
	M10.21[1,2,9]	Drug-induced gout, shoulder
	M10.22[1,2,9]	Drug-induced gout, elbow
	M10.23[1,2,9]	Drug-induced gout, wrist
	M10.24[1,2,9]	Drug-induced gout, hand
	M10.25[1,2,9]	Drug-induced gout, hip
	M10.26[1,2,9]	Drug-induced gout, knee
	M10.27[1,2,9]	Drug-induced gout, ankle and foot
	M10.28	Drug-induced gout, vertebrae
	M10.29	Drug-induced gout, multiple sites
	6th Character meanings for codes as indicated **1 RIGHT 2 LEFT 9 UNSPECIFIED**	
274.01 Acute gouty arthropathy	M10.00	Idiopathic gout, unspecified site
	M10.01[1,2,9]	Idiopathic gout, shoulder
	M10.02[1,2,9]	Idiopathic gout, elbow
	M10.03[1,2,9]	Idiopathic gout, wrist
	M10.04[1,2,9]	Idiopathic gout, hand
	M10.05[1,2,9]	Idiopathic gout, hip
	M10.06[1,2,9]	Idiopathic gout, knee
	M10.07[1,2,9]	Idiopathic gout, ankle and foot
	M10.08	Idiopathic gout, vertebrae
	M10.09	Idiopathic gout, multiple sites
	M10.20	Drug-induced gout, unspecified site
	M10.21[1,2,9]	Drug-induced gout, shoulder
	M10.22[1,2,9]	Drug-induced gout, elbow
	M10.23[1,2,9]	Drug-induced gout, wrist
	M10.24[1,2,9]	Drug-induced gout, hand
	M10.25[1,2,9]	Drug-induced gout, hip
	M10.26[1,2,9]	Drug-induced gout, knee
	M10.27[1,2,9]	Drug-induced gout, ankle and foot
	M10.28	Drug-induced gout, vertebrae
	M10.29	Drug-induced gout, multiple sites
	6th Character meanings for codes as indicated **1 RIGHT 2 LEFT 9 UNSPECIFIED**	

Just as in ICD-9-CM, ICD-10-CM classifies chronic gouty arthropathy by whether a *tophus* is present and further divides the classifications by anatomical site, laterality (where applicable), and cause. The following table is not a complete mapping of all of the types of chronic gouty arthropathy that may occur, but gives the coder an idea of what may be seen in ICD-10-CM. For detailed information on ICD-9-CM to ICD-10-CM mapping, see *Ingenix's ICD-10-CM Mappings*.

 DEFINITIONS

tophus. Calculus that forms in fibrous tissue.

Coding for Chronic Gouty Arthropathy

ICD-9-CM	ICD-10-CM	
274.02 Chronic gouty arthropathy without mention of tophus	M1a.00x0	Idiopathic chronic gout, unspecified site without tophus (tophi)
	M1.a01[**1,2,9**]0	Idiopathic chronic gout, shoulder without tophus (tophi)
	M1.a02[**1,2,9**]0	Idiopathic chronic gout, elbow without tophus (tophi)
	M1.a03[**1,2,9**]0	Idiopathic chronic gout, wrist without tophus (tophi)
	M1.a04[**1,2,9**]0	Idiopathic chronic gout, hand without tophus (tophi)
	M1.a05[**1,2,9**]0	Idiopathic chronic gout, hip without tophus (tophi)
	M1a.20x0	Drug-induced chronic gout, unspecified site without tophus (tophi)
	M1a.21[**1,2,9**]0	Drug-induced chronic gout, shoulder without tophus (tophi)
	M1a.22[**1,2,9**]0	Drug-induced chronic gout, elbow without tophus (tophi)
	6th Character meanings for codes as indicated **1 RIGHT 2 LEFT 9 UNSPECIFIED**	
274.03 Chronic gouty arthropathy with tophus	M1a.a09x1	Idiopathic chronic gout, multiple sites with tophus (tophi)
	M1a.20x1	Drug-induced chronic gout, unspecified site with tophus (tophi)
	M1a.21[**1,2,9**]1	Drug-induced chronic gout, shoulder with tophus (tophi)
	M1a.22[**1,2,9**]1	Drug-induced chronic gout, elbow with tophus (tophi)
	M1a.30x1	Chronic gout due to renal impairment, unspecified site with tophus (tophi)
	M1a.31[**1,2,9**]1	Chronic gout due to renal impairment, shoulder with tophus (tophi)
	M1a.32[**1,2,9**]1	Chronic gout due to renal impairment, elbow with tophus (tophi))
	6th Character meanings for codes as indicated **1 RIGHT 2 LEFT 9 UNSPECIFIED**	

Another common type of arthritis is rheumatoid arthritis (RA). RA is inflammation and destruction of the joint tissues due to an autoimmune disorder. RA can also affect other body systems and organs and is, therefore, sometimes considered a systemic disease.

In ICD-10-CM, it is important to understand the different musculoskeletal manifestations of RA. In ICD-9-CM, a code for RA (714.0) is reported first, followed by a code for any manifestations. The newer classification system expands the categories for RA by anatomical site and common manifestation. Complications identified in ICD-10-CM are myopathy, neuropathy, bursitis, and nodules. Myopathy is any abnormal condition affecting the muscles due to RA; this could be in the form of atrophy, weakness, myalgia, or similar symptoms. Neuropathy can be caused by inflammation and disfigurement of the joints, causing compression and entrapment of nerves. Bursitis, an inflammation of the connective tissue surrounding a joint, in RA is a result of the increased pressure put on joints. And lastly, rheumatoid nodules are firm, rounded masses occurring subcutaneously at areas of pressure, such as the elbows. These occur in approximately 25 percent of patients and are usually associated with more complicated extensions of the disease process.

If there is no manifestation mentioned, documentation specifying whether the patient has an abnormal antibody, called the rheumatoid factor, present in the blood can help in assigning a more detailed code. Rheumatoid factor is present in 80 percent of patients diagnosed with RA. The following table is not a complete mapping of all of the types of rheumatoid arthritis that may occur, but gives the coder an idea of what may be seen in ICD-10-CM. For detailed information on ICD-9-CM to ICD-10-CM mapping, see *Ingenix's ICD-10-CM Mappings*.

Coding for Rheumatoid Arthritis

ICD-9-CM	ICD-10-CM	
714.0 Rheumatoid Arthritis	M05.41[1,2,9]	Rheumatoid myopathy with rheumatoid arthritis, shoulder
	M05.42[1,2,9]	Rheumatoid myopathy with rheumatoid arthritis, elbow
	M05.53[1,2,9]	Rheumatoid polyneuropathy with rheumatoid arthritis, wrist
	M05.54[1,2,9]	Rheumatoid polyneuropathy with rheumatoid arthritis, hand
	M05.75[1,2,9]	Rheumatoid arthritis with rheumatoid factor of hip without organ or system involvement
	M05.76[1,2,9]	Rheumatoid arthritis with rheumatoid factor of knee without organ or system involvement
	M05.77[1,2,9]	Rheumatoid arthritis with rheumatoid factor of ankle and foot without organ or system involvement
	M06.07[1,2,9]	Rheumatoid arthritis without rheumatoid factor, ankle and foot
	M06.08	Rheumatoid arthritis without rheumatoid factor, vertebrae
	M06.1	Adult-onset Stills disease
	M06.26	Rheumatoid bursitis, knee
	M06.27	Rheumatoid bursitis, ankle and foot
	M06.28	Rheumatoid bursitis, vertebrae
	M06.38	Rheumatoid nodule, vertebrae
	M06.39	Rheumatoid nodule, multiple sites
	6th Character meanings for codes as indicated **1 RIGHT 2 LEFT 9 UNSPECIFIED**	

Additional problems can arise when any type of arthritis affects the spine. One of the most common conditions is spinal stenosis, narrowing of a foramen of the spine that puts pressure on the nerves and causes pain, numbness, and weakness of limbs. Stenosis can also be a part of the normal aging process, as the cartilage loses its elasticity and the bones can form spurs, also decreasing the space for the nerves. There are multiple causes of spinal stenosis and ICD-10-CM puts this into perspective by providing categories for narrowing caused by subluxation, bony deformity, connective tissue disorders, intervertebral disc disorders, or any combination of these conditions. It also specifies whether the narrowing is of the vertebral foramen ("neural canal") or the *intervertebral foramen.*

 DEFINITIONS

intervertebral foramen. Opening between vertebrae where the nerves of the spinal cord extend to sites outside of the spine, such as the extremities.

Coding for Spinal Stenosis

ICD-9-CM		ICD-10-CM	
723.0	Spinal stenosis in cervical region	M48.01	Spinal stenosis, occipito-atlanto-axial region
		M48.02	Spinal stenosis, cervical region
		M48.03	Spinal stenosis, cervicothoracic region
		M99.20	Subluxation stenosis of neural canal of head region
		M99.21	Subluxation stenosis of neural canal of cervical region
		M99.30	Osseous stenosis of neural canal of head region
		M99.31	Osseous stenosis of neural canal of cervical region
		M99.40	Connective tissue stenosis of neural canal of head region
		M99.41	Connective tissue stenosis of neural canal of cervical region
		M99.50	Intervertebral disc stenosis of neural canal of head region
		M99.51	Intervertebral disc stenosis of neural canal of cervical region
		M99.60	Osseous and subluxation stenosis of intervertebral foramina of head region
		M99.61	Osseous and subluxation stenosis of intervertebral foramina of cervical region
		M99.70	Connective tissue and disc stenosis of intervertebral foramina of head region
		M99.71	Connective tissue and disc stenosis of intervertebral foramina of cervical region
724.01	Spinal stenosis of thoracic region	M48.04	Spinal stenosis thoracic region
		M48.05	Spinal stenosis thoracolumbar region
		M99.22	Subluxation stenosis of neural canal of thoracic region
		M99.32	Osseous stenosis of neural canal of thoracic region
		M99.42	Connective tissue stenosis of neural canal of thoracic region
		M99.52	Intervertebral disc stenosis of neural canal of thoracic region
		M99.62	Osseous and subluxation stenosis of intervertebral foramina of thoracic region
		M99.72	Connective tissue and disc stenosis of intervertebral foramina of thoracic region
724.02	Spinal stenosis of lumbar region without neurogenic claudication	M48.06	Spinal stenosis lumbar region
		M48.07	Spinal stenosis lumbosacral region
		M99.23	Subluxation stenosis of neural canal of lumbar region
		M99.33	Osseous stenosis of neural canal of lumbar region
		M99.43	Connective tissue stenosis of neural canal of lumbar region
		M99.53	Intervertebral disc stenosis of neural canal of lumbar region
		M99.63	Osseous and subluxation stenosis of intervertebral foramina of lumbar region
		M99.73	Connective tissue and disc stenosis of intervertebral foramina of lumbar region

Deficiencies and Anomalies

Occasionally, bones become soft due to a phosphate or calcium deficiency, known as osteomalacia in adults and rickets in children. Multiple factors can contribute to the insufficient minerals required for normal bone strength, including:

- Vitamin D deficiency due to nutritional deficits or malfunctioning metabolization—vitamin D is imperative to calcium absorption

- Malabsorption possibly due to digestive surgery or disease

- Malnutrition

- Pregnancy

- Pharmaceuticals, such as certain long-term anticonvulsants

- Kidney or liver disorders, which may impact the body's ability to process vitamins and minerals

- Aluminum bone disease—aluminum in high quantities prevents phosphate absorption

There are a couple of differences between ICD-9-CM and ICD-10-CM coding for this condition, most notably the reclassification of osteomalacia from the endocrine, nutritional, and metabolic immunity chapter to the musculoskeletal chapter. ICD-10-CM also differentiates code assignment by the documented cause of the bone softening.

Coding for Osteomalacia

ICD-9-CM		ICD-10-CM	
268.2	Osteomalacia, unspecified	M83.0	*Puerperal* osteomalacia
		M83.1	Senile osteomalacia
		M83.2	Adult osteomalacia due to malabsorption
		M83.3	Adult osteomalacia due to malnutrition
		M83.4	Aluminum bone disease
		M83.5	Other drug induced osteomalacia in adults
		M83.8	Other adult osteomalacia
		M83.9	Adult osteomalacia, unspecified

Another disease that can impact the integrity of the skeletal structure is aseptic necrosis, also known as osteonecrosis and avascular necrosis (AVN). In this condition, the bone lacks a blood supply and the tissue then dies, leaving weakened bones that have the potential to fracture or collapse. There are multiple etiologies for aseptic necrosis, including trauma to blood vessels supplying the area, disease such as sickle cell or lupus, pharmaceuticals, and poor circulation. ICD-10-CM takes into consideration the documented etiology of the aseptic necrosis, as well as anatomical site and laterality. Please note that due to extensive mapping, the table is a sample of the ICD-10-CM codes that represent the various concepts.

DEFINITIONS

puerperal. Pertaining to the time from the end of the third stage of labor until the uterus and other reproductive organs return to their normal state, which is approximately three to six weeks following childbirth.

Coding for Aseptic Necrosis

ICD-9-CM		ICD-10-CM	
733.41	Aseptic necrosis of head of humerus	M87.011	Idiopathic aseptic necrosis of right shoulder
		M87.012	Idiopathic aseptic necrosis of left shoulder
		M87.019	Idiopathic aseptic necrosis of unspecified shoulder
		M87.021	Idiopathic aseptic necrosis of right humerus
		M87.022	Idiopathic aseptic necrosis of left humerus
		M87.029	Idiopathic aseptic necrosis of unspecified humerus
		M87.121	Osteonecrosis due to drugs, right humerus
		M87.122	Osteonecrosis due to drugs, left humerus
		M87.129	Osteonecrosis due to drugs, unspecified humerus
		M87.221	Osteonecrosis due to previous trauma, right humerus
		M87.222	Osteonecrosis due to previous trauma, left humerus
		M87.229	Osteonecrosis due to previous trauma, unspecified humerus
		M87.321	Other secondary osteonecrosis, right humerus
		M87.322	Other secondary osteonecrosis, left humerus
		M87.329	Other secondary osteonecrosis, unspecified humerus
		M87.821	Other osteonecrosis, right humerus
		M87.822	Other osteonecrosis, left humerus
		M87.829	Other osteonecrosis, unspecified humerus
733.44	Aseptic necrosis of talus	M87.074	Idiopathic aseptic necrosis of right foot
		M87.075	Idiopathic aseptic necrosis of left foot
		M87.076	Idiopathic aseptic necrosis of unspecified foot
		M87.174	Osteonecrosis due to drugs, right foot
		M87.175	Osteonecrosis due to drugs, left foot
		M87.176	Osteonecrosis due to drugs, unspecified foot
		M87.274	Osteonecrosis due to previous trauma, right foot
		M87.275	Osteonecrosis due to previous trauma, left foot
		M87.276	Osteonecrosis due to previous trauma, unspecified foot
		M87.374	Other secondary osteonecrosis, right foot
		M87.375	Other secondary osteonecrosis, left foot
		M87.376	Other secondary osteonecrosis, unspecified foot
		M87.874	Other osteonecrosis, right foot
		M87.875	Other osteonecrosis, left foot
		M87.876	Other osteonecrosis, unspecified foot

Sometimes the normal curvatures in the spine become deformed. There are three types of these deformities:

- **Scoliosis,** a lateral curvature of the spine
- **Kyphosis,** an abnormal posterior convex curvature of the spine
- **Lordosis,** an exaggerated inward curvature of the lower back

Figure 3.13: Kyphosis and Lordosis

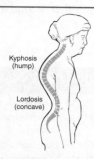

Figure 3.14: Scoliosis and Kyphoscoliosis

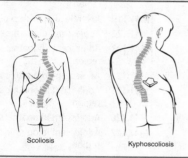

For the most part, ICD-10-CM mimics ICD-9-CM when it comes to coding kyphosis and lordosis, having equivalent one-to-one mapping or, if there is a one-to-many match, the classification is simply divided by spinal region (i.e., cervical, thoracic, or lumbar). However, there are a few distinct differences surrounding the crosswalk for scoliosis and kyphoscoliosis, category 734.3 in ICD-9-CM. In order to appropriately assign a code for (kypho-) scoliosis in ICD-10-CM, the coder must understand the different physiologies of the disease.

There are four major types of scoliosis:

- Congenital

- Neuromuscular, which is due to spinal muscle weakness or nerve damage

- Degenerative

- Idiopathic, which has an unknown cause and is the most common form of the disease. It can be divided by the age of the patient:

    - infantile: birth to 3 months

    - juvenile: 3 months to 9 years

    - adolescent: 10 to 18 years

ICD-9-CM does distinguish between infantile and other types of idiopathic scoliosis, as well as whether the infantile disease is progressive or resolving. In ICD-10-CM, however, the distinction between the age classifications is further specified, and juvenile and adolescent idiopathic scoliosis are also given their own categories, but the detail of whether the disease is progressing or resolving is lost in ICD-10-CM.

In addition to codes clarifying idiopathic scoliosis, codes have been added in ICD-10-CM for neuromuscular and other secondary forms of scoliosis, such as that caused by disc herniation.

Coding for (Kypho-) Scoliosis

ICD-9-CM		ICD-10-CM	
737.30	Scoliosis, idiopathic	M41.112	Juvenile idiopathic scoliosis, cervical region
		M41.113	Juvenile idiopathic scoliosis, cervicothoracic region
		M41.114	Juvenile idiopathic scoliosis, thoracic region
		M41.115	Juvenile idiopathic scoliosis, thoracolumbar region
		M41.116	Juvenile idiopathic scoliosis, lumbar region
		M41.117	Juvenile idiopathic scoliosis, lumbosacral region
		M41.119	Juvenile idiopathic scoliosis, site unspecified
		M41.122	Adolescent idiopathic scoliosis, cervical region
		M41.123	Adolescent idiopathic scoliosis, cervicothoracic region
		M41.124	Adolescent idiopathic scoliosis, thoracic region
		M41.125	Adolescent idiopathic scoliosis, thoracolumbar region
		M41.126	Adolescent idiopathic scoliosis, lumbar region
		M41.127	Adolescent idiopathic scoliosis, lumbosacral region
		M41.129	Adolescent idiopathic scoliosis, site unspecified
		M41.20	Other idiopathic scoliosis, site unspecified
		M41.22	Other idiopathic scoliosis, cervical region
		M41.23	Other idiopathic scoliosis, cervicothoracic region
		M41.24	Other idiopathic scoliosis, thoracic region
		M41.25	Other idiopathic scoliosis, thoracolumbar region
		M41.26	Other idiopathic scoliosis, lumbar region
		M41.27	Other idiopathic scoliosis, lumbosacral region
737.31	Resolving infantile idiopathic scoliosis	M41.00	Other idiopathic scoliosis, site unspecified
		M41.02	Other idiopathic scoliosis, cervical region
		M41.03	Other idiopathic scoliosis, cervicothoracic region
		M41.04	Other idiopathic scoliosis, thoracic region
		M41.05	Other idiopathic scoliosis, thoracolumbar region
		M41.06	Other idiopathic scoliosis, lumbar region
		M41.07	Other idiopathic scoliosis, lumbosacral region
		M41.08	Other idiopathic scoliosis, sacral and sacrococcygeal region
737.32	Progressive infantile idiopathic scoliosis	M41.00	Other idiopathic scoliosis, site unspecified
		M41.02	Other idiopathic scoliosis, cervical region
		M41.03	Other idiopathic scoliosis, cervicothoracic region
		M41.04	Other idiopathic scoliosis, thoracic region
		M41.05	Other idiopathic scoliosis, thoracolumbar region
		M41.06	Other idiopathic scoliosis, lumbar region
		M41.07	Other idiopathic scoliosis, lumbosacral region
		M41.08	Other idiopathic scoliosis, sacral and sacrococcygeal region

ICD-9-CM		ICD-10-CM	
737.39	Other kyphoscoliosis and scoliosis	M41.40	Neuromuscular scoliosis, site unspecified
		M41.41	Neuromuscular scoliosis, occipito-atlanto-axial region
		M41.42	Neuromuscular scoliosis, cervical region
		M41.43	Neuromuscular scoliosis, cervicothoracic region
		M41.44	Neuromuscular scoliosis, thoracic region
		M41.45	Neuromuscular scoliosis, thoracolumbar region
		M41.46	Neuromuscular scoliosis, lumbar region
		M41.47	Neuromuscular scoliosis, lumbosacral region
		M41.50	Other secondary scoliosis, site unspecified
		M41.52	Other secondary scoliosis, cervical region
		M41.53	Other secondary scoliosis, cervicothoracic region
		M41.54	Other secondary scoliosis, thoracic region
		M41.55	Other secondary scoliosis, thoracolumbar region
		M41.56	Other secondary scoliosis, lumbar region
		M41.57	Other secondary scoliosis, lumbosacral region
		M41.80	Other forms of scoliosis, site unspecified
		M41.82	Other forms of scoliosis, cervical region
		M41.83	Other forms of scoliosis, cervicothoracic region
		M41.84	Other forms of scoliosis, thoracic region
		M41.85	Other forms of scoliosis, thoracolumbar region
		M41.86	Other forms of scoliosis, lumbar region
		M41.87	Other forms of scoliosis, lumbosacral region
		M41.9	Scoliosis, unspecified

Summary

The skeletal system is the bony foundation for the human body; its articulations provide movement of this rigid structure. Due to the diversity in structure and location of bones and joints, they can be impacted by various types and severities of disease. ICD-10-CM provides detail in reporting skeletal traumas and disease and, therefore, advanced knowledge of the anatomy and disease processes is imperative.

Chapter 4. **Muscular System**

Anatomic Overview

The muscles and muscle tissue perform five major functions for the human body. This system produces movement (within organs and organ systems as well as external movements), stabilizes posture, reinforces the articulations of the skeleton, helps with storage and regulation of substances within the body, and generates heat.

There are three types of muscle tissue: cardiac, smooth, and skeletal (or striated). Each type shares one or more of the four functional characteristics below that distinguish it as muscle tissue:

- **Excitability:** Ability to receive and react to irritation or stimulation.
- **Contractility:** Ability to reduce in size.
- **Extensibility:** Ability to lengthen or stretch.
- **Elasticity:** Ability to regain its original size and shape after contraction or extension.

Although all three types of tissue have specific attributes that differentiate between them, their general function—providing movement—is the same.

Cardiac Muscle

Cardiac muscle is found only in the heart. It forms the heart walls and performs the contractions that push blood through the vessels of the body. This type of muscle consists of linked fibers (similar to a skeletal muscle) that involuntarily contract (like a smooth muscle) in unison, producing the heartbeat. The movement of this muscle is controlled by electrical impulses sent by the heart's pacemaker. The cardiac muscle is unique because it is *striated* as a skeletal muscle is but involuntarily contracts like a smooth muscle. Because cardiac muscle is found only in the heart, the physiology of this type of muscle will be discussed in the cardiac chapter.

Smooth Muscle

Smooth muscle is involuntary in its movements but is not striated, hence the name "smooth" muscle. This type of muscle lines the hollow organs of the body and contracts to force fluids and other bodily substances through the proper channels. It is found in organs such as the gastrointestinal tract, the uterus, urinary bladder, and blood vessels. Smooth muscle is also responsible for closing these channels to store contents or prevent "backflow" via ring-like bands of muscle called sphincters. Because of the various sites and functions of smooth muscle, the physiology of smooth muscle diseases will be discussed in the chapters coinciding with the location of the organ in which the muscle is found. For example, discussion of the smooth muscle lining the urinary bladder is found in the urinary chapter.

Skeletal Muscle

Skeletal muscle, as its name implies, moves the skeleton. It is responsible for the bumps and bulges under the skin associated with body builders and athletes. Skeletal muscle is striated and moves voluntarily, or consciously. In some cases, such as the movement of the diaphragm for breathing or the muscles that

DEFINITIONS

striated. Something that is striped, marked by parallel lines, or has structural lines.

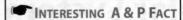

maintain posture, the movement is subconscious but still considered voluntary because a person can consciously cease or change the movement. Each muscle is attached at both ends: the origin (where the muscle is anchored to the bone) and the insertion (the point where the muscle attaches to the bone it moves). Generally, the origin bone does not move but forms an anchor so that when the muscle contracts, the insertion bone is moved toward the origin bone. This will be discussed in more detail later in this chapter. The fleshy contractile part is called the muscle belly.

Due to the various movements skeletal muscles perform depending on their location and function in the body, the structure of each may differ just as with the bones of the skeletal system. However, their basic components are the same. All skeletal muscles are composed of muscle tissue, nerves, blood vessels, and substantial amounts of connective tissue.

There are three kinds of connective tissue associated with muscle structure. Enclosing the entire muscle is a fibrous tissue called the epimysium, which may be commonly referred to as the muscle sheath. This tissue surrounds the outside of the muscle, holding it together. Within the epimysium lies many perimysium, tissue that groups individual muscle fibers together to form bundles called fascicles. Fascicles are the "grain" of the muscle and can be seen with the naked eye, such as in a piece of beef. Surrounding each individual muscle fiber found within these bundles is the endomysium. This complex and layered design allows for each fiber to move somewhat individually.

Also covering the muscle and providing further protection is a dense tissue called fascia. The fascia's main purpose is to hold muscles in place and separate them from surrounding organs or other muscles. It is also important to note that the fascia allows free movement, fills the spaces between muscles, and provides a mechanism for nerves, blood, and lymph vessels to reach the muscles. The space that contains the muscle within the fascia is known as a compartment.

In some cases, the fascia extends past the muscle it surrounds, forming a cord-like structure that attaches to the periosteum of a bone; this cord is referred to as a tendon. Certain tendons are further reinforced by an additional layer of connective tissue referred to as a tendon sheath. In other cases, the fascia extends past its muscle to form broad, thick sheets of connective tissue, called aponeurosis, that connect the muscle to an adjacent muscle.

In certain instances, mainly where muscles and tendons make contact with bone, there are fluid-filled sacs called bursae. A bursa reduces the friction between the muscle or tendon and the bone it moves across.

Figure 4.1: Joint Structures

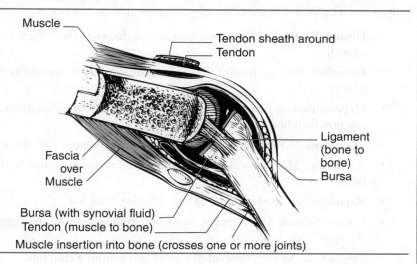

The muscles' movement depends on the origin and insertion of the associated tendons. The origin of a muscle is where the tendon attaches to a stationary bone. For example, when flexing the muscle in the front of the upper arm (bicep), the upper arm/shoulder does not move, making this the origin of the muscle of the upper arm. The bones of the lower arm come closer to the body to cause the contraction in the bicep, making the lower arm the "moveable" attachment, or the insertion. In other words, when a muscle contracts, the insertion is pulled toward the origin.

Also influencing muscle movement is the arrangement of the individual muscle's fascicles. There are five basic shapes the fascicles form:

- **Parallel:** Fascicles follow the long axis of the muscle, forming a strap-like shape.

- **Fusiform:** Fascicles follow the long axis of the muscle but form a belly or bulge in the middle, forming a spindle-like shape.

- **Pennate:** Fascicles are short and feather out from a tendon.

  - **unipennate:** Fascicles attach only to one side of a tendon.

  - **bipennate:** Fascicles attach to both sides of a tendon.

  - **multipennate:** Fascicles attach to all parts of a tendon or both sides of multiple tendons in the same muscle.

- **Convergent:** Fascicles start out broad and end narrow, forming a triangular shape.

- **Circular:** Fascicles are arranged in concentric rings.

Skeletal muscles cause various movements based not only on their origins, insertions, and shape but also coordination with other muscles. Many muscles are in groups that define their actions—when one contracts, another relaxes. The muscle that contracts is called the agonist, and the relaxing muscle is the antagonist. Using the upper arm muscles as an example again, when the bicep contracts, the muscle on the posterior side of the arm (the tricep) relaxes and vice versa. In addition to these obvious muscles, there are also stabilizing muscles that interact with the agonist/antagonist relationship. Known as synergists, these muscles help coordinate the motion or stop unwanted movement. Those that stop unwanted movement are called fixators.

The multiple groups of muscles within the body provide many types of movement. The following terms describe the general body movements:

- **Flexion:** Bending of a joint so that its angle decreases (bending the elbow).
- **Extension:** Straightening of the angle of the joint (straightening at the elbow).
- **Hyperextension:** Extension of the joint beyond its normal anatomical position (bending the head back to look straight up).
- **Abduction:** Movement away from midline (reaching out with the arm).
- **Adduction:** Movement closer to midline (pulling the arm close to the body).
- **Rotation:** Movement around an axis (shaking head "no").
- **Circumduction:** Movement of a part so that the end moves (swinging the arms in circles).
- **Protraction:** Moving forward of a body part (pushing chin out).
- **Retraction:** Movement backward (pulling chin in).
- **Elevation:** Raising of a body part (shrugging the shoulders).
- **Depression:** Lowering of a body part (drooping the shoulders).

It is important to point out that the names of skeletal muscles are based on their basic characteristics: size, shape, action, location, and/or attachments. Many muscle names are formed by using combinations of the basic word roots in medical terminology to describe a distinct attribute of that muscle. Therefore understanding the meaning of a muscle's name gives a clue to that muscle's specific attributes.

Major Skeletal Muscle Groups

There are nearly 700 individual muscles in the body. For ICD-10-CM purposes, only the major muscle groups need to be discussed.

Muscles of the Head

The muscles in the head have three main functions: facial expression, *mastication*, and movement of the eyes.

There are four pairs of major muscles in addition to two single muscles that control facial expression. These muscles are unique in that their insertion points are attached to the skin or muscles of the face and scalp rather than the bones of the skull, making these muscles the most visible in the body.

Starting at the top of the head is the epicranius muscle, which is formed by the two frontalis muscles (over the frontal bone) and two occipitalis muscles (over the occipital bone). These two bundles of muscle tissue are connected by the epicranial aponeurosis. When contracted, this wrinkles the skin of the forehead. Below the bilateral frontalis muscles are two ring-like muscles that circle each of the eyes. The orbicularis oculi causes the eyelids to close or blink. Contracting this muscle causes the skin at the outer edge of the eyes to wrinkle, commonly called "crow's feet." Below the eyes is a pair of zygomaticus muscles, which attach to the cheekbones and lift the corners of the mouth to form a smile or laugh. Beneath the zygomaticus are the buccinators, which form the meaty part of the cheeks; when this muscle contracts, the cheeks "suck" in. Medial to these is the "kissing muscle" encircling the lips. This muscle is known as the orbicularis oris and as its nickname suggests, it is responsible for closing and

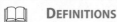

DEFINITIONS

mastication. Process of chewing food to ready it for the digestive system.

puckering the lips. At the bottom of the face, covering the chin and front of the neck, is a thin, sheet-like muscle called the platysma. Its main functions are to pull the corners of the lips down to form a frown and help in lowering the mandible to open the mouth.

Figure 4.2: Muscles of the Face

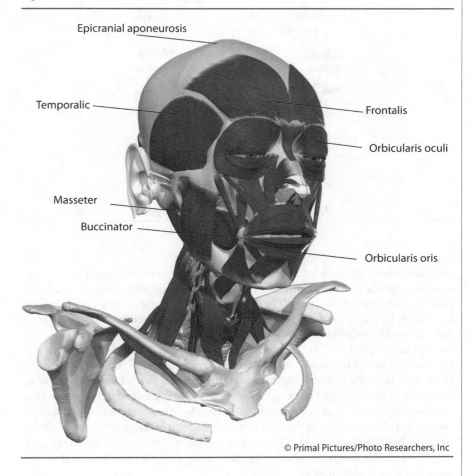

Epicranial aponeurosis

Temporalic

Frontalis

Orbicularis oculi

Masseter

Buccinator

Orbicularis oris

© Primal Pictures/Photo Researchers, Inc

Four pairs of muscles in the face control the chewing process. The three pairs that aid in closing the jaw are the masseter, temporalis, and medial pterygoid. The masseter sits in front of the ear and clenches the jaw by contracting. Sitting just above the ear is the temporalis (covering the temporal bone). The medial pterygoid is found underneath the masseter and aids not only in closing the mouth but also moving the mandible from side to side. The fourth pair of muscles sits adjacent to the medial pterygoid beneath the masseter, attaching the mandible to the sphenoid bone. This muscle is called the lateral pterygoid, and its main purpose is to open the mouth. It also aids in pushing the chin outward and moving the jaw from side to side.

Last, six muscles move each eyeball. These are usually called "extrinsic" eye muscles because they are outside of the eye. They are unique in that their insertion points are on the eyeball itself. The first four muscles, the superior, inferior, lateral, and medial rectus, are aptly named for the direction in which they move the eyeball when contracted. For example, when a person goes cross-eyed, this is the contraction of both medial rectus muscles. The other two

☛ **INTERESTING A & P FACT**

The extrinsic eye muscles are some of the most exact and fastest reacting muscles in the body.

muscles, the superior and inferior obliques, move the eyeballs in the "in between" directions missed by the recti.

Figure 4.3: Eye Musculature

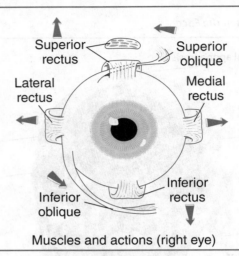

Muscles and actions (right eye)

Muscles of the Neck and Spine

On each side of the neck, running from behind the ear to the top of the sternum, are the sternocleidomastoid muscles. These muscles turn the head and pull the chin toward the chest. They also aid in lifting the sternum during deep breathing. In the back of the neck, there are multiple paired muscle groups. Starting toward midline and working outward are the spinalis capitis, the semispinalis capitis, and the longissimus capitis, which connect various lower cervical and upper thoracic vertebrae to the base of the skull. Lying on top of these muscles is the splenius capitis, a long muscle that extends from the skull to vertebrae in the head and neck. All of these muscles combined act to rotate the head and move the head, as well as hold it upright. Most superior in the back of the neck and connecting to the tops of the shoulders, forming the "crook" of the neck, is the trapezius muscle. This muscle stabilizes and controls movements of the shoulder. Although its superior location is the neck, it extends into the posterior thorax musculature.

Figure 4.4: Associated Regions of Pain due to Neck Injuries

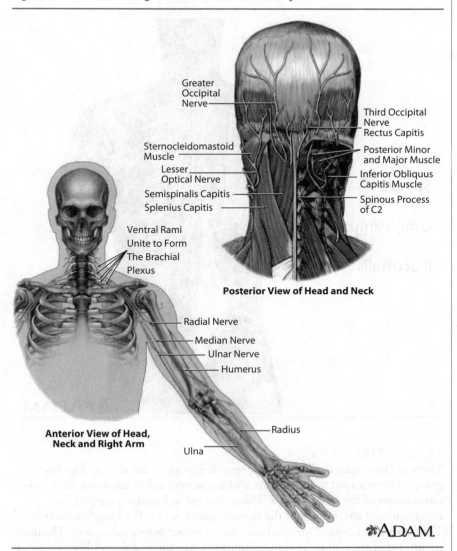

Greater
Occipital
Nerve

Third Occipital
Nerve
Rectus Capitis

Sternocleidomastoid
Muscle

Posterior Minor
and Major Muscle

Lesser
Optical Nerve

Inferior Obliquus
Capitis Muscle

Semispinalis Capitis

Spinous Process
of C2

Splenius Capitis

Ventral Rami
Unite to Form
The Brachial
Plexus

Posterior View of Head and Neck

Radial Nerve

Median Nerve

Ulnar Nerve

Humerus

Radius

**Anterior View of Head,
Neck and Right Arm**

Ulna

❋A.D.A.M.

Further down the vertebrae, the erector spinae muscles run along the bony spine, connecting it to various bones in the axial skeleton. These muscles maintain upright posture and assist in movements. The erector spinae can be divided into three major groups of muscles depending on their proximity to the spine, and then they are divided by their insertion points on the vertebrae. Listed from closest (medial) to the spine to the furthest (lateral), the muscle groups of the erector spinae are:

- **Spinalis:** Spinalis cervitis, spinalis thoracis

- **Longissimus:** Longissimus cervitis, longissimus thoracis

- **Iliocostalis:** Iliocostalis cervitis, iliocostalis thoracis, iliocostalis lumborum

Figure 4.5: Muscles of Erector Spine

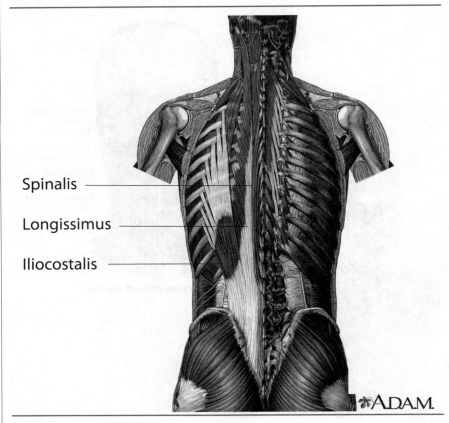

Spinalis

Longissimus

Iliocostalis

Muscles of the Thorax

There are two main functions of the muscle groups in the thorax. The first group of muscles aid in respiration, and the second aid in the movement and stabilization of the thoracic area. Those that aid in breathing control the expansion and contraction of the thoracic cavity, where the lungs are located. The cavity must expand on inhalation and contract during exhalation. The most significant of these muscles is the diaphragm. Serving as a dome-shaped divider between the thoracic and abdominal cavities, this muscle flattens when it contracts, making more space available to the lungs. Also helping to make more space on inspiration, the 11 pairs of external intercostal muscles running between the ribs lift and expand the rib cage. Sitting further inside the rib cage are the internal intercostal muscles, which counteract the external intercostals by compressing the rib cage on expiration.

Figure 4.6: Diaphragm

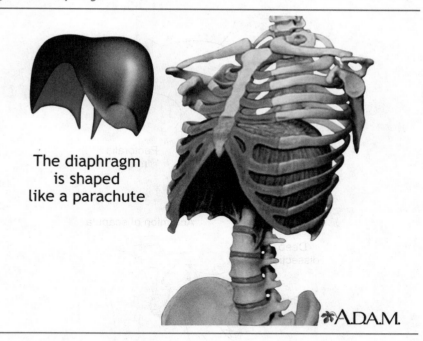

The diaphragm is shaped like a parachute

⚘A.D.A.M.

Anterior to the costal muscles are those muscles that aid in the movement and aesthetics of the chest. The most superficial and exposed muscle in the chest is the pectoralis major, forming bulges on both sides of the sternum. Although this muscle is predominantly seen on the chest, its function is to flex, adduct, and rotate the arm. Lying deep to this muscle is the pectoralis minor, running from the scapula to the second or third to fourth or fifth ribs. This muscle abducts the scapula, pulling the shoulder back, and also contributes to forceful inhalation when needed. Superior to the pectoralis minor, attaching the mid-distal clavicle to the first rib, is the subclavius, whose main function is stabilizing the thorax and shoulder. Wrapping around the sides of the thorax, sitting on top of the superior eight or nine ribs, is the serratus anterior. This muscle acts as an anterior stabilizer for the scapula and pushes the shoulder forward.

Figure 4.7: Pectoralis Major

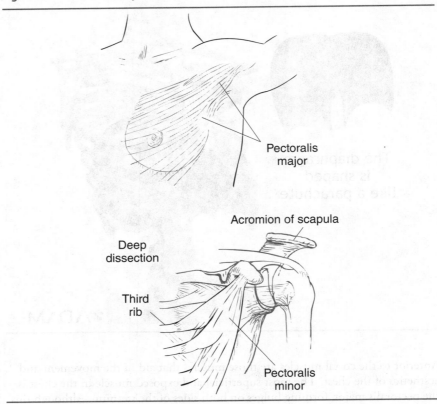

The most superficial muscle in the posterior thorax is also found in the neck, the trapezius. This muscle has origins on the occipital bone and also on the lower cervical and all thoracic vertebrae. The trapezius gets its name from the trapezoid shape of this paired muscle group in the back. Just inferior to the lowest-most portion of the trapezius is the latissimus dorsi. Attached to the lower vertebrae and extending up underneath the arm, this large muscle extends, adducts, and rotates the arm medially. Also lying deep to the trapezius is the rhomboid major and rhomboid minor, which aid in adding force to downward movements of the arms, as well as further stabilizing the scapula.

Figure 4.8: Posterior Thorax

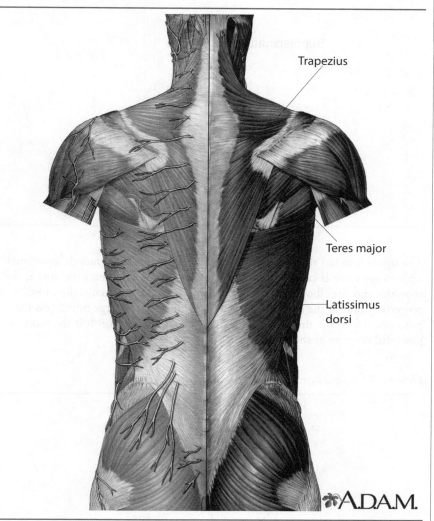

Trapezius

Teres major

Latissimus dorsi

Muscles of the Shoulder and Upper Extremity

Lateral to the rhomboid muscles is the infraspinatus, connecting the scapula to the upper head of the humerus. The infraspinatus muscle connects to the scapula below the spinous process. On the opposite side of the scapula's spinous process is the supraspinatus. Inferior to these muscles are the teres minor and teres major, forming the lower area of the armpit where the back and the arm come together. Sitting on top of these muscles, capping the shoulder, is the deltoid. These muscles all work together to choreograph the various movements of the shoulder joint.

Figure 4.9: Shoulder Muscles

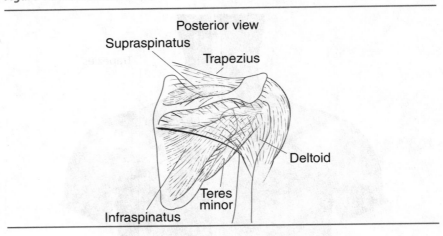

DEFINITIONS

extensor. Any muscle or tendon that extends a joint.

flexor. Muscle or tendon that bends or flexes a limb or part as opposed to extending it.

The upper arm has three major muscles. The anterior-most muscle associated with strong arms is called the biceps brachii. This muscle flexes the arm at the shoulder and the elbow. Just deep to the biceps is the brachialis, the most powerful *flexor* at the elbow joint. And last, there is one large muscle on the posterior side of the upper arm known as the triceps brachii. It is the most powerful *extensor* at the elbow joint.

Figure 4.10: Upper Arm

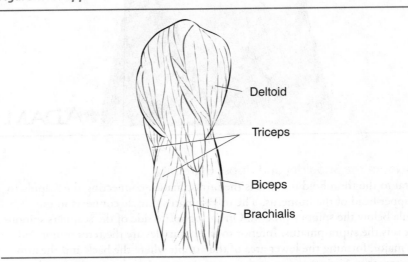

Crossing over the elbow joint, connecting the humerus and ulna to the radius, is a short muscle called the pronator teres. Its main function is to rotate the lower arm medially or to face the palm of the hand down. Performing the opposite action of rotating the forearm laterally and also crossing the elbow joint is the supinator. Also aiding the rotation of the forearm, wrist, and hand is the pronator quadratus, which connects the radius and ulna at the anterior wrist.

Figure 4.11: Forearm

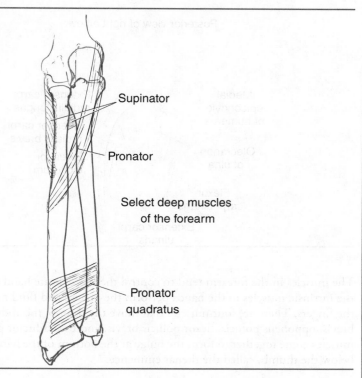

Supinator

Pronator

Select deep muscles
of the forearm

Pronator
quadratus

The rest of the muscles in the forearm can be classified as a flexor or extensor, depending upon the hand movements the muscles are responsible for. The flexors of the lower arm are:

- **Flexor carpi radius:** Located in the anterior medial part of the forearm; it flexes and abducts the hand.

- **Flexor carpi ulnaris:** Located along the pinkie finger side of the lower arm; it flexes and adducts the hand.

- **Palmaris longus:** Between the flexor carpi radius and flexor carpi ulnaris; it flexes the hand at the wrist.

- **Flexor digitorum:** Centrally located and posterior to flexor carpi ulnaris; it flexes the distal phalange joints.

- **Flexor digitorum superficialis:** Centrally located beneath the flexor carpi ulnaris; it flexes fingers and hand.

There are four extensors:

- **Extensor carpi radialis longus:** Located on the thumb side of the forearm; it extends and abducts the hand at the wrist.

- **Extensor carpi radialis brevis:** Medial to the extensor carpi radialis; it extends and abducts the hand at the wrist.

- **Extensor carpi ulnaris:** Located in the medial posterior part of the forearm; it extends and adducts the hand at the wrist.

- **Extensor digitorum:** Located alongside the extensor carpi ulnaris; it extends the fingers.

Figure 4.12: Elbow

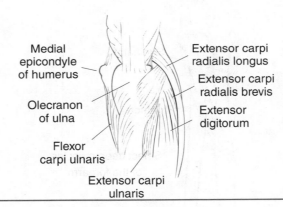

Posterior view of right elbow

Medial epicondyle of humerus

Olecranon of ulna

Flexor carpi ulnaris

Extensor carpi ulnaris

Extensor carpi radialis longus

Extensor carpi radialis brevis

Extensor digitorum

The muscles in the forearm tend to control the less delicate hand movements; the intrinsic muscles in the hands perform the precise and fluid movements of the fingers. There are four muscles that move the thumb: the abductor pollicis brevis, opponens pollicis, flexor pollicis brevis, and the adductor pollicis. These muscles come together to form the bulge at the bottom of the hand on the palm below the thumb, called the thenar eminence.

Figure 4.13: Thumb and Palm

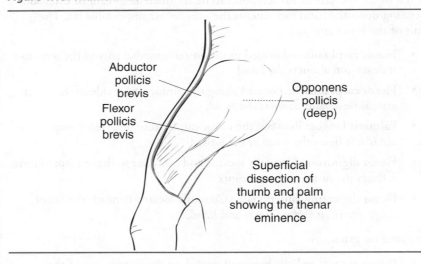

Abductor pollicis brevis

Flexor pollicis brevis

Opponens pollicis (deep)

Superficial dissection of thumb and palm showing the thenar eminence

Moving the little finger (or fifth digit) are three unique muscles as well: the abductor digiti minimi, flexor digiti minimi brevis, and the opponens digiti minimi. The other fingers are controlled by four lumbricals (one laterally flanking the tendons of each finger), three palmar interossei (beside the metacarpal shafts), and four dorsal interossei (on the opposite side of the metacarpal shafts from the palmar interossei).

Figure 4.14: Hand

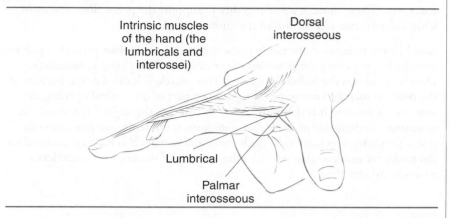

Intrinsic muscles of the hand (the lumbricals and interossei)

Dorsal interosseous

Lumbrical

Palmar interosseous

Muscles of the Abdominal Wall

Looking at the abdominal wall, the image of "six-pack" abdominal muscles comes to mind. Those individual definitions are all parts of one large muscle, called the rectus abdominus, covering the entire abdominal area from the ribs and sternum down to the pubis. This large muscle is covered by aponeuroses. There are three pairs of muscles that form the lateral sides of the abdomen. The most superficial of these is the external obliques, followed by the internal oblique and the transversus abdominus, the deepest.

Figure 4.15: Anatomy of Anterior Abdominal Wall

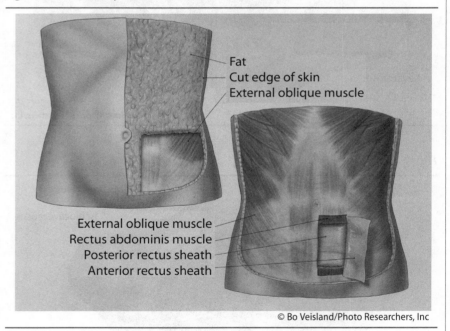

Fat
Cut edge of skin
External oblique muscle

External oblique muscle
Rectus abdominis muscle
Posterior rectus sheath
Anterior rectus sheath

© Bo Veisland/Photo Researchers, Inc

Muscles of the Pelvis

Although male and female anatomy varies significantly in the pelvic area, the muscular structure is surprisingly similar. The muscles in the pelvis can be divided into two distinct classifications based on location. Those that form the pelvic floor are considered part of the deeper pelvic diaphragm, and those that fill the space between the coxal bones are part of the urogenital diaphragm.

There are only two muscles that form the pelvic diaphragm: the levator ani and coccygeus. These muscles come together to support the pelvic floor and assist with the sphincter-like actions of the anus and vagina.

Also helping to support the pelvis is the superficial transversus perinea, a pair of muscles located along the posterior of the urogenital diaphragm. Anterior to these structures is the bulbospongiosus. This muscle is located at the bottom of the penis in men and surrounds the posterior part of the vaginal opening in women. In women, it is the muscle used to contract the vagina. It also aids in urination. To each side of the bulbospongiosus is an ischiocavernosus muscle that assists it with its functions. Both males and females also have a muscle called the sphincter urethrae that encircles the opening of the urethra to restrict or promote urinary flow.

Figure 4.16: Male Pelvic Floor

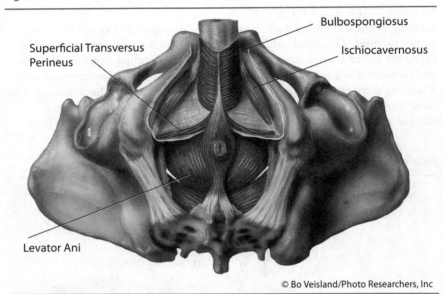

© Bo Veisland/Photo Researchers, Inc

Figure 4.17: Female Pelvic Floor

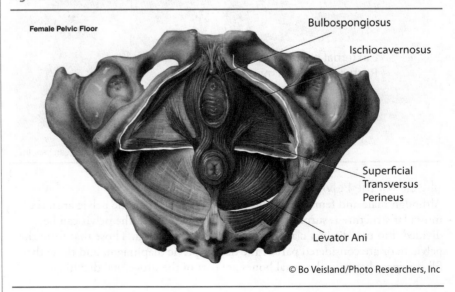

© Bo Veisland/Photo Researchers, Inc

Muscles of the Hips and Lower Extremities

Within the anterior part of the hip region are psoas major and the iliacus. The psoas major is a straplike muscle that connects the lumbar spine to the femur and flexes the upper thigh. The iliacus is a larger, fan-shaped muscle that covers the ilium portion of the pelvic bones. Its main purpose is to assist the psoas major in moving the upper leg in the action of walking. Moving laterally on the hip is the tensor fasciae latae, which sits on the lateral anterior part of the hip.

Figure 4.18: Anterior View of Hip

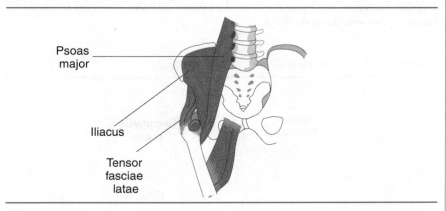

The next muscle moving toward the back of the hip is the gluteus medius, which also covers the gluteus minimus. These two muscles together abduct the thigh and rotate it medially. Partially covering the gluteus medius and forming the buttock is the gluteus maximus; its main functions are to straighten the lower limb and provide the force to stand from a sitting position.

Figure 4.19: Gluteal Muscles

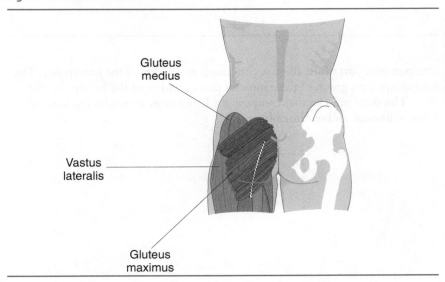

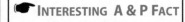
INTERESTING A & P FACT

The gluteus maximus is the largest muscle in the body.

Moving from the medial part of the anterior thigh outward, the first muscle encountered is the gracilis, running from the lower edge of the ischium section of the coxal bones to the tibia, serving to adduct the thigh and flex the knee. The adductor magus and adductor longus are the next two muscles moving medially across the thigh. These muscles adduct the thigh and assist in lateral rotation of the leg. The longus is also a flexor, whereas the magus is an extensor. Cutting across the anterior thigh, connecting the outer hipbone to the medial portion of the knee, is the sartorius muscle. It flexes, abducts, and laterally rotates the thigh.

The group of muscles lateral to the sartorius muscle is sometimes referred to as the quadriceps femoris group. This group of muscles makes up the meaty part of the front and side of the thighs. It consists of four extensor muscles: the rectus femoris, vastus lateralis, vastus medialis, and vastus intermedius. They function together to extend the leg at the knee. The vastus lateralis is covered in a layer of fascia on the outside of the thigh.

Figure 4.20: Anterior View of Thigh

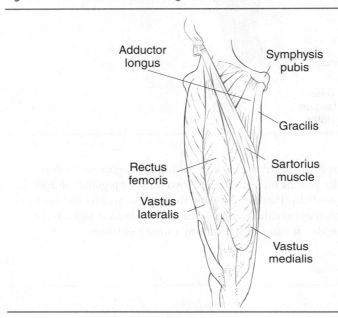

The posterior part of the thigh is commonly referred to as the hamstrings. The hamstrings are a group of three muscles that extend from the ischium to the tibia. The three muscles that compose the hamstrings are the biceps femoris, semitendinosus, and semimembranosus.

Figure 4.21: Gluteus Maximus

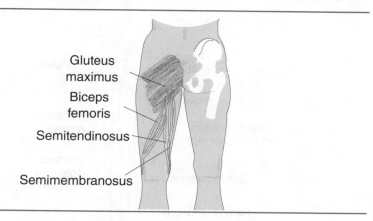

The muscles in the lower part of the leg can be divided by the foot actions for which they are responsible, *dorsiflexion* or *plantar flexion*. Those responsible for dorsiflexion are:

- **Tibialis anterior:** Stretches from the lateral part of the knee to the medial part of the foot; it also assists in *inversion*.
- **Peroneus tertius:** Located on the anterior part of the fibula; it also assists in *eversion*.
- **Extensor digitorum longus:** Between the tibia and fibula; it also assists in eversion and extension of the toes.

The plantar flexors include:

- **Gastrocnemius:** Located in the calf area, it is the most predominant muscle of the posterior lower leg; it also assists in the flexing of the knee.
- **Soleus:** Located underneath the calcaneal tendon, which runs from the gastrocnemius to the calcaneus.
- **Flexor digitorum longus:** Located on the posterior side of the tibia, ending at the distal phalanges of the toes; it also assists in inversion and flexion of the four lateral toes.
- **Tibialis posterior:** Located on the back of the leg and is the deepest muscle; it also assists in inversion.
- **Peroneus longus:** Located on the anterior lateral side of the calf; it also assists in eversion and supports the arch of the foot.

📖 **DEFINITIONS**

dorsiflexion. Bending of the foot upward.

eversion. Movement in which the sole of the foot faces laterally.

inversion. Movement in which the sole of the foot faces medially.

plantar flexion. Bending of the foot downward.

Figure 4.22: Lower Leg

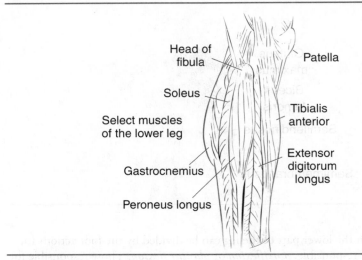

Similar to the hand, the foot has muscles that are responsible for the more specific actions of the foot, such as ambulation and support of the entire body. There is only one muscle on the top of the foot, the extensor digitorum brevis. It extends the toes.

Figure 4.23: Foot

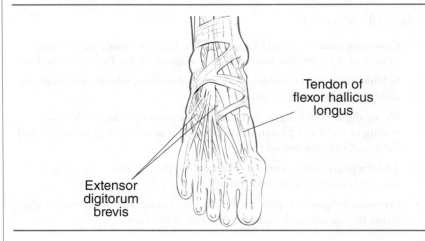

There are four layers of muscles on the plantar side of the foot. The first and most superficial layer includes the abductor hallucis, the flexor digitorum brevis, and the abductor digiti minimi. The next layer includes the quadratus plantae and the lumbricals. There are three muscles in the third layer, the flexor hallucis brevis, adductor hallucis, and flexor digiti minimi brevis. The deepest layer includes the dorsal and plantar interossei, the arrangement of which resembles that of the interossei muscles in the hands.

Figure 4.24: Foot

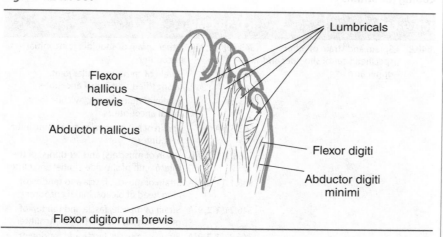

Anatomy and Physiology and the ICD-10-CM Code Set

Knowing the basic anatomy of the muscles is imperative for assigning codes in both ICD-9-CM and ICD-10-CM. To select the appropriate codes in ICD-10-CM, additional, advanced information regarding not only the anatomy but also the action of the skeletal muscles is necessary.

Injuries

Because muscles are soft organs just beneath the subcutaneous tissue and because they absorb and generate force and movement, not only are injuries to them common, but the types of injuries are varied. This chapter highlights the types of injuries for which in-depth knowledge is needed to assign an appropriate code in ICD-10-CM.

It is important to note that ICD-10-CM requires seventh characters to completely describe most traumatic injuries. The most common seventh characters used in conjunction with the muscles are "A"—Initial encounter, "D"—Subsequent encounter, and "S"—Sequela.

A "pulled" muscle, or muscle or tendon strain, is a fairly generic type of injury, and ICD-9-CM treats it as such. In the older classification system, sprains and strains are synonymous; however, physiologically they are very different injuries to a synovial joint. A sprain occurs when there is a stretch or tear of a ligament, the tissue that connects bone to bone. A strain is an injury to a muscle or tendon, usually due to overexertion, twisting, or pulling. ICD-10-CM not only provides separate categories for the two injuries, but also identifies the site and type of action for which the muscle and tendon are responsible.

The differences in the classification systems are best seen when looking at the ICD-9-CM codes for sprains and strains of other specified sites of shoulder and upper arm, 840.8, and sprains and strains of other specified sites of hip and thigh, 843.8.

Coding for Strains

ICD-9-CM		ICD-10-CM	
840.8	Sprain and strain of other specified sites of shoulder and upper arm	S43.49[1,2,9]A	Other sprain of shoulder joint, initial encounter
		S43.60xA	Sprain of sternoclavicular joint, unspecified side, initial encounter
		S43.61xA	Sprain of right sternoclavicular joint, initial encounter
		S43.62xA	Sprain of left sternoclavicular joint, initial encounter
		S46.01[1,2,9]A	Strain of muscle(s) and tendon(s) of the rotator cuff of shoulder, initial encounter
		S46.11[1,2,9]A	Strain of muscle, fascia and tendon of long head of biceps, initial encounter
		S46.21[1,2,9]A	Strain of muscle, fascia and tendon of other parts of biceps, initial encounter
		S46.31[1,2,9]A	Strain of muscle, fascia and tendon of triceps, initial encounter
		S46.81[1,2,9]A	Strain of other muscle, fascia and tendon at shoulder and upper arm level, initial encounter
		S46.91[1,2,9]A	Strain of unspecified muscle, fascia and tendon at shoulder and upper arm level, initial encounter
		6th Character meanings for codes as indicated	
		1 RIGHT 2 LEFT 9 UNSPECIFIED	
843.8	Sprains and strains of other specified sites of hip and thigh	S73.19[1,2,9]A	Other sprain of hip
		S76.01[1,2,9]A	Strain of muscle, fascia and tendon of hip, initial encounter
		S76.21[1,2,9]A	Strain of adductor muscle, fascia and tendon of hip, initial encounter
		S76.31[1,2,9]A	Strain of muscle, fascia and tendon of the posterior muscle group at thigh level, initial encounter
		S76.81[1,2,9]A	Strain of other muscles, fasciae and tendons at thigh level, initial encounter
		S76.91[1,2,9]A	Strain of unspecified muscles, fasciae and tendons at thigh level, initial encounter
		6th Character meanings for codes as indicated	
		1 right 2 left 9 unspecified	

A rotator cuff tear in the shoulder region is a very common injury and is sometimes classified as a sprain. This injury usually involves the supraspinatus muscle but can occur in the other muscles or tendons in the shoulder. In the younger population (younger than 40), the tear is usually due to an earlier trauma to the area, such as a fracture or dislocation, or excessive overhead, repetitive movements required in certain occupations and sports. In the older population, this injury occurs as a result of normal wear and tear on the aging body. The majority of these injuries occur in the older population.

In ICD-9-CM, if rotator cuff tear is the only documentation by the physician, it is assumed to be traumatic, coding to an acute, traumatic injury by default of the volume 2 index. This is the first and most obvious difference between the two classification systems. ICD-10-CM assumes with no further documentation that the injury is nontraumatic, following the clinical findings that the majority of rotator cuff tears are nontraumatic.

Both classification systems give the option to differentiate between the traumatic and nontraumatic if the documentation supports it; however, when the tear is specified as nontraumatic, ICD-10-CM further differentiates the injury by identifying the muscle or type of tendon (flexor or extensor) injured, using the terminology rotator cuff syndrome for a complete or incomplete tear of the supraspinous muscle but giving various codes for tears of the shoulder that do not include this muscle.

ICD-9-CM also describes a degenerative rotator cuff tear with a nonspecific code, whereas ICD-10-CM assumes that degenerative and nontraumatic are the same.

Coding for Rotator Cuff Tears

ICD-9-CM		ICD-10-CM	
840.4	Sprains and strains of rotator cuff (capsule)	S43.421A	Sprain of right rotator cuff capsule, initial encounter
		S43.422A	Sprain of left rotator cuff capsule, initial encounter
		S43.429A	Sprain of unspecified rotator cuff capsule, initial encounter
727.61	Complete rupture of rotator cuff, nontraumatic	M66.211	Spontaneous rupture of extensor tendons, right shoulder
		M66.212	Spontaneous rupture of extensor tendons, left shoulder
		M66.219	Spontaneous rupture of extensor tendons, unspecified shoulder
		M66.811	Spontaneous rupture of other tendons, right shoulder
		M66.812	Spontaneous rupture of other tendons, left shoulder
		M66.819	Spontaneous rupture of other tendons, unspecified shoulder
		M75.10	Rotator cuff syndrome, unspecified shoulder
		M75.11	Rotator cuff syndrome, right shoulder
		M75.12	Rotator cuff syndrome, left shoulder
726.10	Disorders of *bursae* and tendons in shoulder region, unspecified (degenerative rotator cuff tear)	M75.10	Rotator cuff syndrome, unspecified shoulder
		M75.11	Rotator cuff syndrome, right shoulder
		M75.12	Rotator cuff syndrome, left shoulder

 DEFINITIONS

bursa. Cavity or sac containing fluid that occurs between articulating surfaces and reduces friction from moving parts. An anatomical structure frequently referenced in orthopaedic notes, as it may become diseased or need removal.

Another common injury to the muscular system occurs during a laceration, which is usually considered a skin injury. Occasionally, a cut goes below the subcutaneous tissue and severs or injures the fascia, muscle, and tendons. This happens most frequently on injuries of the hand, as the surrounding tissues are thin and don't protect the tendons well.

When assigning a code for tendon injuries in ICD-9-CM, the only necessary information is the site of the injury and tendon involvement. ICD-10-CM goes much farther into the details of the location, not only the anatomical location of the laceration but also the digit the muscle controls. It also differentiates between intrinsic versus extrinsic muscles and tendons, and the movement type (flexor or extensor) of the muscle or tendon that is injured. A detailed crosswalk between ICD-9-CM and ICD-10-CM outlines how to report injuries of the hand.

Coding for Tendon Laceration of the Hand

ICD-9-CM		ICD-10-CM	
882.2	Open wound of hand except finger(s) alone with tendon involvement	S66.929A	Laceration of unspecified muscle, fascia and tendon at wrist and hand level of unspecified side, initial encounter
		S66.021A	Laceration of long flexor muscle, fascia and tendon of right thumb at wrist and hand level, initial encounter
		S66.022A	Laceration of long flexor muscle, fascia and tendon of left thumb at wrist and hand level, initial encounter
		S66.029A	Laceration of long flexor muscle, fascia and tendon of unspecified thumb at wrist and hand level, initial encounter
		S66.12[0-9]A	Laceration of flexor muscle, fascia and tendon of finger at wrist and hand level, initial encounter
		S66.221A	Laceration of extensor muscle, fascia and tendon of right thumb at the wrist and hand level, initial encounter
		S66.222A	Laceration of extensor muscle, fascia and tendon of left thumb at the wrist and hand level, initial encounter
		S66.229A	Laceration of extensor muscle, fascia and tendon of unspecified thumb at the wrist and hand level, initial encounter
		S66.32[0-9]A	Laceration of extensor muscle, fascia and tendon of finger at the wrist and hand level, initial encounter
		S66.421A	Laceration of intrinsic muscle, fascia and tendon of right thumb at wrist and hand level, initial encounter
		S66.422A	Laceration of intrinsic muscle, fascia and tendon of left thumb at wrist and hand level, initial encounter
		S66.429A	Laceration of intrinsic muscle, fascia and tendon of left thumb at wrist and hand level, initial encounter
		S66.52[0-9]A	Laceration of intrinsic muscle, fascia and tendon of other and unspecified finger at the wrist and hand level, initial encounter
		S66.821A	Laceration of other muscle, fascia and tendon at right wrist and hand level, initial encounter
		S66.822A	Laceration of other muscle, fascia and tendon at left wrist and hand level, initial encounter
		S66.829A	Laceration of other muscle, fascia and tendon at unspecified wrist and hand level, initial encounter
		S66.921A	Laceration of unspecified muscle, fascia and tendon at right wrist and hand level, initial encounter
		S66.922A	Laceration of unspecified muscle, fascia and tendon at left wrist and hand level, initial encounter

6th Character meanings for codes as indicated
0 right index 1 left index 2 right middle
3 left middle 4 right ring 5 left ring
6 right little 7 left little 8 other
9 unspecified

Infections and Inflammations

In addition to injuries, tendons and tendon sheaths can suffer from inflammation due to other disease processes such as infection. Inflammation of the tendon and tendon sheath is called tenosynovitis. This occurs most often in the tendons of the wrist, ankle, and feet. A flare-up due to overuse of the tendons of the abductor pollicis longus and extensor pollicis brevis of the wrist at the base of the thumb is called de Quervain tenosynovitis. Because these muscles and tendons cross over the *radial styloid process*, the condition can also be called radial stylus tenosynovitis. Transient tenosynovitis is inflammation of the hip joint in children from 3 to 10 years of age that dissipates within a week.

ICD-9-CM recognizes the most common anatomical locations of tenosynovitis by providing specific codes for the hand and wrist and the foot and ankle, but does not distinguish the cause of the inflammation. In ICD-10-CM, the most common causes of tenosynovitis are given specific categories, each of which includes the major joints of the body, rather than just the most likely joints to be affected.

 DEFINITIONS

radial styloid process. Projection of the distal lateral radial bone.

Coding for Tenosynovitis

ICD-9-CM		ICD-10-CM	
727.04	Radial styloid tenosynovitis	M65.4	Radial styloid tenosynovitis [de Quervain]
727.05	Other tenosynovitis of hand and wrist	M65.831	Other synovitis and tenosynovitis, right forearm
		M65.832	Other synovitis and tenosynovitis, left forearm
		M65.839	Other synovitis and tenosynovitis, unspecified forearm
		M65.841	Other synovitis and tenosynovitis, right hand
		M65.842	Other synovitis and tenosynovitis, left hand
		M65.849	Other synovitis and tenosynovitis, unspecified hand
727.06	Tenosynovitis of foot and ankle	M65.871	Other synovitis and tenosynovitis, right ankle and foot
		M65.872	Other synovitis and tenosynovitis, left ankle and foot
		M65.879	Other synovitis and tenosynovitis, unspecified ankle and foot
727.09	Other synovitis and tenosynovitis	M65.10	Other infective (teno)synovitis, unspecified site
		M65.11[**1,2,9**]	Other infective (teno)synovitis, shoulder
		M65.12[**1,2,9**]	Other infective (teno)synovitis, elbow
		M65.13[**1,2,9**]	Other infective (teno)synovitis, wrist
		M65.14[**1,2,9**]	Other infective (teno)synovitis, hand
		M65.15[**1,2,9**]	Other infective (teno)synovitis, hip
		M65.16[**1,2,9**]	Other infective (teno)synovitis, knee
		M65.17[**1,2,9**]	Other infective (teno)synovitis, ankle and foot
		M65.18	Other infective tenosynovitis other site
		M65.19	Other infective tenosynovitis multiple sites
		M65.80	Other synovitis and tenosynovitis, unspecified site
(Continued on next page)		***6th Character meanings for codes as indicated*** ***1 right 2 left 9 unspecified***	

ICD-9-CM	ICD-10-CM	
727.09 Other synovitis and tenosynovitis *(Continued)*	M65.81[**1,2,9**]	Other synovitis and tenosynovitis, shoulder
	M65.82[**1,2,9**]	Other synovitis and tenosynovitis, upper arm
	M65.85[**1,2,9**]	Other synovitis and tenosynovitis, thigh
	M65.86[**1,2,9**]	Other synovitis and tenosynovitis, lower leg
	M65.88	Other synovitis and tenosynovitis, other site
	M65.89	Other synovitis and tenosynovitis, multiple sites
	M67.30	Transient synovitis, unspecified site
	M67.31[**1,2,9**]	Transient synovitis, shoulder
	M67.32[**1,2,9**]	Transient synovitis, elbow
	M67.33[**1,2,9**]	Transient synovitis, wrist
	M67.34[**1,2,9**]	Transient synovitis, hand
	M67.35[**1,2,9**]	Transient synovitis, hip
	M67.36[**1,2,9**]	Transient synovitis, knee
	M67.37[**1,2,9**]	Transient synovitis, ankle and foot
	M67.38	Transient synovitis, other site
	M67.39	Transient synovitis, multiple sites
	6th Character meanings for codes as indicated **1 right 2 left 9 unspecified**	

Slightly different from tenosynovitis, in that it affects only the tendon without swelling of the tendon sheath, is tendinitis. This condition is usually reported with a vague set of *enthesopathy* ICD-9-CM codes. These code sets include inflammation of the bursa, also called bursitis and various other joint afflictions, such as *osteophytes* and bone spurs, for which ICD-10-CM has assigned specific codes. The table below outlines the more specific conditions that were once reported in a general manner.

Coding for Enthesopathy

ICD-9-CM	ICD-10-CM	
726.30 Unspecified enthesopathy of elbow	M25.721	Osteophyte right elbow
	M25.722	Osteophyte left elbow
	M25.729	Osteophyte unspecified elbow
726.39 Other enthesopathy of elbow region	M70.30	Other bursitis of elbow, unspecified elbow
	M70.31	Other bursitis of elbow, right elbow
	M70.32	Other bursitis of elbow, left elbow
726.4 Enthesopathy of wrist and carpus	M25.731	Osteophyte right wrist
	M25.732	Osteophyte left wrist
	M25.739	Osteophyte unspecified wrist
	M25.741	Osteophyte right hand
	M25.742	Osteophyte left hand
	M25.749	Osteophyte unspecified hand
	M70.10	Bursitis, unspecified hand
	M70.11	Bursitis, right hand
	M70.12	Bursitis, left hand
	M77.20	*Periarthritis* unspecified wrist
	M77.21	Periarthritis, right wrist
	M77.22	Periarthritis, left wrist

 DEFINITIONS

enthesopathy. Disorders that occur at points where muscle, tendons, and ligaments attach to bones or joint capsules.

osteophytes. Bony outgrowth.

periarthritis. Inflammation of tissues around a joint.

ICD-9-CM		ICD-10-CM	
726.5	Enthesopathy of hip region	M25.751	Osteophyte right hip
		M25.752	Osteophyte left hip
		M25.759	Osteophyte unspecified hip
		M70.6[Ø,1,2]	Trochanteric bursitis, hip
		M70.7[Ø,1,2]	Other bursitis of hip
		M76.Ø[Ø,1,2]	Gluteal tendinitis, buttock
		M76.1[Ø,1,2]	Psoas tendinitis, side
		M76.2[Ø,1,2]	Iliac crest spur
		M76.3[Ø,1,2]	Iliotibial band syndrome
		5th Character meanings for codes as indicated 1 unspecified 2 right 9 left	
726.6Ø	Unspecified enthesopathy of knee	M25.761	Osteophyte right knee
		M25.762	Osteophyte left knee
		M25.769	Osteophyte unspecified knee
		M70.5Ø	Other bursitis of knee, unspecified knee
		M70.51	Other bursitis of knee, right knee
		M70.52	Other bursitis of knee, left knee
726.69	Other enthesopathy of knee	M76.899	Other specified enthesopathies of unspecified lower limb, excluding foot
726.7Ø	Unspecified enthesopathy of ankle and tarsus	M25.771	Osteophyte right ankle
		M25.772	Osteophyte left ankle
		M25.773	Osteophyte unspecified ankle
		M25.774	Osteophyte right foot
		M25.775	Osteophyte left foot
		M25.776	Osteophyte unspecified foot
		M76.899	Other specified enthesopathies of unspecified lower limb, excluding foot
		M77.4Ø	*Metatarsalgia* unspecified foot
		M77.41	Metatarsalgia right foot
		M77.42	Metatarsalgia left foot
726.79	Other enthesopathy of ankle and tarsus	M76.7Ø	Peroneal tendinitis unspecified leg
		M76.71	Peroneal tendinitis right leg
		M76.72	Peroneal tendinitis left leg
		M77.5Ø	Other enthesopathy, unspecified foot
		M77.51	Other enthesopathy, right foot
		M77.52	Other enthesopathy, left foot

 DEFINITIONS

metatarsalgia. Foot condition in the metatarsal region of the foot.

Another cause of tendinitis and bursitis is a buildup of calcium deposits within the tissues. ICD-9-CM has a vague code assignment for these conditions, not distinguishing what tissue is affected or the site. ICD-10-CM codes, however, reflect whether the deposits are in the tendon or bursa and the anatomical location.

Coding for Calcium Deposits in the Tendons and Bursa

ICD-9-CM	ICD-10-CM	
727.82 Calcium deposits in tendon and bursa	M65.20	Calcific tendinitis, unspecified site
	M65.22[1,2,9]	Calcific tendinitis, upper arm
	M65.23[1,2,9]	Calcific tendinitis, forearm
	M65.24[1,2,9]	Calcific tendinitis, hand
	M65.25[1,2,9]	Calcific tendinitis, thigh
	M65.26[1,2,9]	Calcific tendinitis, lower leg
	M65.27[1,2,9]	Calcific tendinitis, ankle and foot
	M65.28	Calcific tendinitis, other site
	M65.29	Calcific tendinitis, multiple sites
	M71.40	Calcium deposit in bursa, unspecified site
	M71.42[1,2,9]	Calcium deposit in bursa, elbow
	M71.43[1,2,9]	Calcium deposit in bursa, wrist
	M71.44[1,2,9]	Calcium deposit in bursa, hand
	M71.45[1,2,9]	Calcium deposit in bursa, hip
	M71.46[1,2,9]	Calcium deposit in bursa, knee
	M71.47[1,2,9]	Calcium deposit in bursa, ankle and foot
	M71.48	Calcium deposit in bursa, other site
	M71.49	Calcium deposit in bursa, multiple sites

6th Character meanings for codes as indicated
1 right   2 left   9 unspecified

Most of the other inflammations and infections that affect the muscular system are reported similarly between the two classification systems. The main variance is that in ICD-10-CM, the laterality of the disorder is specified.

Other Abnormalities

Sometimes, muscle tissue becomes more like bone or cartilage and hardens, or ossifies. There are multiple types of this disease, called generally myositis ossificans. The most common type, known as myositis ossificans traumatica, is a localized ossification usually occurring after trauma to the muscle. This disease is most commonly seen in the arms or muscles of the quadriceps. Hardening that occurs locally without mention of trauma is called myositis ossificans circumscripta. Occasionally, second- and third-degree burns cause the muscles in the area of the burns to calcify.

A more serious and often fatal type of muscle hardening is myositis ossificans progressiva. In this rare genetic disease, each muscle progressively becomes ossified until the patient is completely stiff. Most patients with this condition suffer from fatal respiratory infections and pneumonias due to the hardening of the muscles involved in lung function.

It is more important in ICD-10-CM than in ICD-9-CM to know the type or cause of the ossification to assign the code. ICD-9-CM automatically assumes unspecified myositis ossificans is traumatic, as this is the most common type of the condition. ICD-10-CM, however, defaults to a vague code of "other," making understanding the underlying cause important to code selection. Both classification systems distinguish between the three main types of the disease, circumscripta, traumatica, and progressiva, using similar terminology. ICD-10-CM also provides the detail of the body site and laterality for each category, making this a key detail, especially in myositis progressiva, in reporting and tracking the progression of the disease over time. The addition of "in (due to)" in the ICD-10-CM index provides further division of myositis ossificans, clarifying if the condition is due to burn or paralysis.

It is noteworthy that ICD-9-CM treats calcification and ossification as one and the same disease. However, as is clinically correct, ICD-10-CM gives each general term its own category. Ossification is the forming of new bone tissue within the muscles or tendons, whereas calcification is the formation of crystals, usually calcium based, in the soft tissue. The process of calcification occurs during the ossification process, but they are not synonymous. Calcification can occur without ossification.

Coding for Myositis Ossificans

ICD-9-CM		ICD-10-CM	
728.10	Unspecified calcification and ossification	M61.20	Paralytic calcification and ossification of muscle, unspecified site
		M61.21[1,2,9]	Paralytic calcification and ossification of muscle, shoulder
		M61.22[1,2,9]	Paralytic calcification and ossification of muscle, upper arm
		M61.23[1,2,9]	Paralytic calcification and ossification of muscle, forearm
		M61.24[1,2,9]	Paralytic calcification and ossification of muscle, hand
		M61.25[1,2,9]	Paralytic calcification and ossification of muscle, thigh
		M61.26[1,2,9]	Paralytic calcification and ossification of muscle, lower leg
		M61.27[1,2,9]	Paralytic calcification and ossification of muscle, ankle and foot
		M61.28	Paralytic calcification and ossification of muscle, other site
		M61.29	Paralytic calcification and ossification of muscle, multiple sites
		M61.9	Calcification and ossification of muscle, unspecified
		6th Character meanings for codes as indicated *1 right 2 left 9 unspecified*	
728.19	Other muscular calcification and ossification	M61.30	Calcification and ossification of muscles associated with burns, unspecified site
		M61.31[1,2,9]	Calcification and ossification of muscle associated with burns, shoulder
		M61.32[1,2,9]	Calcification and ossification of muscle associated with burns, upper arm
		M61.33[1,2,9]	Calcification and ossification of muscle associated with burns, upper arm
		M61.34[1,2,9]	Calcification and ossification of muscle associated with burns, forearm
		M61.35[1,2,9]	Calcification and ossification of muscle associated with burns, hand
		M61.36[1,2,9]	Calcification and ossification of muscle associated with burns, thigh
		M61.37[1,2,9]	Calcification and ossification of muscle associated with burns, ankle and foot
		M61.38	Calcification and ossification of muscle associated with burns, other site
		M61.39	Calcification and ossification of muscle associated with burns, multiple sites
		M61.40	Other calcification of muscle, unspecified site
		M61.41[1,2,9]	Other calcification of muscle, shoulder
(Continued on next page)		*6th Character meanings for codes as indicated* *1 right 2 left 9 unspecified*	

ICD-9-CM	ICD-10-CM	
728.19 Other muscular calcification and ossification *(Continued)*	M61.42[**1,2,9**]	Other calcification of muscle, upper arm
	M61.43[**1,2,9**]	Other calcification of muscle, upper arm
	M61.44[**1,2,9**]	Other calcification of muscle, forearm
	M61.45[**1,2,9**]	Other calcification of muscle, hand
	M61.46[**1,2,9**]	Other calcification of muscle, thigh
	M61.47[**1,2,9**]	Other calcification of muscle, ankle and foot
	M61.48	Other calcification of muscle, other site
	M61.49	Other calcification of muscle, multiple sites
	M61.5Ø	Other ossification of muscle, unspecified site
	M61.51[**1,2,9**]	Other ossification of muscle, shoulder
	M61.52[**1,2,9**]	Other ossification of muscle, upper arm
	M61.53[**1,2,9**]	Other ossification of muscle, upper arm
	M61.54[**1,2,9**]	Other ossification of muscle, forearm
	M61.55[**1,2,9**]	Other ossification of muscle, hand
	M61.56[**1,2,9**]	Other ossification of muscle, thigh
	M61.57[**1,2,9**]	Other ossification of muscle, ankle and foot
	M61.58	Other ossification of muscle, other site
	M61.59	Other ossification of muscle, multiple sites

6th Character meanings for codes as indicated		
1 right	*2 left*	*9 unspecified*

Some abnormalities in muscle function are considered manifestations of an underlying condition. Many of these are reported with general codes in ICD-9-CM. For example, there are many types of abnormal, involuntary movements. ICD-9-CM lumps all of them into a single code, although these different movements can indicate a disease. ICD-9-CM codes therefore do not convey all of the information about the type of abnormal movement. In contrast, ICD-10-CM has unbundled these symptoms into four unique types of movement:

- **Abnormal head movements:** Include flopping, nodding, tic, chorea, and myoclonic jerks of the head and neck.

- **Tremors:** Involve rhythmic, unconscious contraction and relaxation of one or more muscles.

- **Cramp and spasm:** Contractions of a muscle; the difference is the duration and whether there is associated pain. A spasm is a brief contraction followed by little or no pain, whereas a cramp is more severe in that it is prolonged and painful.

- **Fasciculation:** Small "twitching" of a fascicle.

Understanding these types of movements is key to assigning the correct ICD-10-CM codes that capture the true symptomatology.

Coding for Abnormal Involuntary Movements

ICD-9-CM		ICD-10-CM	
781.0	Abnormal involuntary movements	R25.0	Abnormal head movements
		R25.1	Tremor, unspecified
		R25.2	Cramp and spasm
		R25.3	Fasciculation
		R25.8	Other abnormal involuntary movements
		R25.9	Unspecified abnormal involuntary movements

Abnormal *gait* is another potential symptom of an underlying muscle condition. When a person walks, there are many muscles moving in coordination with one another to produce a fluid and steady motion referred to as *gait*. Any disruption in strength, sensation, coordination, or function of the muscles involved in this process causes an abnormal gait. Because the disruption can be due to a neurological or muscle disorder, it is imperative to know the different ways gait can be altered.

Most prevalent are ataxic- and paralytic-type gait abnormalities. An ataxic gait is represented by a wide stance and unsteady, uncoordinated walking motions. Cerebellar ataxia is considered a neurological disorder and is classified as such in both ICD-9-CM and ICD-10-CM. Paralytic ataxia is caused by hemiparesis or paraplegia due to a cerebrovascular accident, trauma, or disease. Other types of ataxia include scissor gait and antalgic gait, which occurs when the patient avoids a certain movement due to pain. This is usually in response to trauma, osteoarthritis, or hip pain. A scissor gait usually occurs in patients with cerebral palsy.

ICD-9-CM classifies any non-cerebellar gait disturbance to one code, 781.2 Abnormality of gait. However, ICD-10-CM clarifies the different types for clinical as well as research purposes.

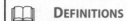

DEFINITIONS

gait. Manner in which a person walks. The phases of the gait cycle include loading, response, mid-stance, terminal stance, pre-swing, initial, mid-swing, and

Coding for Gait Abnormalities

ICD-9-CM		ICD-10-CM	
781.2	Abnormality of gait	R26.0	Ataxic gait
		R26.1	Paralytic gait
		R26.81	Unsteadiness on feet
		R26.89	Other abnormalities of gait and mobility
		R26.9	Unspecified abnormalities of gait and mobility

Summary

Because of the close relationship between the muscles and the skeletal system, the coding and reporting concepts are similar and, in some cases, interrelated, such as with strains and sprains. As demonstrated in this chapter, more extensive knowledge of the size, shape, action, location, and attachments of muscles is important in being able to appropriately assign ICD-10-CM codes as the newer classification system focuses on the specifics of each category.

Chapter 5. **Nervous System**

Anatomic Overview

The nervous system is a complex network of specialized organs, tissues, and cells that coordinate the body's actions and functions. It consists of two main subdivisions: the central nervous system and the peripheral nervous system. The central nervous system includes the brain and the spinal cord, and the peripheral nervous system includes the sense organs and the nerves that link the organs, muscles, and glands to the central nervous system. Nerves designated as cranial nerves originate in the brain and branch through the structures of the head, including the face and cranial sense organs (e.g., eyes, ears). Four groups of peripheral nerves branch from the spinal cord at cervical, thoracic, lumbar, and sacral levels and innervate the corresponding regions of the body.

The central nervous system (CNS) is composed of the brain, the spinal cord, and their associated connective tissues. The brain and spinal cord function as central processing units to receive, integrate, and interpret information, as well as to formulate a response to stimuli.

Figure 5.1: Brain

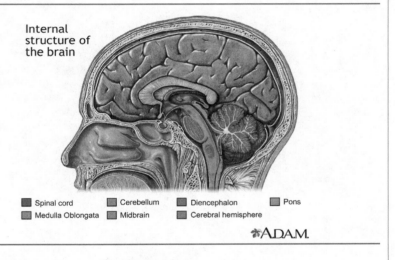

Internal structure of the brain

| ■ Spinal cord | ■ Cerebellum | ■ Diencephalon | ■ Pons |
| ■ Medulla Oblongata | ■ Midbrain | ■ Cerebral hemisphere | |

✸A.D.A.M.

The brain can be divided into several regions:

- **Cerebral hemispheres:** These form the largest part of the brain, occupying the anterior and middle cranial fossae in the skull.

- **Diencephalon:** This includes the thalamus, hypothalamus, epithalamus, and subthalamus, and forms the central core of the brain.

- **Midbrain:** The midbrain is located at the junction of the middle and posterior cranial fossae.

- **Pons:** This part of the brain is in the anterior part of the posterior cranial fossa; fibers within the pons connect the cerebral hemisphere with its opposite cerebellar hemisphere.

- **Medulla oblongata:** This region is continuous with the spinal cord and controls the respiratory and cardiovascular systems.

- **Cerebellum:** The cerebellum overlies the pons and medulla and controls motor functions that regulate muscle tone, coordination, and posture.

The spinal column, which encloses the spinal cord, consists of vertebrae linked by cartilaginous intervertebral discs held together by ligaments. The spinal cord extends from the first lumbar vertebrae to the medulla at the base of the brain. The outer layer of the spinal cord consists of myelin-sheathed nerve fibers that are bundled and that conduct impulses triggered by pressure, pain, heat, and other sensory stimuli or conduct motor impulses activating muscles and glands. The inner layer (i.e., gray matter) is primarily composed of nerve cell bodies. The central canal, within the gray matter, circulates the cerebrospinal fluid.

Three connective layers of meninges wrap around the spinal cord and cover the brain. The pia mater is the innermost layer, the arachnoid lies in the middle, and the dura mater is the outside layer, to which the spinal nerves are attached. The 31 pairs of spinal nerves deliver impulses to the spinal cord, which in turn relays them to the brain. Conversely, motor impulses generated in the brain are relayed by the spinal cord to spinal nerves, which pass the impulses to muscles and glands. Nerve fibers in the spinal cord usually do not regenerate if injured by trauma or disease.

Figure 5.2: Spinal Column

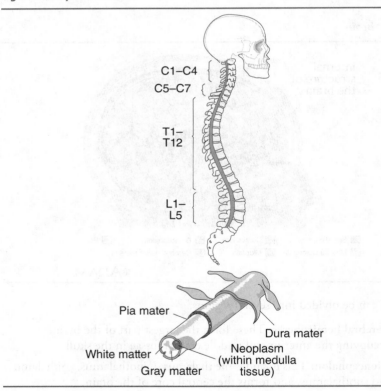

The structures of the peripheral nervous system (PNS) consist of cranial and spinal nerves, which serve as communication lines between the CNS and the rest of the body. The PNS may be subdivided into the autonomic and somatic nervous systems.

The autonomic nervous system facilitates automatic bodily processes—parasympathetic and sympathetic. These processes convey sensory impulses from the blood vessels, heart, and all of the organs in the chest, abdomen, and pelvis through nerves to the central nervous system (specifically the medulla, pons, and hypothalamus within the brain). These impulses are automatic by nature—reflex responses that occur largely without conscious thought. The efferent autonomic nerves affect reactions in the cardiovascular system and organs of the body in response to stimuli, such as environmental temperature, posture, food intake, stressful experiences, and other changes to which all individuals are exposed. The parasympathetic division of the autonomic nervous system controls anabolism (energy storage); an anabolic activity occurs in normal, nonstressful situations, such as initiating digestion after eating. In general, sympathetic processes reverse parasympathetic responses in defense or in response to stress. In defense situations, for example, catabolism (energy use) produces an increased heart rate, an expansion of the lungs to hold more energy, dilated pupils, and blood flow to the muscles and tissues.

Figure 5.3: Peripheral Nervous System

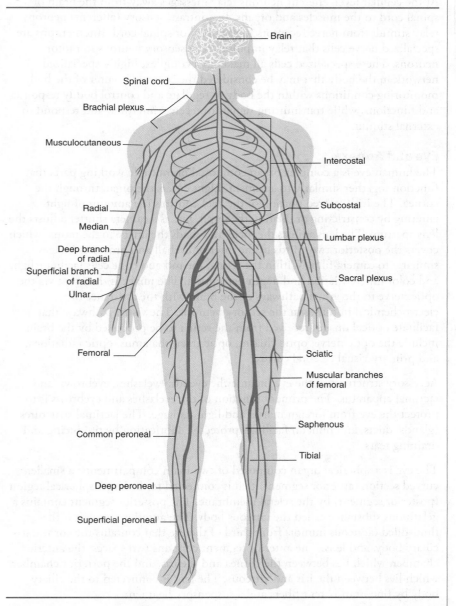

Brain

Spinal cord

Brachial plexus

Musculocutaneous

Intercostal

Radial

Subcostal

Median

Lumbar plexus

Deep branch of radial

Superficial branch of radial

Sacral plexus

Ulnar

Femoral

Sciatic

Muscular branches of femoral

Saphenous

Common peroneal

Tibial

Deep peroneal

Superficial peroneal

As the PNS is composed of nerves that project to the limbs, heart, skin, and other organs outside the brain, it controls the somatic (or bodily) nervous system. This system regulates voluntary control over skeletal muscles in response to stimuli. The SNS processes sensory stimuli and controls voluntary muscle systems within the body by neurotransmission of signals within the efferent, or motor, nerves. This process contrasts with the autonomic nervous system, which generally functions involuntarily, independent of conscious control.

The sympathetic and parasympathetic divisions work together to process and facilitate response to stimuli. These structures control voluntary actions and transmit sensation from the skin (somatic nervous system) and sense organs. Two chemicals, acetylcholine and norepinephrine, act as neurotransmitters that facilitate communication with the autonomic nervous system. Specifically, cholinergic nerve fibers secrete acetylcholine, and adrenergic nerve fibers secrete norepinephrine. In general, whereas acetylcholine causes parasympathetic (inhibiting) effects, norepinephrine causes sympathetic (stimulating) effects.

At the cellular level, efferent neurons relay messages away from the brain or spinal cord to the muscles and organs. In contrast, sensory (afferent) neurons relay stimuli from nerve receptors to the brain or spinal cord. Interneurons are specialized nerve cells that relay impulses from sensory neurons to motor neurons. These specialized cells all make up a complex, highly-specialized network in the body that may be considered the "control" center of the body, monitoring conditions within the body to regulate and control bodily responses and functions, while transmitting signals to receive, interpret, and respond to external stimuli.

Eye and Adnexa

The human eye is a complex organ composed of multiple working parts that function together similarly to a camera. Light enters the organ through the cornea. The iris (colored portion of the eye) controls the amount of light entering by constricting or dilating the pupil, just as a camera shutter adjusts the lens aperture. The lens adjusts the focus and sends the image to the retina, which covers the posterior two-thirds of the interior eyeball and processes images similarly to camera film. Within the retina, the rod and cone cells facilitate light and color differentiation and depth perception. The image is then sent via the optic nerve to the visual pathways of the brain with the assistance of electrochemical impulses in the sensory neurons. The visual pathways that facilitate optical images received from the retina to be processed by the brain include the optic nerve, optic chiasm, optic tract, thalamus, optic radiations, and primary visual cerebral cortex.

Accessory structures of the eye include the eyelids, eyelashes, eyebrows, and lacrimal apparatus. The primary function of the eyelashes and eyebrows is to protect the eye from foreign matter and light damage. The lacrimal structures (glands, ducts, and puncta) facilitate protective lubrication by producing and draining tears.

The eye is a spherical organ composed of two main compartments: a smaller, curved section (anterior segment) that is connected to the larger spherical region (posterior segment) by the scleral membrane. The posterior segment contains a gelatinous substance called the vitreous body. The anterior segment is the fluid-filled (aqueous humor) front third of the eye that contains the cornea, iris, ciliary body, and lens. The anterior segment contains two spaces: the anterior chamber, which lies between the cornea and the iris, and the posterior chamber, which lies between the iris and vitreous. The lens is connected to the ciliary body by fine, transparent fibers and a suspensory ligament.

Figure 5.4: Adnexa

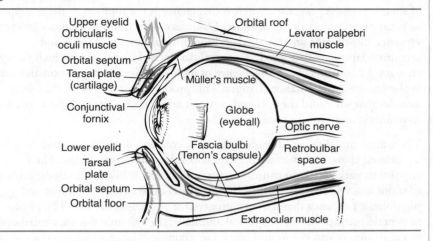

Although the sclera connects the two chambers of the eye, the organ is surrounded by multiple membranes. The outermost layer contains the cornea (anterior segment) and the sclera (posterior segment); the middle layer contains the choroid (vascular layer), ciliary body, and the iris. The innermost layer is the retina, a highly vascularized photosensitive membrane. These inner layers of the eye can be visualized with an ophthalmoscope during dilated eye examination.

The eyes adjust to the motions of the head by a set of extraocular muscles connected to the outer surface of each eye. These muscles allow the eye to focus and receive images, while adjusting to motion on a small area of the retina called the fovea, which facilitates visual acuity. Extraocular muscles include the lateral, medial, and superior recti, and the inferior and superior obliques. These muscles allow the eyes to rotate and are responsible for coordinating and rotating both eyes synchronously. Images are stabilized during movement of the head by the vestibulo-ocular reflex, which allows the image to remain situated at the center of the visual field.

Figure 5.5: Eye Musculature

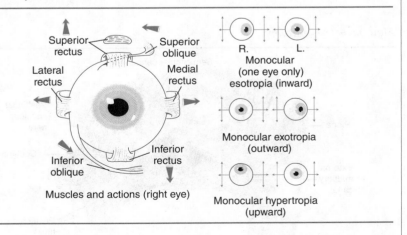

Close-range visual adjustment involves three processes to facilitate image focus on the retina. For two eyes to converge at the same point to visualize an object, the eyes rotate to allow projection of the image on the center of the retina in both eyes. Convergence describes the ability to focus a nearby object by means of rotating the eyes together, whereas divergence is the rotation of the eyes apart to focus on an object in the distance. Disorders of accommodation occur when vergence movements are impaired and the normal process of focus and accommodation are disrupted. Accommodation is the process by which the eye changes the convergence or divergence of light to maintain focus upon an image as the proximity or distance changes. This process is controlled by the ciliary muscles that surround the lens and contract and relax to *refract* light as needed to maintain an object in focus.

There are many diseases, disorders, injuries, congenital anomalies, and age-related changes that affect the eyes and surrounding structures. These conditions vary widely in cause, severity, and onset. While some conditions are of sudden, acute onset (e.g., infection, trauma) others entail anatomic and physiologic processes that follow a progressive or gradual decline. The presence of genetic predisposition, congenital anomalies, or systemic disease contributes to eye disorders and vision problems. For example, diabetes mellitus is a disease increasing in incidence in the United States that can lead to potentially serious retinal damage and precipitate cataract formation and early-onset glaucoma. The natural aging process also contributes to certain degenerations within the ocular structures that facilitate vision, the most common of which include eyelid laxity, liquefaction of the vitreous with opacification, retinal degeneration, cataract formation, and normal age-related pupillary changes. Although the cause of myopia may be multifactorial if not uncertain, it has been estimated that the prevalence of near-sightedness in the United States affects one out of 10 children and two out of 10 adults.

Ear

In human anatomy, the ear detects sound and facilitates equilibrium of balance and body position. The ear can be anatomically divided into external, middle, and inner sections. The outer ear (also called the pinna or auricle) is made up of cartilaginous and cutaneous tissue. It acts as a funnel for sound waves, which travel through the pinna into the external auditory canal, a short tube that terminates at the tympanic membrane, or eardrum. The external auditory canal contains tiny hairs and specialized sebaceous (oil) glands that secrete a protective, waxy substance called cerumen.

Figure 5.6: Ear Anatomy

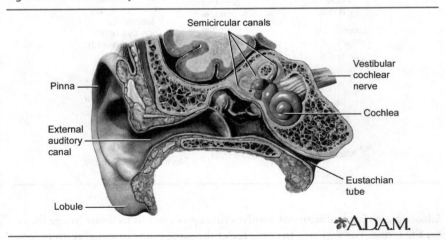

The middle ear is an air-filled cavity behind the tympanic membrane. Three tiny ear bones (ossicles) vibrate in response to sound waves. These bones include the malleus (hammer), incus (anvil), and stapes (stirrup), which vibrate and strike against the tympanic membrane to amplify the sound waves. The malleus resembles a hammer, in that it contains a long process that is attached to the mobile portion of the tympanic membrane (eardrum). The incus connects the malleus and stapes. The three bones are arranged so that movement of the tympanic membrane causes movement of the malleus, which causes movement of the incus, which causes movement of the stapes. Two tiny ligaments (tensor tympani, tensor stapedius) adjust the tension of the tympanic membrane to protect the inner ear from loud noises. The stapes strikes against the oval window, which is in front of another membranous opening, the round window. The movement of the stapes against these membranes moves the fluid within the cochlea (a portion of the inner ear). The vibrations of the ossicles stimulate the fluid-filled cochlea of the inner ear to transform sound into nerve impulses that are passed on to the brain via the eighth cranial (auditory) nerve.

Also within the middle ear is the eustachian (auditory) tube, the primary functions of which are to drain fluid from the middle ear into the pharynx and to equalize pressure between the outer and middle ears. It is a hollow, tubular structure that normally remains collapsed but expands in response to changes in air pressure.

The inner ear contains a series of canals: the cochlea, the vestibule, and the semicircular canals. These structures are encased within the temporal bone of the skull. The cochlea is a spiral-shaped (snail-like) structure filled with fluid. The semicircular canals (labyrinths) contain receptor cells to facilitate balance together with the vestibular apparatus (semicircular ducts, utricle, and saccule). Specialized epithelial and ciliary cells (microscopic hairs) within the cochlea release chemical neurotransmitters to a portion of the temporal lobe within the cerebral cortex that processes sound sensory input. The eighth cranial (auditory) nerve originates from the brainstem, with its point of insertion in the inner ear. Sound waves are received by the structures of the external ear, pass through the vibrating structures within the middle ear, and are transferred to the oval window of the cochlea in the inner ear, as described above. The fluid inside the ducts flows against specialized sensory cells in the organ of Corti, which is situated on the basilar membrane in the cochlea and stimulates the auditory nerve to transmit the information to the brain. The stimulation of thousands of tiny, specialized hair cells in the semicircular canals not only plays a part in auditory processing, but is also key in the sensation of equilibrium. The hair cells, microvilli, release neurotransmitters to the sensory neurons, which are passed to the vestibulocochlear nerve. These impulses are then passed on to the brainstem, cerebellum, thalamus, and cerebral cortex for processing, translation, and stimulation of responsive mechanisms.

> ☞ **INTERESTING A & P FACT**
>
> The stapes is the smallest bone that has a name in the human body.

Anatomy and Physiology and the ICD-10-CM Code Set

The nervous system can be affected by many types of disease. The tissues that make up or protect portions of the nervous system are susceptible to degeneration, neoplasm, infection, and other pathology.

The nervous system works closely with other organ systems within the body to maintain homeostatic function. For example, the nervous system sends and receives information from the endocrine system to produce and inhibit secretion of hormones to perform a variety of bodily functions, including regulating metabolism. For this reason, endocrine manifestations may be commonly associated with certain nervous system diseases, and vice versa. Additionally, the nervous system is vulnerable to infectious agents such as bacteria, parasites, and viruses, resulting in conditions such as encephalomyelitis, meningitis, and certain infectious neuropathies.

See the *ICD-10-CM Draft Official Guidelines for Coding and Reporting* for specific guidance regarding coding certain nervous system disorders, including pain, and reporting conditions that affect the ***dominant*** versus the ***nondominant*** side.

Inflammatory Diseases of the Central Nervous System

As in ICD-9-CM, certain conditions are described by multiple codes or the codes describing them must be sequenced in a particular way. However, because ICD-10-CM has greater data granularity, there are fewer manifestation code edits. For example, code section G00–G09 Inflammatory diseases of the central nervous system, contains only five codes in ICD-10-CM, down from 18 such codes in ICD-9-CM. A manifestation code is not allowed to be reported as a principal or first-listed diagnosis because it describes a manifestation of some other underlying disease, not the disease itself. This is important to understand when reporting CNS infections, since additional codes often are assigned for the causal infection or organism. Certain CNS infections represent a primary infection, one originating within the central nervous system. Other CNS infections present as secondary sites from an infection that originated elsewhere within the body. Therefore, it is important to understand the clinical terminology as it applies to many of the disease classifications included in this chapter.

Generally, the ICD-10-CM code set describes conditions in a more clinically or anatomically specific manner than the ICD-9-CM system. However, it is interesting to note that at the time of this publication, there are some instances in which ICD-10-CM is less specific than ICD-9-CM:

ICD-9-CM

320.81 **Anaerobic meningitis**
Bacteroides (fragilis)
Gram-negative anaerobes

ICD-10-CM

G00.8 **Other bacterial meningitis**
Meningitis due to Escherichia coli
Meningitis due to Friedländer's bacillus
Meningitis due to Klebsiella
Use additional code to further identify organism (B96.-)

In this example, ICD-9-CM provides a single, specific classification code for anaerobic meningitis, whereas ICD-10-CM reclassifies the condition to a general "other" category, requiring an additional code to identify the organism. In this example, ICD-10-CM requires multiple codes, and ICD-9-CM classifies the condition to a single, specific classification code. Certain conditions represented with unique classification codes in ICD-9-CM require more than one code in ICD-10-CM. In these instances, manifestation-etiology edits indicate that the manifestation code must be sequenced secondary to the underlying disease or condition:

DEFINITIONS

dominant (side). Exercising the most influence or control (left-handed versus right-handed).

nondominant (side). Pertaining to that with the least influence or control.

Coding for Meningitis

ICD-9-CM		ICD-10-CM	
321.1	Meningitis in other fungal diseases	G02	Meningitis in other infectious and parasitic diseases classified elsewhere
321.2	Meningitis due to viruses not elsewhere classified	G02	Meningitis in other infectious and parasitic diseases classified elsewhere
321.3	Meningitis due to trypanosomiasis	G02	Meningitis in other infectious and parasitic diseases classified elsewhere
321.4	Meningitis in sarcoidosis	G02	Meningitis in other infectious and parasitic diseases classified elsewhere

ICD-10-CM:

G02 **Meningitis in other infectious and parasitic diseases classified elsewhere**
Code first underlying disease, such as:
Poliovirus infection (A80.-)

The examples above illustrate reclassification of infectious meningitis to the causal infectious disease code in chapter 1 of ICD-10-CM, thereby conserving space within the classification for future expansion and minimizing redundancies. The less specific code description in ICD-10-CM does not mean that coders do not need to be knowledgeable about these other infectious and parasitic diseases. In fact, it means that coders must watch for additional information in the medical record to make sure the underlying disease is coded first. Now instead of one combination code, two or more codes must be used.

Certain ICD-10-CM classifications differentiate specific conditions that were previously classified together. For example, 323.9 Unspecified causes of encephalitis, myelitis, and encephalomyelitis, is equivalent to two possible codes in ICD-10-CM:

ICD-9-CM

323.9 **Unspecified causes of encephalitis, myelitis, and encephalomyelitis**

ICD-10-CM

G04.90 **Encephalitis and encephalomyelitis, unspecified**

G04.91 **Myelitis, unspecified**

When coding and reporting conditions classified to section G00–G09 Inflammatory diseases of the central nervous system, it is important to distinguish between the site and type of infection as specified in the diagnosis. For this reason, a clear understanding of the terminology associated with central nervous system inflammatory conditions is essential.

Infections and inflammatory conditions of the CNS are serious and potentially fatal. The associated cerebral edema can cause irreversible brain damage or intracerebral hemorrhage. Infections included in this code section include *meningitis, encephalitis, encephalomyelitis,* and *myelitis.*

- **Meningitis:** Meningitis is inflammation of the CNS meninges, the protective membranes surrounding the brain and spinal cord. Causal factors include toxic effects viruses, bacteria, or other microorganisms, and infection with viruses, bacteria, or other microorganisms. Presenting symptoms include headache, cervicalgia, fever, confusion, photophobia, nausea, and vomiting.

 DEFINITIONS

encephalitis. Inflammation or infection of the brain.

encephalomyelitis. Inflammation or infection of the brain and spinal cord.

meningitis. Inflammation or infection of the cerebrospinal meninges.

myelitis. Inflammation or infection of the spinal cord.

- **Encephalitis:** This is an inflammatory condition of the brain and is most commonly caused by a viral infection. Primary encephalitis is a direct viral infection of the brain, whereas secondary encephalitis occurs as a result of an infection originating elsewhere in the body.

- **Myelitis:** This condition is inflammation of the spinal cord most commonly caused by viral infection. Symptoms vary by region of the spinal cord affected and most commonly include fever, headaches, neuralgia, paresthesia, or impaired bladder or bowel control.

- **Encephalomyelitis:** This is a general term describing an inflammatory condition of the brain and spinal cord. Presenting symptoms overlap those of other CNS infections. Treatment focuses on eradicating the causal infection or stabilizing the causal condition.

- *Encephalopathy:* Encephalopathy is a nervous system dysfunction due to toxicity, trauma, disease, or other pathology affecting the brain. It may be permanent or reversible and varies widely in severity, depending on the etiology. The most common symptom is altered mental state, which may be accompanied by a host of additional neurological signs and symptoms.

ICD-10-CM requires coders to understand anatomy, physiology, and pathology to code accurately. Code section GØØ–GØ9 contains certain codes that require multiple coding, as do many of their ICD-9-CM counterparts. In general, code structure within this rubric is similar between systems, with a few exceptions.

Coding for Cerebral Cryptococcus

ICD-9-CM		ICD-10-CM	
117.5	Cryptococcus	B45.1	Cerebral cryptococcus
321.Ø	Cryptococcal meningitis	B45.1	Cerebral cryptococcus

Understanding the terminology and pathological disease processes inherent in the nervous system is vital to understanding the process of ICD-10-CM coding, especially in making the switch from ICD-9-CM.

Lipoidosis is a general term describing several inherited disorders of fat metabolism. These disorders are characterized by the abnormal accumulation of specific lipids (fat cells) in the body that result in progressive debility due to the associated destruction of the brain and nervous system tissue. Leukodystrophy is a condition in which inherited deficiencies in protein synthesis disrupt the growth or maintenance of the myelin sheath. The myelin (e.g., myelin sheath) is a fatty-appearing insulating membrane that covers and protects nerve axons while serving as a conducting mechanism for transmitting electrical signals between nerve cells. In effect, disorders of the myelin sheath can be loosely equated to problems with electrical wire insulation. These disruptions cause multiple deleterious nervous system effects.

Depending on the causal metabolic abnormality, deficiency of certain fat metabolizing enzymes cause various multisystemic disease processes. Codes have been created based on causal genetic defects and associated systemic manifestations.

DEFINITIONS

encephalopathy. Disease or disorder of the brain.

CLINICAL NOTE

Cryptococcal infection occurs due to contact with a rare pathogen, most commonly caused by inhaling the spores into the lungs, resulting in pneumonia. It can also affect the CNS, manifesting as meningitis or focal brain lesions (cryptococcomas), which may cause hydrocephalus, seizures, and focal neurological deficits.

Coding for Cerebral Lipoidoses and Leukodystrophies

ICD-9-CM		ICD-10-CM	
330.0	Leukodystrophy	E75.23	Krabbe disease
		E75.25	Metachromatic leukodystrophy
		E75.29	Other sphingolipidoses
330.1	Cerebral lipoidoses	E75.00	GM2 *gangliosidosis,* unspecified
		E75.01	Sandhoff disease
		E75.02	Tay-Sachs disease
		E75.09	Other GM2 gangliodiosis
		E75.11	*Mucolipoidosis* IV
		E75.4	Neuronal ceroid *lipofuscinosis*

Specific codes have been created in ICD-10-CM for certain cerebral degenerative diseases of childhood onset to reflect medical advances in identifying genetic links to disease.

Coding for Degenerative Diseases

ICD-9-CM		ICD-10-CM	
330.8	Other specified cerebral degenerations in childhood	F84.2	Rett's syndrome
		G31.81	Alpers disease
		G31.82	Leigh's disease

Rett's syndrome is an inherited disorder caused by mutations in the X chromosome linked MECP2 gene and therefore occurs almost exclusively in females. Onset of symptoms occurs most commonly between 6 and 18 months of age and includes progressive problems with movement, coordination, and communication. Additional symptoms include breathing problems, arrhythmias, seizures, and constipation. Genetic testing establishes the diagnosis, which is often evasive and may be confused with autism, cerebral palsy, or other developmental delay.

Leigh's disease is an inherited neurometabolic disorder of the central nervous system that occurs due to mutations of the mitochondrial DNA (mtDNA). These mutations impair the growth and development of essential brainstem cells, which inhibits motor skills. The disease is characterized by the patient's inability to control movement. In infants, early symptoms include poor sucking ability, inability to control head movements, and seizure. As the disease progresses, organ function and development are delayed or regress, resulting in failure to thrive. Prognosis varies widely in accordance with age of onset and severity.

Alpers disease is an inherited autosomal recessive disorder caused by mutations in the mtDNA, specifically identified as the POLG gene. Initial symptoms in infancy include developmental delay, hypotonia, and spasticity. Disease progression is marked by progressive paralysis, dementia, and mental retardation. Myoclonic seizures are characteristic of Alpers disease. Diagnostic imaging of the central nervous system often displays status spongiosis degeneration of the cerebrum. Prognosis is poor. Patients often expire within the first decade of life.

Alzheimer's and Parkinson's Disease and Related Syndromes
ICD-9-CM contains a specific code for Alzheimer's disease; ICD-10-CM has been expanded to provide information regarding onset within the code set itself.

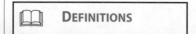

DEFINITIONS

gangliosidosis. Abnormal harmful accumulation of certain lipids (gangliosides) due to enzyme deficiency, causing progressive destruction of nervous system tissues.

lipofuscinosis (ceroid). Abnormal accumulation of lipopigments in the nervous system tissues causing neurodegeneration.

mucolipidosis. Abnormal harmful accumulation of lipids in cells manifested by damage to the motor nerve and ocular tissues.

Coding for Alzheimer's Disease

ICD-9-CM		ICD-10-CM	
331.0	Alzheimer's disease	G30.0	Alzheimer's disease with early onset
		G30.1	Alzheimer's disease with late onset
		G30.8	Other Alzheimer's disease
		G30.9	Alzheimer's disease, unspecified

Alzheimer's disease is a chronic, progressive form of dementia caused by the destruction of subcortical white matter in the brain with plaque formations. Diagnostic imaging typically reveals shrinkage of white matter and an increase in the size of the ventricles.

In a normally functioning process, the ends of nerve cells (synapses) release neurotransmitter molecules that bind to neurotransmitter receptors, thus converting a nerve impulse into a chemical signal. The neurotransmitter receptor receives the transmitter signal and, in turn, generates a responsive nerve impulse. In Alzheimer's disease, there is a deficit in the levels of acetylcholine and degeneration of cholinergic neurons, neurotransmitter proteins, and cells within the brain. The debilitating and ultimately fatal disease is manifested by cognitive and memory decline and other neuropsychiatric symptoms and behavioral dysfunctions. Patients exhibit progressive behavioral changes, including loss of interest and memory problems. The associated frustration and aggressiveness can be treated with sedative or neuroleptic therapies.

Figure 5.7: Neuromuscular Junction

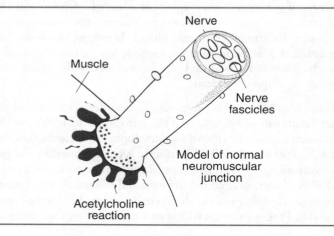

Parkinson's disease (paralysis agitans) is an idiopathic neurological condition marked by degeneration and dysfunction within the basal ganglia, clusters of nerve cells (neurons) at the base of the cerebrum, on both sides of the thalamus, above the brainstem. The basal ganglia may also be referred to as separate structures that include the caudate nucleus, putamen, and globus pallidus. This disease involves the degeneration of the nigral neurons, a group of specialized cells in the midbrain that contain neuromelanin and manufacture the neurotransmitter dopamine. When 75 to 80 percent of the dopamine innervation is destroyed, signs and symptoms of parkinsonism begin to manifest. These symptoms include tremor, rigidity, shuffling gait, drooling, "pill rolling" hand movement, and impaired control of facial muscles.

Figure 5.8: Parkinson's Disease

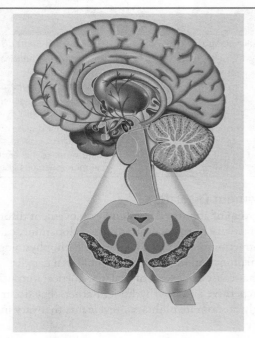

© J. Bavosi/Photo Researchers, Inc

Secondary parkinsonism occurs due to the adverse effects of certain disease processes, drugs, or chemicals. These may include exposure to toxic chemicals, adverse effects of anesthesia, and overdose or prolonged use of certain medications or drugs, including narcotics. Additional causal factors include secondary effects of infectious or inflammatory disease (e.g., encephalitis, meningitis), cerebrovascular disease (stroke), or diseases that damage dopamine neurons. ICD-10-CM expands to a number of codes for diseases of the basal ganglia. Certain related conditions may be classified elsewhere (e.g., 31.83 Lewy body disease). Whereas ICD-9-CM provided a single code for secondary parkinsonism, ICD-10-CM differentiates between certain causal factors.

Coding for Parkinsonism

ICD-9-CM	ICD-10-CM	
332.1 Secondary parkinsonism	G21.11	Neuroleptic induced parkinsonism
	G21.19	Other drug induced secondary parkinsonism
	G21.2	Secondary parkinsonism due to other external agents
	G21.3	Postencephalitic parkinsonism
	G21.8	Other secondary parkinsonism
	G21.9	Secondary parkinsonism, unspecified

ICD-10-CM can be much more specific than ICD-9-CM when it comes to clinical differentiation of conditions. For example:

Coding for Degenerative Diseases of the Basal Ganglia

ICD-9-CM		ICD-10-CM	
333.0	Other degenerative diseases of the basal ganglia	G23.0	*Hallervorden-Spatz disease*
		G23.1	Progressive supranuclear ophthalmoplegia
		G23.2	*Striatonigral degeneration*
		G23.8	Other specified degenerative diseases of the basal ganglia
		G23.9	Degenerative disease of basal ganglia, unspecified
		G90.3	Multi-system degeneration of the autonomic nervous system

📖 **DEFINITIONS**

extrapyramidal. Neural pathways situated outside of or independent from corticospinal pyramidal tracts.

Hallervorden-Spatz disease. Demyelination of the nerves between the stratum and pallidum.

Huntington's chorea. Fatal hereditary disease in which degeneration of the cerebral cortex and basal ganglia result in chronic, progressive mental deterioration; dementia and death occur within 15 years of onset.

motor cortex. Regions of the cerebral cortex of the brain that coordinate and control motor functions.

neuroleptic (drug). Antipsychotic, tranquilizing medication.

striatonigral degeneration. Neurodegeneration caused by localized abnormalities in the striatum and substantia nigra (mesencephalon) causing difficulty with balance and movement.

Chorea and Movement Disorders

Chorea describes a group of abnormal involuntary movement disorders characterized by overactivity of the neurotransmitter dopamine, causing irregular muscle contractions known as dyskinesias. Pathophysiology is thought to originate from a malfunction in the regulation of basal ganglia neurotransmission that causes an excess of thalamo-cortical output. The movements are nonrepetitive and nonrhythmic. Rather, they occur as irregular, abrupt, and seemingly random involuntary movements that vary in severity and affected anatomic site.

Mild cases may manifest as restlessness or fidgeting, whereas more severe movements may include wild, violent flinging of the extremities (ballism). Multiple types of chorea have been identified, including certain inherited forms (e.g., *Huntington's chorea*), those due to adverse effects of drugs (e.g., hormonal therapies, neuroleptics), and underlying endocrine disease (e.g., thyroid).

Associated contributing factors include pregnancy (e.g., chorea gravidarum), infection (e.g., rheumatic fever), or autoimmune disease (e.g., systemic lupus erythematosus). Certain choreas can interfere with speech, swallowing, gait, or posture and may become exacerbated during periods of anxiety or stress, abating during rest or sleep. Prognosis and treatment options vary, depending on the type of chorea, causal factors, and associated disease processes. Symptomatic treatment may include neuroleptic medications, dopamine inhibitors, and benzodiazepines.

Disorders specified as "*extrapyramidal*" affect the areas of the brain that coordinate muscle movement. They are so named for the complex pathways and feedback loops that lie outside the tracts of the *motor cortex*, which extend through the pyramid-shaped regions of the medulla. Certain pyramidal pathways innervate motor neurons of the brainstem or spinal cord, whereas the extrapyramidal tracts conduct and modulate motor activity indirectly, transmitting nerve impulses from the pons and medulla of the brain using motor neurons of the basal ganglia, cerebellum, and thalamus to the spinal cord. These pathways help regulate automatic movements that affect muscle tone, balance, and posture. The complexity of the neural circuitry that indirectly achieves motor control through routes other than the direct innervation of the pyramidal system has made it difficult to establish a cohesive, collaborative definition of the extrapyramidal pathways.

Figure 5.9: Pyramidal Pathways

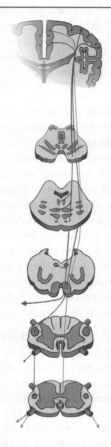

© BSIP/Photo Researchers, Inc

Many of these conditions are identified in association with the anatomic location of the disease or disease characteristics. In general, extrapyramidal symptoms may be described as *akathisia*, *akinesia*, and muscle spasms. Causal factors may include adverse effects of antipsychotic or other medications (e.g., neuroleptics), or as sequelae of brain injury. Unique codes have been established throughout this chapter to differentiate drug-induced nervous system disorders from those otherwise specified, including extrapyramidal and abnormal movement disorders.

ICD-10-CM:

G25.1	Drug-induced tremor
G25.61	Drug-induced tics
G25.4	Drug-induced chorea
G24.02	Drug-induced acute dystonia
G24.09	Other drug-induced dystonia
G25.70	Drug-induced movement disorder
G25.71	Drug-induced akathisia
G25.71	Other drug-induced movement disorders

 DEFINITIONS

akathisia. Motor restlessness.

akinesia. Inability to initiate movement.

DEFINITIONS

diplopia. Double vision.

disseminated. Widely spread or distributed; dispersed throughout a large area or region.

Demyelinating Diseases

Demyelinating diseases of the central nervous system previously coded to categories 340–341 in ICD-9-CM have been expanded in the ICD-10-CM coding system, and will have their own distinct section (rubric), G35–G37. Included within these categories are multiple sclerosis (G35), acute *disseminated* demyelination (G36), and other demyelinating disease of the central nervous system (G37).

Demyelinating diseases affect both the central and peripheral nervous systems. Pathogenesis of demyelination may be summarized as the abnormal loss of myelin, the protective white matter substance that insulates nerve endings and facilitates neuroreception and neurotransmission. When this substance is damaged, nerve function is short-circuited, resulting in impaired or loss of function. As a result, patches of scar tissue (sclerosis) develop where the protective myelin has been damaged at the nerve endings. Although healing remyelination can occur in certain disease processes, there could be permanent damage in the form of sequelae and long-term effects. The anatomic location of demyelination may be associated with certain types or manifestations of disease. For example, patients with transverse myelitis usually exhibit demyelination at the thoracic spine level, with associated lower extremity, bowel, and bladder impairments. Causal factors include genetic predisposition, certain infections, autoimmune disease, and exposures to certain drugs or chemicals.

Multiple sclerosis is a chronic demyelinating disease affecting the white matter of the spinal cord and brain. It is characterized by the breaking down of the myelin fibers of the nervous system; patches of scarred nervous fibers develop at these sites. The etiology is unknown, but recent studies suggest the condition may be a cell-mediated autoimmune disease due to an inherited disorder of immune regulation. The disease affects adults between ages 20 and 40 and occurs more often in women. Signs and symptoms of multiple sclerosis include vision disturbances (e.g., acute optic neuritis, *diplopia*), poor muscle control and coordination (e.g., clumsiness, stumbling, or falling), incontinence, paresthesias, and mental changes. Therapies include corticosteroids to lessen the intensity and duration of acute exacerbations, physical and occupational therapy to preserve muscle strength and maintain motor function, and muscle relaxant and transcutaneous electrical nerve stimulation (TENS) units to treat spasm and pain.

Figure 5.10: Myelin and Nerve Structure

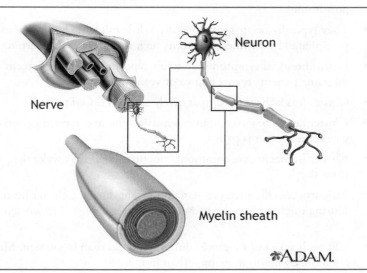

Headache, Migraine, and Epilepsy

Classifications for *epilepsy, migraine,* and headache are generally similar between systems. However, ICD-10-CM includes expanded subclassifications that differentiate headache as "*intractable*" or "not intractable," by type similar to existing classifications for epilepsy and migraine. A note at category G40 Epilepsy and recurrent seizures, and G43 Migraine, provides synonymous terms for the classification of "intractable," including:

- Pharmacoresistant (pharmacologically resistant)
- Treatment resistant
- Refractory (medically)
- Poorly controlled

Coding for Cluster Headache

ICD-9-CM		ICD-10-CM	
339.00	Cluster headache syndrome, unspecified intractable	G44.001	Cluster headache syndrome, unspecified, intractable
		G44.009	Cluster headache syndrome, unspecified, not intractable
339.01	Episodic cluster headache	G44.011	Episodic cluster headache, intractable
		G44.019	Episodic cluster headache, not intractable
339.02	Chronic cluster headache	G44.021	Chronic cluster headache, intractable
		G44.029	Chronic cluster headache, not intractable

Differentiating between the various types of headache, such as cluster headache and migraine, can be difficult. To further complicate matters, patients may experience overlapping types of headache, such as a migraine and cluster headache combination. However, cluster headaches can be differentiated from migraine in that:

- There are no discernible phases (i.e., prodrome, aura, headache, and postdrome).
- They typically occur spontaneously, while migraine headaches are often precipitated by sentinel symptoms such as aura or other warning.
- Gastrointestinal symptoms are rarely reported, while 40 percent of migraine patients report nausea or vomiting symptoms.
- Cluster headaches are comparatively short in duration.
- Cluster headaches may go into remission for an extended period of time where the patient is pain-free.
- Cluster headaches are commonly nocturnal and may wake the patient from sleep.
- Patients generally prefer to remain upright during a cluster headache. During migraine attacks, movement is often reported to worsen the pain.
- Cluster headaches are more common in men than in women. Migraines are more common in women than in men.

ICD-10-CM classifications for headache syndromes map directly to their ICD-9-CM counterparts, with the exception of a sixth-digit severity indicator that differentiates between intractable versus not intractable presentations. However, there are many clinical variations of headache pain with distinct characteristics and treatments. Treatment relies on accurate diagnosis; therefore, differentiation between headache syndromes is essential. Classification distinctions include the following:

- **Cluster headaches:** Incorporating a "clock" mechanism, cluster headaches occur most frequently at night and are associated with rapid eye movement (REM). Approximately half of cluster headache patients are awakened from sleep by paroxysmal pain, usually within two hours of falling asleep.
- **Drug-induced headache:** Headaches caused by the frequent use of certain over-the-counter (OTC) or prescription drugs. When the effect of one dose wears off, a withdrawal effect occurs, triggering the next headache and another round of medication, perpetuating the cycle.
- **Hemicrania continua:** Previously defined as a persistent primary unilateral headache of unknown causation, this type of headache is characteristically responsive to indomethacin, differentiating hemicrania continua from migraine or cluster headache. Other medications, including Triptans, are not effective.
- **New daily persistent headache (NDPH):** Developing rapidly (over less than three days), this new, unrelenting headache occurs daily at the same time. NDPH is not a continuum of a migraine or tension headache but may present with similar features. The cause is unknown, but it may be associated with viral infection. NDPH is typically unresponsive to traditional medical therapies.
- **Post-traumatic headache:** This type of headache occurs commonly following head trauma. Although the headache has the potential to persist for months or even years, frequency and severity of post-traumatic headache usually resolve within six to 12 months of injury. Associated symptoms may include dizziness, insomnia, difficulties in concentration, and mood and personality changes. Chronic headache after trauma is commonly caused by sustained muscle

contractions of the neck and scalp or by vascular changes caused by previous injury. Emotional stress and reactions to the headache occurrences and initial injury can complicate treatment by creating a situational anxiety cycle.

- **Tension type (or stress) headaches:** The most common type of headache among adults, tension headaches are *idiopathic* but may be triggered by or associated with various factors, including stress, sleep habits, and emotional state.

- **Trigeminal autonomic cephalgia (TAC):** This group of primary headache disorders is characterized by unilateral distribution of pain along the fifth cranial nerve occurring in association with characteristic autonomic ipsilateral cranial features.

Epilepsy is a disorder characterized by recurrent transient disturbances of the cerebral function. An abnormal paroxysmal neuronal discharge in the brain usually causes convulsive seizures but may result in loss of consciousness, abnormal behavior, and sensory disturbances in any combination. Epilepsy may be secondary to prior trauma, hemorrhage, intoxication (toxins), chemical imbalances, anoxia, infections, neoplasms, or congenital defects. Signs and symptoms of epilepsy include momentary interruption of activity, staring, and mental blankness. More severe symptoms include complete loss of consciousness, sudden momentary loss or contracture of muscle tone, rolling of the eyes, stiffness, violent jerking movements, and incontinence.

Clinical classification of seizures is based on whether the origin or source of the seizure is localized (partial or focal, involving one part of the brain) or generalized (distributed throughout multiple areas of the brain). These classifications can progress or overlap, in which case certain seizures may manifest as partial and progress to generalized. Localized or partial seizures are further differentiated by the extent to which consciousness is affected. For example, consciousness is impaired in a complex partial seizure, whereas in simple localized seizures, consciousness is unaffected. Although all generalized seizures lead to impairment or loss of consciousness, ICD-10-CM differentiates among them by specifying whether they are idiopathic in origin, associated with an underlying cause (e.g., drugs, hormones), or distinguished as inherent to certain identifiable syndromes (e.g., *Lennox-Gastaut, West's*).

Although coding for migraine is generally similar between systems, ICD-10-CM includes expanded subclassifications that differentiate certain identifiable migraine variants.

Coding for Migraine

ICD-9-CM		ICD-10-CM	
346.21	Variants of migraine, NEC without status migrainosus	G43.819	Other migraine, intractable, without status migrainosus
		G43.A19	Cyclical vomiting, intractable, without status migrainosus
		G43.B19	Opthalmoplegic migraine, intractable, without status migrainosus
		G43.C19	Periodic headache syndromes in child or adult, intractable, without status migrainosus

Migraine is a common type of vascular headache. Migraine headaches appear to be caused by blood vessels that overreact to various triggers, such as stress, or an

DEFINITIONS

idiopathic. Self-originating or of unknown cause.

Lennox-Gastaut syndrome. Severe epilepsy with onset in early childhood; seizures occur frequently and vary in type.

West's syndrome. Serious severe infantile epilepsy often due to anoxic brain injury, birth trauma, or other disease process; characterized by a triad of infantile spasms, specific EEG pattern changes, and developmental regression.

DEFINITIONS

aura. Warning symptoms that precede migraine headache or seizure.

photophobia. Sensitivity to light.

scotoma. Blind spot within the visual field or an area of lost or diminished vision.

allergic reaction that creates vasoconstrictive spasm. The spasm reduces blood flow and therefore oxygen supply to the brain. In response, vasodilation occurs, triggering the release of pain-producing substances called prostaglandins. The result is a throbbing pain in the head. Diagnosis of migraine may be made based on clinical presentation.

Status migrainosus describes a severe migraine attack that lasts for more than 72 hours and is often associated with nausea and vomiting. Certain symptoms, collectively known as "*aura*," may include flashing lights, bright spots, loss of part of one's field of vision, *scotoma*, geometric visual patterns, or numbness or tingling in the hand, tongue, or side of the face. Aura may precede various types of migraine, including classical or common migraine. Other symptoms may include:

- Moderate to severe throbbing pain for up to 72 hours; pain may be localized to a specific part or region of the head

- Nausea, with or without vomiting

- Sensitivity to light (*photophobia*) and sound

- Visual or auditory hallucinations

Common migraine pain can last three to four days. In addition to classic and common, migraine headache can take several other forms:

- **Basilar artery migraine:** Disturbance of the basilar artery; occurs primarily in adolescent and young adult women.

- **Hemiplegic migraine:** Characterized by temporary paralysis on one side of the body. Familial hemiplegic migraine (FHM) has been linked to mutations of specific genes on chromosomes 1 and 19. Sporadic hemiplegic migraine (SHM) is FHM without the familial connection and that particular genetic mutation.

- **Menstrual migraine:** Associated with hormonal changes inherent to the menstrual cycle.

- **Ophthalmoplegic migraine:** Presents with pain around the eye; often is associated with a droopy eyelid, double vision, and other visual problems.

Migraine complications may include associated cerebral infarction in which the migraine adversely disrupts circulation, resulting in significant ischemia with subsequent infarction (stroke).

Neurological Effects of Vascular Conditions

Many vascular conditions with neurologic effects previously coded as circulatory conditions in ICD-9-CM will now be coded as nervous system conditions. Conversely, paralytic sequelae of cerebral infarct/stroke are classified in ICD-10-CM to chapter 9, "Diseases of the Circulatory System." Code categories G45 and G46 contain expanded subclassifications that include specific types of vascular conditions with updated terminology. In some cases, conditions previously separately classified have been combined and in other cases conditions previously classified to other specified (.8) codes or "ill-defined" codes in ICD-9-CM have been assigned unique codes in ICD-10-CM. These reclassifications provide greater specificity by which to differentiate certain TIA syndromes by type or affected anatomic site.

Coding for Neurovascular Effects of Vascular Conditions

ICD-9-CM		ICD-10-CM	
435.8	Other specified transient cerebral ischemias	G45.1	Carotid artery syndrome
		G45.2	Multiple and bilateral *precerebral artery* syndromes
435.2	Subclavian steal syndrome	G45.8	Other transient cerebral ischemic attacks and related syndromes
435.8	Other transient cerebral ischemias	G45.8	Other transient cerebral ischemic attacks and related syndromes
		G46.0	Middle cerebral artery syndrome
		G46.1	Anterior cerebral artery syndrome
		G46.2	Posterior cerebral artery syndrome
437.8	Other ill-defined cerebrovascular disease	G46.3	Brain stem stroke syndrome
		G46.4	Cerebellar stroke syndrome
		G46.5	Pure *motor lacunar* syndrome
		G46.6	Pure *sensory* lacunar syndrome
		G46.7	Other lacunar syndromes
		G46.8	Other vascular syndromes of brain in cerebrovascular diseases

Transient cerebral ischemia or attack (TIA) describes episodes of focal neurological symptoms. A typical transient ischemic event may last between two and 15 minutes, yet resolve within 24 hours. The most common cause of a TIA-type event is *embolization* due to cardiovascular causes, including rheumatic heart disease, arrhythmia, valve disease, endocarditis, and myocardial infarction. Transient cerebral ischemia may be identified by affected vessel, such as the *basilar* or *vertebral* arteries. The primary function of the vertebral and basilar arteries is to supply the brain with oxygen-rich blood. The paired vertebral arteries (right and left) together with the basilar artery are often referred to as the vertebrobasilar system. These vessels connect with the *circle of Willis*, a vascular network of five bilateral arteries.

Figure 5.11: Circle of Willis

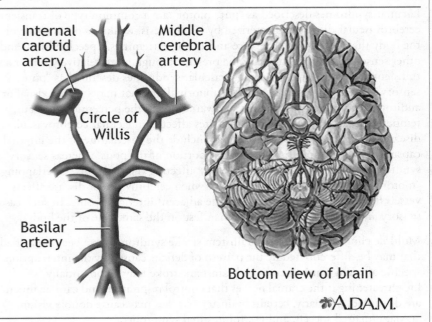

Internal carotid artery

Middle cerebral artery

Circle of Willis

Basilar artery

Bottom view of brain

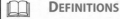

📖 **DEFINITIONS**

basilar artery. Major cerebral artery (origin) inferior to the pons that (insertion) divides into the posterior cerebral arteries and the superior cerebellar artery.

circle of Willis. Circular network of arteries that supply blood to the brain.

embolization. Forming of a circulatory obstruction out of circulating matter or particle (e.g., blood clot or plaque) and associated physiologic disruptions.

lacunar. Pertaining to discontinuity of space within an anatomical structure; pits, depressions, or hollows.

motor. Of or relating to a motor nerve; one that causes or imparts motion.

precerebral artery. Artery that flows to the cerebrum but is not located within the cerebrum.

sensory. Of or relating to the senses; including vision, hearing, tactile sense, or taste.

vertebral artery. Major cervical artery (origin) branching from the subclavian arteries to (insertion) the basilar artery.

Vascular syndromes specified as middle, anterior, or posterior artery in nature indicate conditions in which the blood supply from the affected artery is restricted, leading to a reduction of the function of the portions of the brain supplied by that vessel. Presenting symptoms are often represented by impairment in the brain functions performed by the affected area of the brain. For example, cerebellar stroke syndrome is so named for the characteristic manifestations associated with cerebellum-mediated functions. When disease compromises the vasculature of the cerebellum, the associated physiological functions of the cerebellum that control hearing and balance are disrupted, resulting in hearing loss, dizziness, and ataxia.

Lacunar strokes, ischemic attacks, and other vascular syndromes originate due to disease processes in intracerebral vessels, most commonly occlusions of the branches of a larger artery (e.g., middle cerebral, posterior cerebral, basilar). Lacunar cerebrovascular events tend to occur in the deeper, smaller vessel branches within the brain.

Figure 5.12: Cerebrovascular Arteries

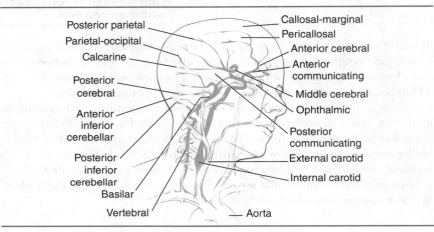

Lacunar syndromes described as "pure motor" are a common type of transient cerebrovascular disease characterized by hemiparesis, weakness on one side of the body that may include the face and/or the extremities. Speech, vision, and other sensory symptoms may also be present, though often relatively minor and transient. By contrast, those cerebrovascular syndromes described as "pure sensory" are characterized by sensory abnormalities that may include visual or auditory disturbances, numbness, and variations in the perceptions of pain, temperature, and pressure. Anatomic sites affected in lacunar cerebrovascular disease with motor manifestations may include the vasculature of the internal capsule or the basis pontis, the anterior portion of the pons, whereas sensory syndromes typically arise from pathology affecting the thalamus. Overlapping "motor" and "sensory" symptoms occur when cerebrovascular disease affects vessels that supply the thalamus and the adjacent interior capsule. In such cases, sensory and motor symptoms may manifest on the same side of the body.

Multiple clinical variations of brainstem stroke syndrome have been identified that may be differentiated by the pattern of deficits caused by the interruption of specific affected cranial nerves. A brainstem stroke may be potentially life-threatening if the cranial nerves that control respiration and cardiac function are disrupted. Similarly, certain brainstem strokes may cause double vision, ataxia, impaired speech, and gastrointestinal symptoms.

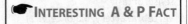

INTERESTING A & P FACT

The term "cerebellum" may be translated to mean "little brain." Situated posterior to the cerebrum, above the medulla oblongata, its main function is to coordinate fine motor skills and learning, equilibrium, and balance.

Certain syndromes identified elsewhere in ICD-9-CM will be coded as cerebrovascular syndromes in ICD-10-CM. For example, ICD-10-CM code G46.3 Brain stem stroke, includes:

- Benedikt's, Foville's, Weber, and Millard-Gubler syndromes (344.89), and Claude syndrome (352.6), characterized by oculomotor nerve palsy, contralateral hemiparesis, ataxia, and hemiplegia of the face and upper extremities

- Paraplegia and anesthesia over part of the body caused by lesions in the brain or spinal cord

- Wallenberg syndrome (436), characterized by dysphagia, hoarseness, loss of taste, and paralysis of the ipsilateral vocal cord and tongue due to lesions of the glossopharyngeal (IX) & vagus (X) nerves.

Figure 5.13: Trigeminal and Facial Nerve Branches

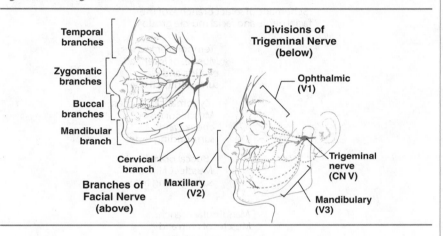

Facial Nerve Disorders

Although many codes are mapped directly between the systems (e.g., trigeminal neuralgia is coded as 350.1 in ICD-9-CM and G5Ø.Ø in ICD-10-CM), ICD-10-CM provides unique codes to identify certain facial nerve disorders that were previously included in "other specified" (.8) ICD-9-CM classifications.

Coding for Facial Nerve Disorders

ICD-9-CM		ICD-10-CM	
351.8	Other facial nerve disorders	G51.2	Melkersson's syndrome
		G51.3	Clonic hemifacial spasm
		G51.4	Facial myokymia
		G51.8	Other disorders of facial nerve

Melkersson (-Rosenthal) syndrome is a genetic condition with onset in childhood or adolescence. It is characterized by chronic facial swelling, localized particularly to the lips, and recurrent facial palsy. Recurrent attacks may become permanent, with a hardening, discoloration, and cracking of labial tissue. Associated conditions include fissured tongue and ophthalmic symptoms, including lagophthalmos, blepharochalasis, corneal opacities, retrobulbar neuritis, and exophthalmos.

☞ **INTERESTING A & P FACT**

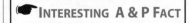

Clonic derives from the Greek word klonos, which means "turmoil."

DEFINITIONS

clonic. Neuromuscular abnormality characterized by rapidly alternating muscular contraction and relaxation.

myokymia. Involuntary, spontaneous muscle contractions characterized by undulating or rippling-appearing muscle spasms.

Facial *myokymia* may be described as a form of involuntary movement, or "quivering," in which the affected muscle appears to spasm in continuous, rippling motions. Causal conditions include neoplasm (typically a brainstem glioma), demyelinating diseases (e.g., multiple sclerosis), or certain polyneuropathies (e.g., Guillain Barré syndrome).

Clonic facial spasm is an idiopathic disorder with onset in the fifth or sixth decade of life. Presentation is most commonly unilateral, although bilateral presentations have been observed in severe cases. Characteristic clonic facial muscle spasm occurs on one side of the face, with abnormally rapid periods of alternating muscular contractions and relaxations. Facial muscles typically affected include the corrugator, frontalis, orbicularis oris, platysma, and zygomaticus.

Figure 5.14: Facial Nerves

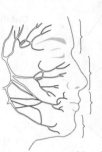

Schematic of select branches of the facial nerve and facial muscle groups

Temporal branches: Muscles of forehead, eyelids, and surrounding tissue

Zygomatic branches: Muscles of nose, cheeks, and surrounding tissue

Buccal branches: Muscles of lips and surrounding tissue

Mandibular branch: Muscles of chin and surrounding tissue

Sustained tonic contractions can result in chronic irritation of the facial nerve, hyperexcitability, and disruptions in neurotransmission. Causal conditions include compressive lesions (e.g., tumor), stroke, multiple sclerosis, and infection.

Eye and Adnexa

ICD-10-CM separates the nervous system disease classifications from those of the sense organs (eye and ear), creating three separate chapters. Perhaps one of the most significant changes in the ICD-10-CM system is the incorporation of laterality; that is, the codes reflect paired organs and anatomic sites. Some code classifications indicate right, left, bilateral, and unspecified laterality. This is particularly evident in chapter 7, "Diseases of the Eye and Adnexa (H00-H59)."

ICD-10-CM associates certain ophthalmic diseases with closely related manifestations separately. For example, parasitic endophthalmitis has been expanded to include separate classifications for parasitic cyst, by affected anatomic site. Previously, ICD-9-CM provided a single code for parasitic endophthalmitis and parasitic cyst, regardless of affected site.

Coding for Endophthalmitis

ICD-9-CM		ICD-10-CM	
360.13	Parasitic endophthalmitis, NOS	H21.331	Parasitic cyst of iris, ciliary body or anterior chamber, right eye
		H33.121	Parasitic cyst of retina, right eye
		H44.121	Parasitic endophthalmitis, unspecified, right eye

Figure 5.15: Anterior Chamber

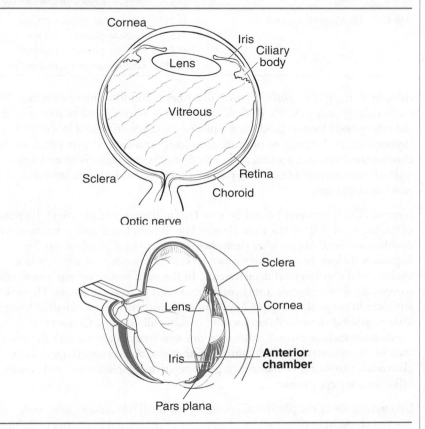

Endophthalmitis is an infection or inflammation of the tissues and internal structures of the eye. The anterior or posterior chamber, or both, may be affected. Parasitic endophthalmitis describes an infection of the eye due to invasion by a parasitic microorganism through direct exposure to the parasite or through blood-borne transportation to the eye or adjacent structures. There are multiple parasites that can invade the eye that for coding purposes may be classifiable elsewhere, depending on the nature of the organism and anatomic site of infection. Signs of infection include white nodules on the lens capsule, iris, retina, or choroid, or inflammation of all of the ocular tissues, which leads to a globe of full, purulent exudates. General symptoms may include impairment of visual acuity and the visual field, pain, excessive tearing, ocular discharge, and photophobia. If the infection is inadequately treated, inflammation may spread to the orbital soft tissue.

Some ICD-10-CM code descriptions have been updated to reflect current clinical terminology and in response to a better understanding of conditions through advancing medical technologies. For example, the diagnoses blind hypotensive eye and blind hypertensive eye have been revised to atrophy of the globe and absolute glaucoma, respectively.

Coding for Hypotensive and Hypertensive Eyes

ICD-9-CM		ICD-10-CM	
360.41	Blind hypotensive eye	H44.521	Atrophy of globe, right eye
		H44.522	Atrophy of globe, left eye
		H44.523	Atrophy of globe, bilateral
		H44.529	Atrophy of globe, unspecified eye
360.42	Blind hypertensive eye	H44.511	Absolute glaucoma, right eye
		H44.512	Absolute glaucoma, left eye
		H44.513	Absolute glaucoma, bilateral
		H44.519	Absolute glaucoma, unspecified eye

Atrophy of the globe (*phthisis* bulbi) describes vision loss due to extremely low intraocular pressure (IOP). Phthisical eye occurs when disease or damage causes the ciliary body to stop producing aqueous fluid, resulting in a loss of IOP (hypotony). Prolonged low pressure can distort and cause degeneration of the chorioretinal vascular, cornea, and optic disc. Phthisis bulbi is an end-stage severity presentation of ocular hypotony characterized by a soft, atrophic, and nonfunctional eye.

Normal IOP is between 10 and 20 mm Hg (millimeters of mercury). Hypotony of the eye is an IOP of less than 10 mm Hg, although it may not be considered problematic until the pressure drops below 6 mm Hg. Causal factors for hypotony include postsurgical wound leak, inflammatory eye diseases (e.g., uveitis), and chorioretinal detachments. In the past, hypotony was a common complication of trabeculectomy procedures used to treat glaucoma. However, advances in surgical technique have rendered incidence to minimal, although leakage around the scleral flap incision occasionally occurs. Certain eye conditions, such as chronic inflammations and retinal defects, alter the osmotic state of the eye, resulting in hypotony. Other associated conditions include glaucoma, neoplasm, ocular injury, postoperative complications, and certain inflammatory eye diseases.

Characteristics of the phthisical eye include a small, shrunken globe with marked thickening of the sclera, metaplasia of the retinal pigment epithelium, displacement or atrophy of the intraocular contents, and ossification. At the advanced stages inherent to phthisis bulbi, prognosis is poor, resulting in a small shrunken globe of tissue with no function. Treatment options include *enucleation* with replacement of the globe or fitting a scleral shell prosthesis.

The ciliary body produces aqueous humor, which is integral to maintaining intraocular pressure. The lens and anterior eye structures separate the aqueous humor from the posterior segment of the eye. The anterior segment is divided into the anterior and posterior chambers. The aqueous humor flows into the posterior chamber through the pupil of the iris and the anterior chamber. It proceeds through the trabecular meshwork to enter the normal body circulation. Ocular hypertension, or increased IOP, may be caused by increased production or decreased outflow of aqueous humor.

Ocular hypertension is a significant finding of multifactorial etiology. Patients with a history of myopia or diabetes have an increased incidence of elevated IOP. Although ocular hypertension is not typically synonymous with glaucoma, increased IOP is a characteristic sign of glaucoma. Ocular hypertension is

DEFINITIONS

atrophy. Wasting away or decrease in the size of a body organ or part due to malnutrition or other damage.

enucleation. Surgical removal of the eye.

phthisis. Wasting disease; a disease or condition characterized by wasting.

typically defined as an IOP greater than 21 mm Hg, with absolute glaucoma representing vision loss due to the severity and progression of ocular hypertension.

In its initial stages, ocular hypertension is quiescent; it often has no discernible signs or symptoms. It is often noted upon routine eye exam by tonometry. Not all patients with increased IOP develop glaucoma—ocular hypertension is a physical finding and glaucoma represents a myriad of intraocular diseases characterized by increased IOP. General symptoms may include vision loss, eye pain, increased eye pressure sensation and an abnormally hardened texture to the globe. The diagnosis of "blind hypertensive eye" represents the end stage of intraocular hypertensive disease, whereby the ocular structures have sustained irreparable damage.

ICD-10-CM includes unique codes for conditions not previously identified by ICD-9-CM. In the classification of retinoschisis and retinal cysts, new subcategory codes have been created to specifically identify cyst ora serrata, the junction between the retina and the ciliary body.

☛ INTERESTING A & P FACT

Increased IOP is a characteristic sign of glaucoma but does not necessarily indicate the disease.

Coding for Cyst Ora Serrata

ICD-9-CM		ICD-10-CM	
361.19	Other retinoschisis and retinal cysts	H33.111	Cyst of ora serrata, right eye
		H33.112	Cyst of ora serrata, left eye
		H33.113	Cyst of ora serrata, bilateral
		H33.119	Cyst of ora serrata, unspecified eye

Subcategory H33.1 classifies acquired retinoschisis and other retinal cysts. These include primary and secondary retinal cysts and pseudocysts, similar to ICD-9-CM. However, ICD-10-CM includes a unique code subcategory to identify ora serrata cysts. In normal anatomy, the ora serrata is the serrated junction between the retina and the ciliary body. The ciliary body is part of the uvea and connects anteriorly to the root of the iris and posteriorly to the choroid at the ora serrata retinae. It is divided into the pars plana and the pars plicata. Cysts in this area of the eye may form as part of a degenerative retinoschisis, which typically originates at the periphery of the retina and extends into the ora serrata as the condition progresses. However, primary and secondary retinal cysts increase the patient's risk for retinal detachment. Secondary cysts form as a result of other (primary) ophthalmic disease. Pseudocyst describes an area of fluid accumulation without an encasing membranous lining. Retinoschisis, which can be hereditary or acquired, is an abnormal splitting of the retinal layers. It most commonly occurs in the outer plexiform layer of nervous tissue, causing vision loss in the affected area. Degenerative retinoschisis (e.g., flat, bullous) is the most common presentation. It is easily confused with retinal detachment but must be differentiated, since the management and treatment options are different.

Coding for Diabetic Ophthalmic Disease

ICD-9-CM		ICD-10-CM	
362.01	Background diabetic retinopathy	E10.311	Type 1 diabetes mellitus with unspecified diabetic retinopathy with macular edema
		E10.319	Type 1 diabetes mellitus with unspecified diabetic retinopathy without macular edema
366.41	Diabetic cataract	E10.36	Type 1 diabetes mellitus with diabetic cataract
		E11.36	Type 2 diabetes mellitus with diabetic cataract
362.07	Diabetic macular edema	E10.311	Type 1 diabetes mellitus with unspecified diabetic retinopathy with macular edema
		E10.321	Type 1 diabetes mellitus with mild nonproliferative diabetic retinopathy with macular edema
		E11.341	Type 2 diabetes mellitus with severe nonproliferative diabetic retinopathy with macular edema

In the example above, the ICD-10-CM chapter 4 code (E00–E88) includes the causal disease (diabetes mellitus), type of disease, specific ophthalmic manifestation, and associated conditions or complications. ICD-10-CM codes for diabetes mellitus no longer indicate whether the disease is controlled. See the *ICD-10-CM Draft Official Guidelines for Coding and Reporting* for specific guidance regarding coding and reporting diabetes.

Diabetes mellitus is a complex metabolic disorder with multisystemic manifestations. It can be a primary disease or occur secondary to infection, drug or chemical exposures, or other disease processes. Diabetes is clinically categorized as Type 1 or Type 2. Type 1 indicates inadequate secretion of insulin by the pancreas, whereas Type 2 is the body's inability to respond to insulin, called insulin resistance. Both have similar symptoms, including excessive thirst, hunger, and urination. Laboratory tests that detect glucose in the urine and elevated levels of glucose in the blood usually confirm the diagnosis.

Diabetes may manifest in a wide range of problems that affect the eyes, in particular the retina, lens, and trabecular meshwork. Visual changes can be minimal to severe and temporary or permanent depending on the type, location, and extent of damage.

Diabetic retinopathy (DR) is a frequent and common complication of the retinal vasculature that eventually affects most diabetic patients. Leakage and scar tissue caused by damaged retinal vessels distort and blur vision. The retina is sensitive nervous tissue that sends messages via the optic nerve to the brain and one of three layers of the eyeball. The outer, white layer is the sclera, which is the true wall of the eyeball. Lining the sclera is the choroid, a thin membrane that supplies nutrients to part of the retina. The retina, the innermost layer, begins posterior to the iris, just behind the area called the pars plana, and lines the inner wall of the eye. The central portion of the retina is the macula, which is roughly the area inside of the arcade vessels that extend from the optic nerve and around the macula. The *macula* is the area of the retina where central vision is the clearest for color and reading vision. The true focal point of the eye is the foveal avascular zone (FAZ), which is only 400 microns wide (0.4 mm). The

 DEFINITIONS

macula. Central part of the retina that provides sharp vision, the ability to discern fine detail, and color.

single-layer retinal pigment epithelium (RPE) outside the retina provides nutrients to the photoreceptors; it is also dark with melanin, which decreases light scatter within the eye. The rods and cones are photoreceptors; the cone system dominates vision in daytime, whereas the rod system dominates night vision. Below the RPE is a multilayered membrane called Bruch's membrane, which separates the RPE and retina from the choroid, a vascular layer that provides most of the oxygen to the photoreceptors and RPE. The vitreous is a clear, gel-like substance that fills up most of the inner space of the eyeball. It lies behind the lens and is in contact with the retina.

Diabetic retinopathy represents a continuum of disease, a progression of pathologic changes in the retina due to microvascular complications inherent in diabetes mellitus. Nonproliferative diabetic retinopathy indicates early stage of the disease. Microaneurysms form, retinal hemorrhages occur, and blind spots are characteristic. Increased vessel leakage occurs as the disease progresses, resulting in further vision impairment. The disease progresses from mild to moderate to severe nonproliferative retinopathy and becomes proliferative in its more advanced stage, characterized by new blood vessel formation in the retina due to significant ischemia from the damaged vessels. Diabetic macular edema (DME) occurs when leakage from the blood vessels causes swelling of the central portion of the retina, which impairs vision. Exudates or plaques may develop in the posterior pole of the retina due to the breakdown of retinal vasculature, which can precipitate vision loss.

Retinal vascular occlusion is a potentially blinding blockage that occurs in any of the blood vessels in the retina, the light-sensitive membrane in the back of the eye. Central retinal artery occlusion is blockage of the central retinal artery. The blockage is often caused by a tiny embolus in the bloodstream that obstructs circulation and oxygen supply to the retina, causing sudden, complete vision loss. In some cases, antecedent amaurosis fugax has been reported before complete occlusion and loss of vision. In the past, the term amaurosis fugax referred to symptomatic temporary blindness. However, clinical studies suggest that the underlying anatomic origin of retinal *ischemia* should be distinguished from the pathophysiologic origin to ensure optimal treatment. Recently, amaurosis fugax has been attributed in the majority of cases to internal carotid artery stenosis. This condition is considered a risk factor for permanent occlusion of the central retinal artery and stroke.

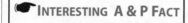

☞ INTERESTING A & P FACT

Diabetic retinopathy is the third leading cause of legal blindness in adults in the United States.

📖 DEFINITIONS

ischemia. Decrease in blood supply to the organs or tissues.

Figure 5.16: Posterior Segment of Eye

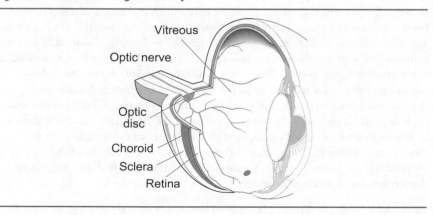

The central retinal artery enters the eye through the optic disc and divides into multiple branches to perfuse the inner layers of the retina. If circulation remains in the cilioretinal arteries to supply the macula, central vision may be preserved. However, there is a small window of opportunity to treat central retinal artery occlusion, as irreversible retinal damage occurs rapidly after onset. Occlusion of a branch of the retinal artery is often caused by a tiny embolus in the bloodstream that blocks circulation and oxygen supply to the retina, resulting in visual field loss. Loss of visual acuity indicates *foveal* involvement.

Disease progression for retinal artery occlusion is determined by the anatomical location, area of supply, drainage, arterial or venous supply, and the extent of occlusion. For central retinal artery occlusion, outcomes improve dramatically if treatment is sought within 24 hours of onset. If vision does not improve after 72 hours, the retina may have infarcted (tissue died because of partial occlusion of a vessel), in which case blindness may be permanent. Studies suggest that early detection and pathogenic differentiation between transient and permanent eye and brain ischemic syndromes can lead to more effective mechanisms for stroke prevention.

Coding for Retinal Degeneration

ICD-9-CM		ICD-10-CM	
362.34	Senile reticular degeneration of the peripheral retina	H34.00	Transient retinal artery occlusion, unspecified eye
		H34.01	Transient retinal artery occlusion, right eye
		H34.02	Transient retinal artery occlusion, left eye
		H34.03	Transient retinal artery occlusion, bilateral

ICD-10-CM classifications for retinal dystrophies primarily involving the Bruch's membrane have been reclassified as choroidal degenerations and atrophies. The alphabetic index directs the coder to "see choroid" for conditions affecting the Bruch's membrane.

The Bruch's membrane is the stratified inner layer of the choroid that separates the choroid from the pigmented layer of the retina (RPE) and the *endothelial* cells of the choriocapillaris. It has inner and outer collagenous layers rich in elastin and elastin-associated proteins.

In normal anatomy, the retinal pigment epithelium transports metabolic waste from the photoreceptors across Bruch's membrane to the choroid. Similar to the age-related forms of disease, the Bruch's membrane thickens abnormally and the transportation of metabolites becomes less efficient, which may lead to *drusen* or age-related macular degeneration. As a result, certain inflammatory and neovascular processes may occur as the membrane fragments, leading to destruction of the retinal architecture with progressive vision loss. Conditions such as pseudoxanthoma elasticum, myopia, and trauma can also cause defects in Bruch's membrane, with associated choroidal neovascularization. As the Bruch's membrane thickens, accumulation of debris and calcification (hardening) commonly occurs. Complications may include the formation of drusen and basal *laminar* deposits.

In ICD-10-CM, conditions previously classified separately as preglaucoma or borderline glaucoma are now classified to a single ICD-10-CM code.

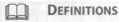

DEFINITIONS

drusen. Accumulation of extracellular material on the Bruch's membrane of the choroid.

endothelial. Related to flat cells that make up the inner linings of cavities and organ structures.

foveal. Related to the center of the retinal macula, where light falls directly on the cones.

laminar. Having to do with a thin, flat membrane or layer of a larger structure.

Coding for Glaucoma

ICD-9-CM		ICD-10-CM	
365.00	Unspecified preglaucoma	H40.0	Glaucoma suspect
365.01	Borderline glaucoma, open angle with borderline findings		
365.02	Borderline glaucoma with anatomical narrow angle		
365.03	Borderline glaucoma with steroid responders		
365.04	Borderline glaucoma with ocular hypertension		

The diagnosis of "glaucoma suspect" describes a patient with borderline signs and symptoms of glaucoma, such as a suspicious-looking optic nerve, a borderline high IOP (intraocular pressure), and associated visual field deficits. Ocular hypertension is an increase in the pressure inside the eye (IOP) and is higher than normal. Normal eye pressure ranges from 10 to 21 mm Hg. Eye pressure is measured in millimeters of mercury (mm Hg). The eye pressure for ocular hypertension is greater than 21 mm Hg. Code H40.0 describes high intraocular pressures, including those with no apparent cause, that may create a minor block in aqueous outflow from the eye when a definitive diagnosis of glaucoma is suspected but has not yet been established.

Conditions once coded separately in ICD-9-CM as pseudoexfoliation glaucoma (365.51) are now coded as open angle, primary *capsular glaucoma.* The alphabetic index directs the coder accordingly.

📖 **DEFINITIONS**

capsular glaucoma. Glaucoma occurring in association with widespread deposit of cellular organelles on the lens capsule, ocular blood vessels, iris, and ciliary body.

Figure 5.17: Glaucoma

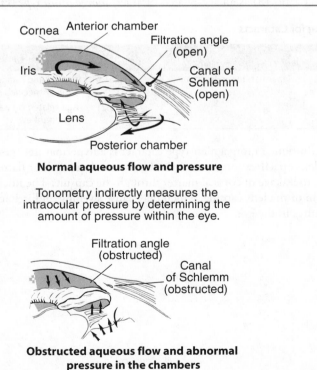

Normal aqueous flow and pressure

Tonometry indirectly measures the intraocular pressure by determining the amount of pressure within the eye.

Obstructed aqueous flow and abnormal pressure in the chambers

In glaucoma, pseudoexfoliation of the lens capsule is characterized by small, grayish particles deposited on the pupillary margin of the iris, anterior chamber, and lens. This occurs when cells within the eye release dandruff-like flakes as the outer layers of the lens slough off and block normal flow of the aqueous humor. Material deposited on the front surface of the lens in the eye may be partially rubbed off as the pupil moves over the lens. This exfoliation may occlude the outflow track (trabecular meshwork) and cause intraocular pressure to rise. Left untreated, this condition could lead to subsequent damage to the optic nerve, causing visual field loss and progressive blindness. Pseudoexfoliation syndrome-associated glaucoma commonly affects elderly patients with coexisting cataracts. It typically presents unilaterally but can progress to a bilateral presentation within several years.

Primary angle-closure glaucoma occurs when aqueous outflow is obstructed by occlusion of the trabecular meshwork, resulting in optic nerve damage and visual field loss. The pressure from secretion of aqueous into the posterior chamber by the ciliary body pushes the peripheral iris anteriorly, closing the angle. Clinical presentation varies from gradual and progressive to rapid and emergent. Symptoms of open-angle glaucoma include progressive loss of peripheral vision over a span of years, blurred or foggy vision, seeing halos around lights, reduced night vision, and aching in the eyes.

ICD-10-CM code descriptions for cataract classifications have been updated (as with other ocular disorders) by replacing the term "senile" with "age-related," where appropriate, since the term "senile" has been confused with an age-related dementia, cognitive decline, or other degenerative mental health conditions beyond that associated with the normal aging process. ICC-10-CM has also revised terminology within the cataract classification categories, changing *"after-cataract"* to "secondary cataract" and denoting hypermature senile cataract (366.18) as an age-related cataract, *morgagnian type* (H25.2-).

Coding for Cataracts

ICD-9-CM		ICD-10-CM	
366.18	Hypermature senile cataract	H25.20	Age-related cataract morgagnian type, unspecified eye
		H25.21	Age-related cataract morgagnian type, right eye

By definition, a morgagnian-type cataract is a hypermature, age-related cataract with lens opacification characterized by a soft, liquefied, or flattened lens that is prone to leakage of cortical matter through the capsule. The nucleus shifts to the bottom of the lens capsule, which may cause swelling and irritation of other structures in the eye.

DEFINITIONS

after-cataract. Cataract characterized by opacifications of the posterior capsule occurring subsequent to extracapsular cataract extraction.

morgagnian-type cataract. Mature, age-related cataract with lens opacification and a soft, liquefied or flattened fragile lens, causing nuclear shifts to the bottom of the lens capsule.

Figure 5.18: Cataract

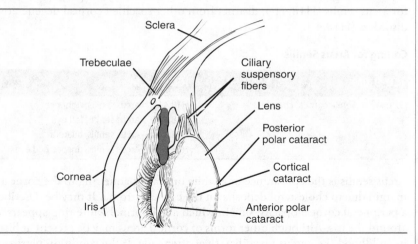

A senile (age-related) cataract involves partial or total opacity of the lens due to degenerative changes associated with the aging process. Age-related cataracts form gradually and often bilaterally in patients 55 to 70 years of age. Signs and symptoms of a senile cataract include a slow, progressive, and painless loss of vision, leukocoria (white reflection from the pupil), difficulty in night driving, altered color perception, and strabismus. Cataracts can be clinically classified by the zones of the lens involved in the opacity: anterior and posterior cortical, equatorial cortical, and supranuclear and nuclear. Age-related cataracts may include specific types of cataract, including cuneiform, nuclear, or posterior subcapsular cataract, or those with overlapping characteristics. Most age-related cataracts are identified by increased opacity of the lens followed by its softening and shrinkage associated with degeneration.

ICD-9-CM required two codes in specific sequence to report ophthalmic infection with *Acanthamoeba,* whereas ICD-10-CM has a single code:

Coding for *Acanthamoeba* Infection

ICD-9-CM		ICD-10-CM	
136.21	Specific infection due to Acanthamoeba	B60.13	Keratoconjunctivitis due to Acanthamoeba
370.8	Other forms of keratitis		
136.21	Specific infection due to Acanthamoeba	B60.12	Conjunctivitis due to Acanthamoeba
372.15	Parasitic conjunctivitis		

Diseases caused by the free-living (not parasitic) ameboid protozoan *Acanthamoeba* include amoebic keratoconjunctivitis and meningoencephalitis. *Acanthamoeba* infection is a rare but potentially blinding affliction of the cornea. It primarily affects otherwise healthy persons who improperly store, handle, or disinfect their contact lenses (e.g., by using tap water or homemade solutions for cleaning). Symptoms are similar to those of other eye infections, but targeted treatment is necessary to be effective. Complications include corneal scarring and vision loss. Long-term therapy and management are often required.

Certain ICD-10-CM code descriptions have been updated and code classifications further specified by creating unique codes for conditions once listed as inclusion terms under less-specific ICD-9-CM codes. For example, ICD-9-CM listed *arcus senilis* as an inclusion term under code 371.41 Senile

 DEFINITIONS

arcus senilis. Abnormal white or gray opaque ring appearing at the periphery of the corneal margin; occurring in older adults and often associated with hypercholesterolemia.

corneal changes. ICD-10-CM has created a separate subcategory classification for arcus senilis (H18.41-), distinct from other specified corneal degenerative disorders (H18.4-).

Coding for Arcus Senilis

ICD-9-CM		ICD-10-CM	
371.41	Senile corneal changes	H18.411	Arcus senilis, right eye
		H18.412	Arcus senilis, left eye
		H18.413	Arcus senilis, bilateral
		H18.419	Arcus senilis, unspecified eye

Arcus senilis is the appearance of a white or gray opaque ring in the corneal margin due to cholesterol deposits on the corneal stroma. It may be described as a peripheral corneal opacity, one in which an abnormal white ring appears around the iris. Although other forms of corneal arcus may be present at birth or in childhood (i.e., arcus juvenilis), they often fade. If the condition persists earlier in life, it may herald an underlying lipid disorder. In the aged population, arcus senilis is commonly due to hypercholesterolemia but may also occur as a sign of corneal ischemia secondary to other ocular disease. Normally, arcus senilis does not adversely affect vision or require treatment other than to precipitate treatment of the underlying disease (e.g., ischemia, lipid disorder).

Figure 5.19: Arcus Senilis

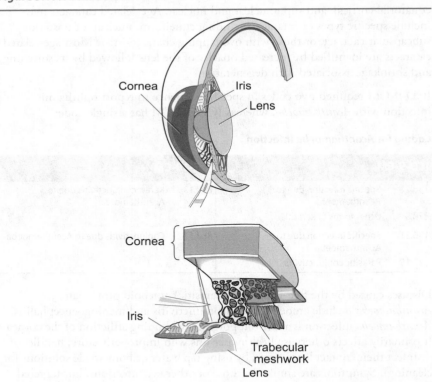

The cornea is the transparent tissue that covers the front of the eye and is composed of three layers:

1. The epithelium blocks the passage of foreign material and provides a smooth surface that absorbs oxygen and other needed cell nutrients that are contained in tears.

2. The stroma gives the cornea its strength and elasticity, and the protein fibers of the stroma produce the cornea's light-conducting transparency.

3. The endothelium pumps excess water out of the stroma.

Unlike most tissues in the body, the cornea contains no blood vessels to protect it against infection. The cornea is a physical barrier that shields the inside of the eye from germs, dust, and other foreign objects. It also acts as the eye's outermost lens; when light strikes the cornea, it refracts the incoming light onto the crystalline lens. The lens focuses the light onto the retina. Although much thinner than the lens, the cornea provides about 65 percent of the eye's power to bend light. Most of this power resides in the center of the cornea, which is rounder and thinner than the outer part of the tissue and is better suited to bending light waves.

Although certain ICD-10-CM codes that separate conditions according to severity of presentation are similar to those of ICD-9-CM, terminology has been updated to reflect current clinical language. For example, keratoconus was previously classified as unspecified (371.60), stable (371.61), or with acute hydrops (371.62). In ICD-10-CM, the term "unstable" replaces the less frequently documented "acute hydrops."

Coding for Keratoconus

ICD-9-CM		ICD-10-CM	
371.62	Keratoconus, acute hydrops	H18.621	Keratoconus unstable, right eye

Keratoconus causes the normally round shape of the cornea to thin and take on a bulging, cone-shaped appearance. It is a progressive, noninflammatory, usually bilateral disease of the cornea. Onset may occur in the teens and early 20s, progressing for five to 15 years, and sometimes longer. When progression stops, the disease is considered stable and typically remains so for the remainder of the patient's life. During rapid progression, sudden visual disturbances can spontaneously occur. In acute or unstable presentations, a break in *Descemet's membrane* allows aqueous to drain into the cornea, resulting in an immediate edema, corneal opacification, and reduced visual acuity. Vision loss is attributed primarily to resultant *astigmatism*, *myopia*, and secondary corneal scarring.

Certain conditions affecting the eyelids have been differentiated in ICD-10-CM not only by laterality, but by anatomic site: upper eyelid or lower eyelid. For example, the following ophthalmic conditions have been further specified in ICD-10-CM by creating unique codes for conditions once listed as inclusion terms under less-specific ICD-9-CM codes, specifying both laterality and anatomic site. *Chloasma, vitiligo* and *madarosis* were previously listed as inclusion terms under comparatively general ICD-9-CM code descriptions.

 DEFINITIONS

astigmatism. Condition causing blurred vision due to the irregular shape of the cornea or curvature of the lens.

chloasma. Patchy tan to brown skin discolorations, often secondary to melanocyte stimulation; may be associated with hormonal fluctuation or imbalance.

Descemet's membrane. Collagenous inner layer of the corneal endothelium.

madarosis. Loss of eyelashes, congenital or acquired; most commonly occurs secondary to other medical conditions.

myopia. Impairment of distant vision; nearsightedness.

vitiligo. Tan to white patches of skin discoloration from the loss or impairment of cutaneous melanocytes.

Coding for Eyelid Disorders

ICD-9-CM		ICD-10-CM	
374.52	Hyperpigmentation of eyelid	H02.711	Cholasma of right upper eyelid and periocular area
374.53	Hypopigmentation of eyelid	H02.731	Vitiligo of right upper eyelid and periocular area
374.55	Hypotrichosis of eyelid	H02.721	Madarosis of right upper eyelid and periocular area

Ear and Mastoid Process

ICD-10-CM classifies disorders of the ear and mastoid process by anatomic site, according to those conditions that affect the external (H60–H62), middle (H65–H75), or inner (H80–H83) ear. Additional classification sections group together other disorders of ear (H90–H94) and intraoperative or postprocedural disorders (H95). In addition, code titles were revised to uniquely classify certain types of disease previously included within a code category.

Coding for Otitis Media

ICD-9-CM		ICD-10-CM	
381	Nonsuppurative otitis media and eustachian tube disorders	H65	Nonsuppurative otitis media
382	Suppurative and unspecified otitis media	H66	Suppurative and unspecified otitis media
		H67	Otitis media in diseases classified elsewhere
		H68	Eustachian salpingitis and obstruction
		H69	Other and unspecified disorders of the eustachian tube

These unique codes enable conditions to be more specific, making the granularity of data greater than in the ICD-9-CM system. This is particularly evident in ICD-10-CM classification of ear infections, in which code categories have been differentiated and expanded, not only to further specify site, laterality, and severity of presentation (i.e., acute, chronic, unspecified), but also to distinguish between specific types and characteristics of infection.

Coding for Ear Infections

ICD-9-CM		ICD-10-CM	
380.10	Unspecified infective otitis externa	H60.01	**Abscess** of right external ear
		H60.11	**Cellulitis** of right external ear
		H60.311	**Diffuse** otitis externa, right ear
		H60.321	**Hemorrhagic** otitis externa, right ear
380.22	Other acute otitis externa	H60.511	Acute actinic otitis externa, right ear
		H60.521	Acute chemical otitis externa, right ear
		H60.531	Acute contact otitis externa, right ear
		H60.541	Acute eczematoid otitis externa, right ear
		H60.551	Acute reactive otitis externa, right ear

Furthermore, ICD-10-CM separately classifies recurrent acute otitis media. ICD-9-CM does not identify recurrent acute conditions specifically.

📖 **DEFINITIONS**

abscess. Enclosed, localized collection of pus.

cellulitis. Inflammation of the cells caused by infection of the tissue just below the skin surface.

diffuse. Scattered or spread throughout an area.

hemorrhagic. Characterized by bleeding (hemorrhage).

ICD-10-CM, however, describes certain recurrent forms of allergic otitis media in code category H65.11 Acute and subacute allergic otitis media. Separately classified as mucoid, sanguinous, or serous in ICD-9-CM, acute otitis media is identified instead by laterality and presentation (recurrent or nonrecurrent) in ICD-10-CM.

Coding for Otitis Media

ICD-9-CM		ICD-10-CM	
381.01	Acute serous otitis media	H65.01	Acute serous otitis media, right ear
		H65.04	Acute serous otitis media, recurrent, right ear
381.02	Acute mucoid otitis media	H65.111	Acute and subacute allergic otitis media, right ear
		H65.114	Acute and subacute allergic otitis media, recurrent, right ear
381.03	Acute sanguinous otitis media	H65.111	Acute and subacute allergic otitis media, right ear
		H65.114	Acute and subacute allergic otitis media, recurrent, right ear
381.04	Acute allergic serous otitis media	H65.111	Acute and subacute allergic otitis media, right ear
		H65.114	Acute and subacute allergic otitis media, recurrent, right ear
381.05	Acute allergic mucoid otitis media	H65.111	Acute and subacute allergic otitis media, right ear
		H65.114	Acute and subacute allergic otitis media, recurrent, right ear
381.06	Acute allergic sanguinous otitis media	H65.111	Acute and subacute allergic otitis media, right ear
		H65.114	Acute and subacute allergic otitis media, recurrent, right ear

Disorders of the external ear include those of the auricle (pinna) and external auditory meatus. The auricle consists of the helix, anthelix, scapha, concha, tragus, antitragus, intertragic notch, and lobule. The auricle is a single, elastic cartilage covered in skin and normal adnexal features (hair follicles, sweat glands, and sebaceous glands). The ridges in the auricle channel sounds into the acoustic meatus. The semicircular depression leading to the ear is named the concha, Latin for shell. The external auditory meatus consists of cartilaginous and osseous portions with the canal lined with epidermis, hair, and ceruminous glands that extend to the tympanic membrane.

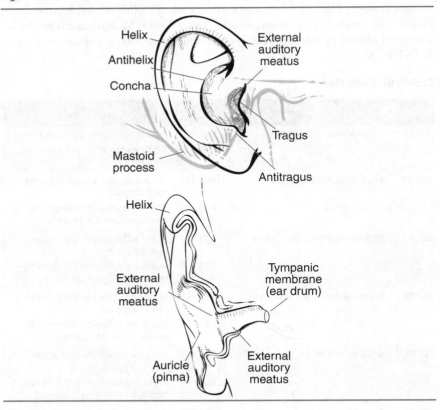

Figure 5.20: External Ear

 DEFINITIONS

meatus. Body opening or passage (e.g., the external opening of a canal).

otitis externa. Inflammation or infection of the auricle and external auditory meatus.

psoriasis. Chronic, painful skin disease characterized by inflamed, reddened patches on the skin and thickened, silvery scales.

seborrheic. Characterized by the overproduction of sebum, the oily secretion of sebaceous glands.

Otitis externa is an inflammation or infection of the auricle and external *meatus*. Although otitis externa is most commonly caused by infection, it may also be associated with noninfectious local or systemic conditions. Infective otitis externa indicates the presence of bacteria as the etiology of the inflammation. Causal organisms may include *Pseudomonas, Proteus vulgaris, Streptococci,* and *Staphylococcus aureus,* or fungal infections such as *Candida albicans.* Bacterial overgrowth can often be attributed to excessive exposure to moisture or trauma, both of which compromise the natural homeostasis within the ear. Cerumen provides a natural defense against the overgrowth of bacteria and creates a barrier for excess moisture; however, an imbalance in the amount of cerumen can impair these defensive processes and create an environment vulnerable to pathogenesis. Signs and symptoms of infective otitis externa include pain, redness, and swelling that can obstruct the meatus, serous or purulent drainage, external ear tenderness, and enlarged regional lymph nodes. Diagnostic tests include culture and sensitivity to identify the infective organism. An otoscopy reveals inflammation and ceruminous impaction. Therapies include antimicrobials (topically, systemically, or both), heat therapy to relieve pain, and gentle ear cleansing.

Noninfectious *otitis externa* can precipitate infectious otitis externa or occur independently of infection. Both systemic and local dermatologic conditions can result in an inflammation of the ear. Causal conditions may include certain types of dermatitis (e.g., eczematous, atopic, contact, *seborrheic*), lupus erythematosus, *psoriasis,* and acne. Similarly, localized inflammation can occur secondary to exposures to allergens or other irritants. Allergic dermatitis is commonly acute in presentation, with characteristic redness, pruritus, and edema. Contact dermatitis is often similar in presentation but with epidermal thickening and hardening. Tissue irritation due to noninfectious causes can precipitate secondary bacterial infection. Treatment depends on identifying and removing the irritant. Topical steroids are often beneficial in reducing inflammation and facilitating healing.

Disorders of the middle ear affect the structures inside the tympanic membrane, extending to the oval window of the cochlea. The middle ear (tympanic cavity) lies within the temporal bone and contains the ossicles, the trio of auditory bones connected by synovial joints and suspended by specialized ligaments and muscles. The eustachian tube connects the tympanic and nasal cavities to help equalize pressure within the cavities with the atmospheric pressure. Equalized pressure allows the tympanic membrane to vibrate freely. Disproportionate pressure can result in severe pain, hearing impairment, "ringing" in the ears, and vertigo. Middle ear infections often occur as a result of pathogens migrating from the nasopharynx through the eustachian tube to the auditory canal.

Figure 5.21: Middle and Inner Ear

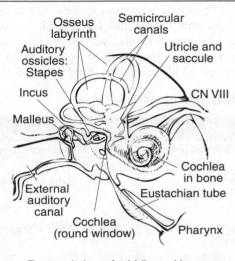

Exposed view of middle and inner ear

Otitis media is a painful inflammation of the tympanic membrane characterized by a build-up of fluids in the middle ear. Signs and symptoms may be similar to an upper respiratory infection and include chills and fever, malaise, deep throbbing ear pain, nausea and vomiting, dulled or impaired hearing, ear drainage, bulging of tympanic membrane, and a tender, swollen mastoid process. Untreated otitis media can progress to a suppurative presentation in which the tympanic membrane becomes thinned and *necrotic* and perforates.

Suppurative otitis media is most commonly caused by a bacterial infection (e.g., *Streptococcus pneumoniae, Haemophilus influenza, Moraxella catarrhalis*). Complications of otitis media are often associated with chronic or subacute disease. Acute and chronic otitis media infection may spread beyond the temporal bone and cause intratemporal (e.g., mastoiditis, petrositis, labyrinthitis, and facial nerve paralysis) and intracranial (e.g., extradural abscess, brain abscess, subdural abscess, otic hydrocephalus, and meningitis) complications. Associated conditions include adenoiditis or tonsillitis, colds or sinusitis, cholesteatoma, adhesions or scarring of middle ear structures, conductive hearing loss, abscesses, and jugular vein thrombosis.

 DEFINITIONS

necrotic. Pertaining to the deterioration or death of tissue in response to disease or injury.

suppurative. Characterized by the formation and discharge of pus.

DEFINITIONS

ankylosis (ossicles). Abnormal stiffness, adhesion, rigidity, or hardening of the auditory ossicles, decreasing mobility and conduction.

tympanosclerosis. Characterized by the accumulation of hardened, dense tissue or plaque in the middle ear, adversely affecting the mobility of the tympanic membrane and ossicles.

Tympanosclerosis is a common sequela after acute and chronic otitis media; the pathological calcified plaques are found in the tympanic membrane and the middle ear ossicles. These accumulation of plaques decreases the mobility of the tympanic membrane (tympanic sclerosis) and of the ossicles (*ankylosis*), impairing hearing.

Diagnosis includes use of a pneumatoscopy to ascertain whether there is fluid behind the eardrum or an otomicroscopy using the operating microscope to visualize depth and three-dimensional structure. Antibiotics are usually prescribed for infection. Once osteitis is diagnosed, mastoidectomy is generally warranted to remove the infected, often necrotic bone. If there is an abscess, surgery is performed to drain pus and remove the infected bone.

Therapies include systemic antibiotics, nasal decongestants, and analgesics such as aspirin to control pain and fever, and myringotomy with aspiration of the middle ear fluid if the tympanic membrane is in danger of rupture. Surgery may be performed (tympanoplasty, myringoplasty, mastoidectomy, excision of cholesteatomas) for chronic otitis media.

Although ICD-10-CM generally is far more specific than ICD-9-CM, certain classifications have been made less specific. For example, certain forms of vertigo, labyrinthitis, labyrinthine fistula, and dysfunction once separately classified according to type have been grouped together within revised subcategories and are instead identified by general diagnosis and laterality.

Coding for Vertigo, Labyrinthitis, and Fistula

ICD-9-CM		ICD-10-CM	
386.19	Other and unspecified peripheral vertigo	H81.311	Aural vertigo, right ear
386.31	Serous labyrinthitis	H83.01	Labyrinthitis, right ear
386.32	Circumscribed labyrinthitis		
386.33	Suppurative labyrinthitis		
386.41	Round window fistula	H83.11	Labyrinthine fistula, right ear
386.42	Oval window fistula		
386.43	Semicircular canal fistula		
386.51	Hyperactive labyrinth, unilateral	H83.2x	Labyrinthine dysfunction, right ear
386.55	Loss of labyrinthine reactivity unilateral	H83.2x1	Labyrinthine dysfunction, right ear

The inner ear consists of a system of fluid-filled tubes and sacs called the labyrinth, as well as the nerves that connect the labyrinth to the brain. Impulses for equilibrium are transmitted along the vestibular cochlear nerve to the brain. The vestibular system lies within the temporal bone of the skull and contains the labyrinth and the cochlea. The cochlea contains fluid-filled channels and membranes that transmit sound vibrations via thousands of tiny, specialized hairs to the vestibulocochlear nerve. The vestibular apparatus of the inner ear contains the semicircular ducts, utricle, and saccule, which work together to maintain dynamic equilibrium. The nerve impulses transmitted to the brain are relayed to the medulla, pons, and cerebellum. The cerebellum receives the sensory information from the vestibular apparatus and makes the corrective adjustments to maintain static and dynamic equilibrium.

Figure 5.22: Schematic of Labyrinth and Semicircular Ducts

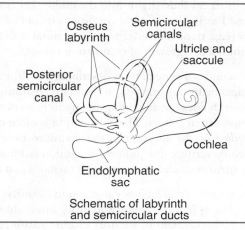

Schematic of labyrinth
and semicircular ducts

Classification systems differentiate between aural vertigo and Ménière's disease, although clinical definitions for both conditions overlap. For classification purposes, vertigo specified as "aural" or "otogenic" describes peripheral vertigo of inner ear origin, not specified as Ménière's disease. Peripheral vertigo refers to a group of conditions in which the vertigo symptoms are of inner-ear origin, whereas "central" vertigo refers to a group of conditions in which the symptoms originate in the central nervous system.

Ménière's disease is a disorder of the inner ear that causes episodes of vertigo, tinnitus, a feeling of fullness or pressure in the ear, and fluctuating hearing loss that can last two to four hours. Episodes may occur in clusters, or weeks, months, or years may pass between episodes. Between the acute attacks, most people are free of symptoms or note only mild imbalance and tinnitus. Between attacks, medication may be prescribed to help regulate the fluid pressure in the inner ear, reducing the severity and frequency of episodes. Treatment includes medical or surgical measures to relieve the pressure on the inner ear or to block the transmission of information from the affected ear to the brain.

Labyrinthitis and neuronitis are inflammatory conditions of the inner ear commonly caused by viral or bacterial infection. Inflammation of the cochlea can cause disturbances in hearing, such as tinnitus. Dizziness, unsteadiness, or imbalance when walking and nausea are the most common symptoms of vestibular disorders. Because the vestibular system interacts with other parts of the nervous system, concurrent visual disturbances, cognitive difficulties, amnesia, and motor function impairment may occur with such disorders. Patients with vestibular disorders often report fatigue, loss of stamina, and an inability to concentrate. Trauma and ear infections (e.g., otitis media, labyrinthitis) may reduce blood flow to the inner ear, which can damage the vestibular apparatus. High doses or long-term use of certain antibiotics can also cause permanent damage to the inner ear. Other drugs, such as aspirin, caffeine, alcohol, nicotine, sedatives, and tranquilizers can cause temporary dizziness but do not permanently damage the vestibular system.

Benign paroxysmal positional vertigo is commonly induced upon repositioning the head or body (e.g., getting out of bed, standing up from a sitting or lying position) and is often attributed to calcium-impacted inner ear canals. Treatment includes removing the impaction.

DEFINITIONS

cholesteatoma. Abnormal overgrowth of granulation tissue in the middle ear and/or mastoid process.

oscillopsia. Illusion that the environment is moving caused by disrupted neurotransmission from the labyrinth to the brain.

Labyrinthine fistula is an abnormal opening between the inner and middle ear through which the inner ear fluid drains into the middle ear cavity. Symptoms include dizziness and hearing loss. Causal conditions include dislocation of the inner ear structures (e.g., trauma or infection), congenital malformation, or *cholesteatoma* (abnormal overgrowth of granulation tissue).

Labyrinthine dysfunction is a general term describing a malfunction of the labyrinth that disrupts neurotransmission to the brain regarding body position. As a result, the labyrinth does not respond properly to movement. Trauma and infection are common causal factors. The dysfunction is often characterized by the sensation of *oscillopsia*, the illusion that the environment is moving. Symptoms may include vertigo, disequilibrium, motion sickness, nausea and vomiting, visual disturbances, and difficulty with memory and concentration.

ICD-10-CM codes for abnormal auditory perception disorders separately identify certain conditions (e.g., temporary auditory threshold shift), whereas other conditions (e.g., impairment of auditory discrimination) are grouped into general code subcategories such as H93.29 Other abnormal auditory perceptions.

Coding for Auditory Misperception

ICD-9-CM		ICD-10-CM	
315.32	Central auditory processing disorder	H93.25	Central auditory processing disorder
388.40	Unspecified abnormal auditory perception	H93.241	Temporary auditory threshold shift, right ear
		H93.291	Other abnormal auditory perceptions, right ear
388.43	Impairment of auditory discrimination	H93.299	Other abnormal auditory perceptions, unspecified ear
388.45	Acquired auditory processing disorder		

The ear has a number of defense mechanisms that protect its complex sensory structures from damage. For example, vasoconstriction of the auditory blood vessels in response to loud sound reduces the blood supply to the organ of Corti, thereby reducing the sensitivity and response of the sensory hair cells and protecting these structures from damage. Under normal conditions, the ear's sensitivity adjusts according to sound exposure. Sound vibrations are detected by the sensory apparatus of the inner ear and transmitted to the brain where they can be interpreted to yield meaningful information. Advances in diagnostic medicine continue to identify certain disorders pertaining to physiological interpretation and processing of sound, which were previously overlooked or misdiagnosed. These conditions may overlap or coexist with those classified elsewhere, such as ototoxic disorders secondary to adverse effects of medication, trauma, infection, or other systemic disease.

In auditory medicine, the term "auditory perception" may be defined as the ability to identify, interpret, and attach meaning to sound. Disorders of auditory perception can be difficult to diagnose because they can occur independently or secondary to infection, stroke, trauma, or other health problems. In children, these auditory perception and processing disorders may be associated with learning difficulties and therefore may be misdiagnosed as attention deficit disorder or certain forms of autism.

Auditory processing and perception disorders are not synonymous with deficits in general attention, language, or cognitive function, although such conditions may coexist or overlap. For example, individuals with auditory discrimination difficulties are unable to denote the differences between sounds, which is integral to language development. Auditory discrimination also is necessary in distinguishing between foreground and background noise. If this process is not functioning properly, the individual may become confused or overwhelmed when they are unable to ignore irrelevant noise. This state can impair learning and be misinterpreted as an inability to focus or concentrate.

Auditory synthesis facilitates language comprehension by combining sounds into understandable units. The term "auditory sequencing" may also refer to the process by which one understands and remembers the order in which sounds occur. Auditory synthesis and sequencing are integral to auditory perception and memory.

Disorders of auditory perception may be congenital or acquired. The onset of either form in early childhood can pose learning challenges. Individuals with impaired auditory perception may seem not to respond well to auditory or verbal cues or understand what they hear, or require that auditory cues be repeated before giving the desired response. These conditions are generally attributed to a disorder or dysfunction of the auditory nerve, which most appropriately identifies the underlying physiological causal factors.

Auditory processing disorder is a general term describing various disorders that often arise from impaired neural function. Manifestations may include problems differentiating between related speech sounds, and speech and environmental sounds; or relating spoken word with intent. Coping mechanisms may include depending on visual cues such as body language, eye contact, or lip reading.

Diplacusis describes a cochlear dysfunction in which the patient hears a single auditory stimulus as two sounds. This condition may be colloquially described as being "tone deaf." Acquired diplacusis may be attributed to allergies, head trauma, infection, exposure to toxins, or neoplasms (e.g., leukemia, acoustic neuromas).

Hyperacusis is a condition of acute hearing sensitivity that may or may not be accompanied by pain. Causal conditions include migraine, Asperger syndrome, Bell's Palsy, and many other conditions.

Auditory recruitment describes the abnormal perception of volume of speech or sound. It is often associated with certain degrees of sensorineural hearing loss or labyrinthitis, in which hearing is not sensitive to quiet sounds, yet is overly sensitive to loud sounds.

Auditory threshold shift is the process by which the ear protects itself by adjusting its sensitivity when exposed to noise. When this occurs, only sounds louder than a certain level are heard. Also known as "aural fatigue," the duration of shift can be temporary or permanent. Temporary auditory threshold shift often implies a temporary hearing loss to low-level sounds and may be associated with tinnitus. If the sensory hair cells of the inner ear are not allowed to recover through reduced exposure to loud sounds, they can become permanently damaged.

Coding for Conductive Hearing Loss

ICD-9-CM		ICD-10-CM	
389.03	Conductive hearing loss, middle ear	H90.0	Conductive hearing loss, bilateral
		H90.11	Conductive hearing loss, right ear, unilateral, unrestricted contralateral side
		H90.12	Conductive hearing loss, left ear, unilateral, unrestricted contralateral side

Conductive hearing loss arises from external or middle ear problems, which are often mechanical. There are various causes for conductive hearing loss, including otitis media and otosclerosis. The most common cause of conductive hearing loss in children is otitis media infection in the middle ear cavity. The most common cause in adults is otosclerosis, fixation of the stapes (the third bone in the middle ear) so that sounds cannot be transported to the inner ear. Conductive hearing loss can be temporary or permanent and is treatable with medication or surgery.

Sensory hearing losses are due to disorders in the inner ear, specifically, the cochlea. This type of loss may be congenital, resulting from abnormal cochlea development or inherited conditions, or the loss may be the result of an acquired condition, such as meningitis, an infection of the fluid around the brain often extending into the inner ear.

Neural hearing loss arises from a problem with the auditory nerve, often caused by an acoustic neuroma, a benign tumor that grows on the vestibular nerve and presses upon the auditory nerve. Early detection and prompt removal of the tumor is curative and may prevent future hearing loss. One way to test for neural hearing loss is to measure the acoustic reflex, the contraction of the stapedius, a small muscle attached to the stapes, in response to any loud sound, thus protecting the ear. The level of sound required to elicit this acoustic reflex can be used as a rough measure of hearing sensitivity. If the middle ear is normal, absence of the acoustic reflex may indicate a neural type of hearing loss, which is also characterized by a greater loss of speech discrimination than with sensory loss.

Sensorineural hearing loss is usually permanent loss of hearing sensitivity, often occurring more in the high frequencies than in the lower frequencies. Involving not only a reduction in sound level, sensorineural hearing loss also affects speech, cognition, and the ability to hear clearly and understand conversations. Damage to the cochlea (inner ear) or to the nerve pathways from the inner ear to the brain causes this type of hearing loss. This damage could be due to birth injury, diseases, toxic drugs, genetic syndromes, head trauma, exposure to noise, viruses, tumors such as acoustic neuroma or meningioma, and aging. Asymmetrical hearing loss is bilateral but more pronounced in one ear, while unilateral hearing loss affects only one side. If a sensorineural cause is suspected, electrocochleography and auditory brainstem response tests are performed to measure the activity of the cochlea, auditory nerve, and brain. Occasionally, a conductive hearing loss occurs in combination with a sensorineural hearing loss in that damage occurs in the outer or middle ear, as well as in the inner ear (cochlea) or auditory nerve. This type of hearing loss is referred to as a mixed hearing loss.

Central auditory dysfunction refers to auditory impairment resulting from problems in the brain and is uncommon. While it causes communication difficulties, the dysfunction does not cause deafness because it usually affects only one side of the brain—both sides of the brain are involved in hearing. Central auditory dysfunction can result from aging, Alzheimer's disease, and other uncommon problems.

Summary

The nervous system, as well as the special sense organs of the eyes and ears, is an area of great detail and growth under the ICD-10-CM code set. It is important and necessary to pay close attention to the differences between the two coding systems from an anatomy and pathology perspective. The additional detail and specificity afforded by the ICD-10-CM coding system is certainly a benefit, though it is clear that proper code selection rests on thoroughly understanding the new terms referenced and how certain ICD-9-CM categories break out in ICD-10-CM.

Chapter 6. **Endocrine System**

Anatomic Overview

The endocrine system comprises *glands* that produce and secrete *hormones* with a varied array of vital functions. These hormones are chemical substances released by organs or individual cells within an organ. The hormones are then carried through the bloodstream to other organs or tissues. A hormone's purpose is varied and includes the regulation of growth, metabolism, and sexual development and function. Hormones are often referred to as the "chemical messengers" because they transfer information from one set of cells to another to synchronize the body's functions.

The major glands of the endocrine system are the hypothalamus, pituitary, thymus, thyroid, parathyroid, adrenal, pineal body, ovaries, testes, and pancreas. Many organs and tissues within the body work with the endocrine system even though they are not fully functioning parts of the system. These organs and tissues contain cells that also secrete hormones, including but not limited to adipose tissue, heart, liver, kidneys, placenta, skin, small intestine, and stomach.

The endocrine system is made up of two different types of glandular tissue: exocrine and endocrine. Exocrine glands release secretions into ducts, which distribute the secretions to other areas of the body. Exocrine glands include digestive, mucus, oil, and sweat glands. Endocrine glands secrete hormones into the fluid surrounding the secretory cells. The blood then carries the hormones throughout the body.

Approximately 50 hormones are produced within the endocrine system. Hormones move throughout the body but can react only with certain cells, referred to as *"target cells."* These cells contain specific protein receptors that allow the hormone to chemically bind to the cells. Receptors are continuously being created and broken down within the body. When certain hormone imbalances occur, the body may produce excessive amounts of a hormone. The receptors automatically respond by reducing the number of receptors reacting to the target cells and by making the target cells less sensitive to the hormone. When there is a decrease in hormone production, the target tissue becomes more sensitive and more receptors appear in the cells.

Hormones are released when the body is stimulated by the nervous system (e.g., anxiety, fear, or stress) or from chemical changes in the blood, such as sugar level. For example, after ingesting a meal, glucose levels rise and the pancreas responds by releasing the hormone insulin into the bloodstream. The insulin circulates throughout the body until glucose levels return to normal.

Hormones are divided into different classifications based on chemical structure. Some are soluble in water, and others are soluble in fats or lipids. Water-soluble hormones typically include *amines* and *peptide* hormones. Lipid-soluble hormones include steroids, thyroid hormones, and nitric oxide.

Examples of water-soluble hormones grouped to amines include:

- Epinephrine (Epi) (adrenaline)
- Histamine
- Melatonin

INTERESTING A & P FACT

The endocrine glands are sometimes referred to as ductless glands.

DEFINITIONS

amines. Chemical compound that is derived from ammonia and contains nitrogen.

endocrine glands. Group of glands that secrete hormones directly into the blood and not through a duct.

hormone. Chemical substance produced by the body that has a regulatory effect on the function of its specific target organ(s).

peptide. Molecule consisting of two or more amino acids.

target cell. Specific collection of cells that responds to a given hormone treatment or tissue against which any type of immunity is directed.

DEFINITIONS

amino acid. One of the building blocks of protein that contains a basic amino (NH2), an acidic carboxyl (COOH), and a variable side chain (R) attached to an alpha carbon atom.

- Norepinephrine (NE) (noradrenaline, NA)
- Serotonin (5-HT)

Peptide hormones are the largest class of hormones and include all of the hormones secreted by the hypothalamus, pituitary, heart, kidneys, thymus, digestive tract, and pancreas. Peptide and protein hormones are grouped together depending upon the number of *amino acids* the hormone contains.

A few examples of these types of hormones include:

- Alpha-fetoprotein
- Antidiuretic hormone (vasopressin)
- Erythropoietin (EPO)
- Follicle stimulating hormone (FSH)
- Gastrin
- Glucagon
- Growth hormone (GH)
- Human chorionic gonadotropin
- Insulin
- Luteinizing hormone (LH)
- Oxytocin
- Prolactin
- Secretin
- Somatostatin
- Thyrotropin (TSH)

Examples of lipid-soluble hormones include:

- Steroids:
  - aldosterone
  - ardrogen
  - calcitriol
  - cortisol
  - estrogen
  - progesterone
  - testosterone
- Thyroid hormones:
  - triiodothyronine (T^3)
  - thyroxine (T^4)
- Gas:
  - nitric oxide (NO)

Figure 6.1: Endocrine System

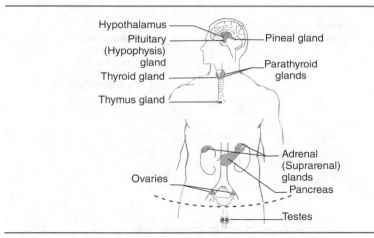

Pancreas Gland

The pancreas is a fish-shaped gland that extends horizontally behind the stomach from the curve of the duodenum to the spleen. The pancreas has two types of glandular tissue: the exocrine, which secretes digestive enzymes, and the endocrine, which produces hormones. However, it is primarily an exocrine organ.

The major part of the pancreas, called the exocrine pancreas, secretes digestive enzymes into the gastrointestinal tract. Distributed through the pancreas are clusters of endocrine cells that secrete insulin, glucagon, and somatostatin. These specialized cells are needed to maintain stable blood sugar levels in the body. Insulin helps body cells use glucose for energy, therefore reducing the amount of sugar in the bloodstream. At the same time, the hormone glucagon stimulates the liver to release its stored sugar into the blood, which raises the blood sugar levels.

Figure 6.2: Pancreas

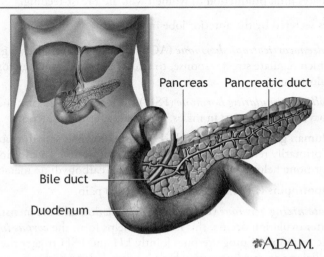

📖 DEFINITIONS

pancreatitis. Inflammation of the pancreas that may be acute or chronic, symptomatic or asymptomatic, due to the autodigestion of pancreatic tissue by its own enzymes that have escaped into the pancreas, most often as a result of alcoholism or biliary tract disease such as calculi in the pancreatic duct.

Figure 6.3: Pituitary Gland

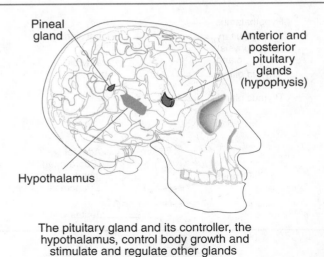

The pituitary gland and its controller, the hypothalamus, control body growth and stimulate and regulate other glands

DEFINITIONS

adrenocorticotropic hormone. Hormone secreted by the anterior pituitary that acts on the adrenal cortex and its secretion of corticosteroids. ACTH is used in hormone replacement therapy and as a diagnostic aid.

corpus luteum. Yellowish mass of endocrine tissue in the ovary that secretes progesterone, formed by a mature follicle that has released its ovum. The corpus luteum dissolves after about 10 days if there is no fertilization but persists for several months if the ovum is impregnated.

follicle-stimulating hormone. Gonadotropic hormone secreted by the anterior lobe of the pituitary gland. In women, it stimulates growth and maturation of the ovum and its enclosing cells, the production of estrogen, and the endometrial changes that occur in the first phase of the menstrual cycle. In men, the hormone stimulates the production of sperm.

luteinizing hormone. Gonadotropic hormone secreted by the pituitary gland. In women, it promotes ovulation, the release of the egg from the ovary, and sustains the luteal (second) phase of the menstrual cycle. It also promotes the secretion of progesterone. In men, the hormone stimulates the development of testicular Leydig's cells.

Pituitary Gland

The pituitary gland, also referred to as hypophysis, is a pea-shaped structure located in the sella turcica of the sphenoid bone in the skull. The gland is attached to the undersurface of the hypothalamus by a short, slender stalk called the infundibulum. The pituitary gland contains endocrine cells surrounded by an extensive capillary network. It is also part of the hypophyseal portal system and provides entry into the circulatory system. It secretes several hormones that control the function of the other endocrine glands and regulates growth and fluid balance.

The pituitary gland is divided into two parts: the anterior and posterior lobes, each having separate functions. It is further subdivided into the distal part pars distalis and the intermediate part pars intermedia. The majority of the endocrine cells are found in the pars distalis. The anterior lobe regulates the activity of the thyroid, adrenal, and reproductive glands. It also regulates the body's growth and stimulates milk production in women who are breast-feeding.

Hormones secreted by the anterior lobe include:

- *Adrenocorticotropic hormone* (**ACTH**): Triggers the adrenal glands, which regulate stress response, to release hormones such as cortisol and aldosterone.

- *Follicle-stimulating hormone* (**FSH**): In females, this hormone controls oocyte development; in males, it triggers sperm production.

- **Human growth hormone** (**HGH**): Also known as somatotropin, HGH is primarily responsible for growth and maturation. In addition, this hormone helps control protein, lipid, and carbohydrate metabolism.

- **Lipotropins** (**LPH**): Reduces sensitivity to pain.

- *Luteinizing hormone* (**LH**): Controls ovulation and the menstrual cycle. After ovulation occurs, this hormone helps form the *corpus luteum* and the secretion of progesterone. Jointly LH and FSH trigger the ovarian follicle to secrete estrogen, which is needed along with progesterone for implantation of the fertilized ovum into the uterus.

- **Melanocyte-stimulating hormone** (**MSH**): This hormone stimulates melanocytes of the skin.

- **Prolactin:** Stimulates milk production.

- **Thyrotropic hormone (TSH):** Stimulates the thyroid gland to release thyroid hormones. These hormones control the basal metabolic rate and play an important role in growth and maturation.

The posterior lobe of the pituitary gland contains the nerve endings (axons) from the hypothalamus, which stimulate or suppress hormone production. This lobe secretes antidiuretic hormones (ADH), which control water balance in the body. ADH secretion is stimulated by a rise of electrolytes or a decrease in blood volume or blood pressure. Also secreted is oxytocin, which controls muscle contractions in the uterus. In males, oxytocin stimulates muscle contraction of the prostate gland, which is essential in the release of semen before ejaculation.

Hypothalamus Gland

The hypothalamus controls the pituitary gland from deep within the brain. Although it is part of the brain, the hypothalamus is considered part of the endocrine system because it secretes several hormones. It is the primary link between the brain and the pituitary gland, and the primary link between the endocrine and nervous systems. The hypothalamus contains nerve cells that control the pituitary gland by producing chemicals that stimulate or suppress hormone secretions from the pituitary. Many factors, such as emotions and seasonal changes, can influence the production and secretion of pituitary hormones. This information (such as environmental temperature, light exposure patterns, and feelings) is sensed by the brain and relayed by the hypothalamus to the pituitary.

The hypothalamus also regulates blood sugar levels, body temperature, metabolism, and body rhythms (e.g., activity and rest, appetite and digestion, sexual behavior, and menstrual and reproductive cycles).

Pineal Gland

The pineal gland is a small, cone-shaped gland located in the middle of the brain. It secretes only one hormone, melatonin, which regulates the body's *circadian* rhythm. The gland's production of melatonin varies according to the time of day and with age, with production dramatically increased during the nighttime hours and decreased during the day. Melatonin contributes to the release of female reproductive hormones. It helps determine when a woman starts to menstruate, the frequency and duration of the menstrual cycle, and when a woman enters *menopause.* It has been found that melatonin levels drop significantly just before puberty and are lower still in adults. Melatonin seems to suppress a child's body from undergoing sexual maturation, since sex hormones such as luteotropin that play a role in the development of sexual organs emerge only after melatonin levels have declined.

📖 **DEFINITIONS**

circadian. Relating to a cyclic, 24-hour period.

menopause. Cessation of menstruation involving four physical stages: premenopause, in which periods may be irregular but without classic menopausal symptoms; perimenopause, the onset of symptoms that indicate a drop in estrogen, such as erratic periods, hot flashes, and vaginal dryness—this stage lasts approximately four years, counting the first two years before and after the last period; menopause, referring to the final menstrual period, marked once the female has had no periods for one year; and postmenopause, the phase in which a woman has been free of periods for at least one year.

Figure 6.4: Thyroid

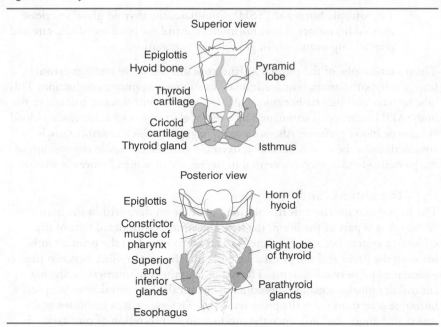

Thyroid Gland

The thyroid gland is located in the front part of the lower neck. Its right and left lobes lie on each side of the trachea, connected in the middle by a mass of tissue called the isthmus. The thyroid is filled with microscopic circular sacs called thyroid follicles that store the thyroid hormones. It derives its blood supply from the superior and interior thyroid arteries. Although a separate gland, the thyroid is controlled by the pituitary gland. When thyroid hormone levels decrease, the pituitary gland sends a signal to the thyroid by producing thyroid-stimulating hormone (TSH), which in turn stimulates the thyroid gland to produce more hormones. Under the influence of TSH, the thyroid manufactures and secretes thyroxine (T4) and triiodothyronine (T3). These hormones regulate growth and metabolism and play a role in brain development during childhood.

Nestled between the thyroid follicles are parafollicular cells. These cells produce calcitonin, which lowers the concentration of calcium in the blood when it rises above the normal value.

Figure 6.5: Dorsal View of Parathyroid Glands

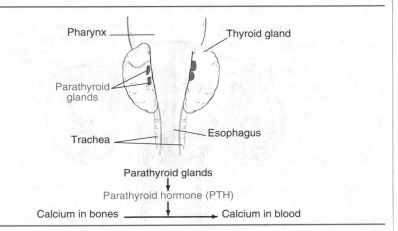

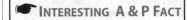

Parathyroid Gland

The parathyroid is located behind the thyroid gland at the front of the neck. There are four glands: a superior pair and an inferior pair.

There are two types of cells in the parathyroid glands: oxyphil cells and chief cells. Oxyphil cells appear at the onset of puberty, although their function is unknown. The chief cells are responsible for producing the parathyroid hormone (PTH), which regulates the level of calcium in the bones and the rest of the body. Calcium is the primary element that causes muscle contraction and is also very important to the normal conduction of electrical currents along nerves. The PTH hormone is responsible for the bones releasing calcium into the bloodstream, which keeps the calcium in the blood at a normal level. If there is too much PTH, the bones release excessive amounts of calcium and leave the bones with too little calcium, leading to conditions such as *osteopenia* and *osteoporosis.*

Another way PTH acts to increases calcium in the blood is through the intestines. The PTH makes the lining of the intestine more efficient at absorbing calcium found in foods. In addition to regulating the amount of calcium in the blood from bone and intestine, PTH also controls the excretion of calcium in urine, thus conserving calcium in blood.

Adrenal Glands

The adrenal glands, also called suprarenal glands, are located on the top of each kidney and have two distinct parts. The outer part, called the adrenal cortex, produces a variety of hormones called corticosteroids. Chief among the corticosteroids is cortisol, which regulates salt and water balance in the body, prepares the body for stress, regulates metabolism, interacts with the immune system, and influences sexual function. The inner part, the adrenal medulla, is considered an extension of the sympathetic nervous system (SNS); therefore, the hormones it secretes are called sympathomimetic hormones. The medulla produces catecholamines, epinephrine (adrenaline), and norepinephrine (noradrenaline). During times of stress these hormones increase blood pressure and heart rate, they facilitate blood flow to the muscles and brain, cause relaxation of *smooth muscles,* and help with conversion of glycogen to glucose in the liver.

☞ INTERESTING A & P FACT

As many as 14 percent of the population have five parathyroid glands; and a few are known to have six.

📖 DEFINITIONS

osteopenia. Decreased calcification that is less severe than that resulting from osteoporosis, caused by the resorption of bone at a rate that exceeds bone synthesis.

osteoporosis. Bone degeneration caused by the breakdown of the bony matrix without equivalent regeneration, resulting in a weak, porous, fragile bone structure.

smooth muscle. Thin layers of muscle tissue that move involuntarily as part of the body's natural processes. Smooth muscle lines the walls of hollow organs, such as the uterus and gastrointestinal

---

Figure 6.6: Uterus and Ovaries

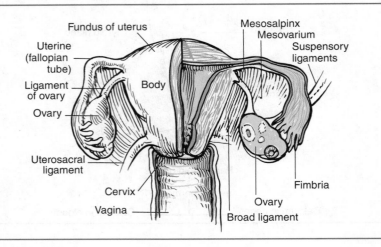

DEFINITIONS

androgen. Male sex hormone. Testosterone is the primary androgen. In the fetus, androgens cause the formation of external male genitalia.

estrogen. Group of estrus-stimulating hormones produced by the ovaries, possibly the adrenal cortex and testes, that have different functions in both sexes. They are the main female sex hormones (estradiol, estrone, and estriol) responsible for the maturation and development of female secondary sex characteristics and that act on the reproductive organs to prepare for fertilization, implantation, and nourishment of the embryo. Estrogens also have nonreproductive actions such as minimizing calcium loss from bones by antagonizing the effects of parathyroid hormone and promoting blood clotting.

progesterone. Steroid hormone, secreted by the corpus luteum of the ovary and by the placenta, that acts to prepare the uterus for implantation of the fertilized ovum, to maintain pregnancy, and to promote development of the mammary glands.

testes. Male gonadal paired glands located in the scrotum that secrete testosterone and contain the seminiferous tubules where sperm is produced.

Gonad Gland

The gonads are the main source of sex hormones. Female gonads (ovaries) secrete sex hormones in response to stimulation from the pituitary gland. Located in the pelvis, the ovaries produce eggs. They also secrete female sex hormones, *estrogen* and *progesterone,* which regulate development of the reproductive organs, female secondary sex characteristics, and menstruation and pregnancy.

Male gonads (*testes*) are located in the scrotum. They produce sperm and secrete *androgens*. The androgens, the most important of which is testosterone, regulate the sexual and reproductive functions in males. Among other things, testosterone also regulates body changes associated with puberty, including enlargement of the penis, the growth spurt that occurs during puberty, and characteristics such as deepening of the voice, growth of facial and pubic hair, and the increase in bone and muscle mass.

Figure 6.7: Male Pelvic Organs

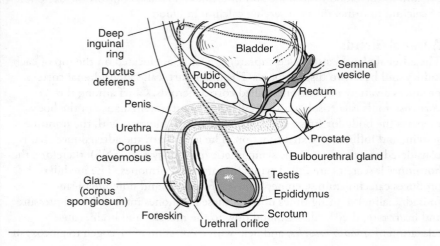

More information regarding the ovaries and testes can be found in the reproductive chapter of this publication.

Figure 6.8: Thymus Gland

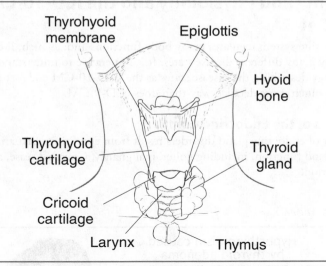

Labels: Thyrohyoid membrane, Epiglottis, Hyoid bone, Thyrohyoid cartilage, Thyroid gland, Cricoid cartilage, Larynx, Thymus

Thymus Gland

The thymus gland is located just under the breast bone in the anterior, superior mediastinum, and is composed of lymphatic and epithelial tissue (Hassall's corpuscles). It has two lobes, each divided into lobules by a *septum.* Hormones produced within the gland are collectively known as thymosins. These hormones play a key role in the development and maintenance of immune defenses by controlling white blood cell maturation. White blood cells (WBC), known as *lymphocytes,* pass through the thymus and are transformed into T cells. The T cells' primary role is to fight infection. The role of the thymus is not entirely understood, though it seems to be most important from infancy through puberty, after which the lymphatic tissue diminishes and is replaced by fat. In adults, the thymus can be removed without a significant health impact.

 DEFINITIONS

lymphocytes. White blood cells formed in the body's lymph system.

septum. Anatomical partition or dividing wall.

Anatomy and Physiology and the ICD-10-CM Code Set

The endocrine system regulates many body functions and, as such, it can be affected by many different disease states. It is imperative to understand the terminology describing the disease states as the ICD-10-CM code set describes them in a much more detailed way than does ICD-9-CM.

Disorders of the Endocrine Gland

A number of endocrine gland disorders result from conditions that affect thyroid gland function, including goiter, malignancy, Grave's disease, and inflammation.

Figure 6.9: Goiter

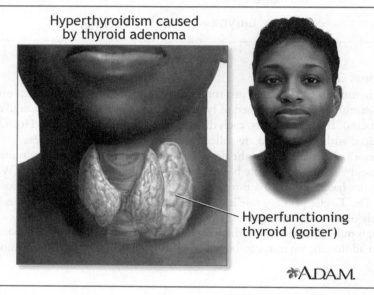

Hyperthyroidism caused by thyroid adenoma

Hyperfunctioning thyroid (goiter)

✿A.D.A.M.

Goiter

A goiter is an abnormal enlargement of the thyroid gland commonly caused by a deficiency of dietary iodine. Goiters can be simple or nontoxic nodular. If a goiter has enough mass, it may cause compression that may lead to airway restriction, swallowing difficulty, or problems with venous flow.

In simple goiter, the thyroid gland is enlarged, but the thyroid hormone secretions are still within normal limits and not associated with malignancy. A simple goiter can have several causes, such as iodine deficiency. The thyroid of a person whose diet has insufficient iodine, which is essential to thyroid hormone secretion, becomes enlarged so that it can produce more of the hormone. Iodine deficiency is the most common cause of simple goiter, but as there is no deficiency in the United States, this cause is rarely seen here. Simple goiter can also occur during puberty, pregnancy, or during menses as a result of hormonal imbalances.

An endemic goiter is the swelling of the thyroid gland due to inadequate amounts of dietary iodine. This deprivation leads to diminished production and secretion of thyroid hormone by the gland. Endemic goiter occurs from time to time in adolescents at puberty and widely in population groups in geographic areas in which limited amounts of iodine are present in soil, water, and food. This type of goiter is without apparent signs of hyperthyroidism or hypothyroidism of the gland.

Coding for Goiters

ICD-9-CM		ICD-10-CM	
240.0	Goiter, specified as simple	E04.0	Nontoxic diffuse goiter
240.9	Goiter, unspecified	E01.0	Iodine-deficiency related diffuse endemic goiter
		E01.2	Iodine-deficiency related endemic goiter unspecified
		E04.9	Nontoxic goiter, unspecified

In a nontoxic nodular goiter, the thyroid gland exhibits palpable nodules that do not affect thyroid hormone secretion. Goiters are classified as having a singular nodule or multiple nodules. This type of goiter may be malignant.

Coding for Goiter

ICD-9-CM		ICD-10-CM	
241.0	Nontoxic uninodular goiter	E04.1	Nontoxic single thyroid nodule
241.1	Nontoxic multinodular goiter	E01.1	Iodine-deficiency related multinodular (related) goiter
		E04.2	Nontoxic multinodular goiter
241.9	Unspecified nontoxic nodular goiter	E04.8	Other specified nontoxic goiter
		E04.9	Nontoxic goiter, unspecified

Hyperthyroidism

Hyperthyroidism is a broad term referring to the production of too much of the thyroid hormone thyroxine (T4) and/or triiodothyronine (T3). Hyperthyroidism has several causes, including thyroid nodules, *thyroiditis,* and Grave's disease. Another cause of hyperthyroidism is ingestion of too much iodine or overmedicating with synthetic thyroid hormone used to treat hypothyroidism.

Grave's disease, also referred to as *toxic diffuse goiter,* is an autoimmune disease. It is the most common cause of hyperthyroidism. In this disease, the immune system produces an antibody called thyroid stimulating immunoglobulin (TSI), which acts much like TSH and causes the thyroid to produce too much thyroid hormone.

A nodule, or fluid-filled cyst, is a growth within the thyroid that can be benign or malignant. Nodules have many causes, including *Hashimoto's disease,* genetic defects, a lack of iodine, and radiation treatments.

Thyrotoxicosis is a toxic condition caused by an excess of thyroid hormones in the blood. It is often related to hyperthyroidism, where the thyroid gland is overproducing hormones. There are many factors that can contribute to thyrotoxicosis, including goiters, benign tumors, and thyroid adenomas, which can become toxic and cause excess hormones to be produced. Medications and radiation may also lead to this condition.

A thyrotoxic crisis or storm is a sudden, life-threatening crisis in which symptoms of hyperthyroidism are exacerbated and new symptoms develop. It is most likely to occur at the time of infection, surgical procedure, or trauma in a patient with undertreated or untreated hyperthyroidism. The patient may

DEFINITIONS

diffuse toxic goiter. Diffuse thyroid enlargement seen mostly in women that stems from the autoimmune process. It is accompanied by the secretion of excessive thyroid hormone, goiter, and bulging eyes.

ectopic. Relating to an organ or other structure that is aberrant or out of place.

Hashimoto's disease. Autoimmune disorder marked by goiter, chronic inflammation of the thyroid, and often hypothyroidism.

thyroiditis. Inflammation of the thyroid gland.

develop a fever, emotional instability or psychosis, heart complications, and an enlarged liver.

Coding for Thyrotoxicosis

ICD-9-CM		ICD-10-CM	
242.00	Toxic diffuse goiter without mention of thyrotoxic crisis or storm	E05.00	Thyrotoxicosis with diffuse goiter without thyrotoxic crisis or storm
242.01	Toxic diffuse goiter with mention of thyrotoxic crisis or storm	E05.01	Thyrotoxicosis with diffuse goiter with thyrotoxic crisis or storm
242.10	Toxic uninodular goiter without mention of thyrotoxic crisis or storm	E05.10	Thyrotoxicosis with toxic single thyroid nodule without thyrotoxic crisis or storm
242.11	Toxic uninodular goiter with mention of thyrotoxic crisis or storm	E05.11	Thyrotoxicosis with toxic single thyroid nodule with thyrotoxic crisis or storm
242.20	Toxic multinodular goiter without mention of thyrotoxic crisis or storm	E05.20	Thyrotoxicosis with toxic multinodular goiter without thyrotoxic crisis or storm
242.21	Toxic multinodular goiter with mention of thyrotoxic crisis or storm	E05.21	Thyrotoxicosis with toxic multinodular goiter with thyrotoxic crisis or storm
242.30	Toxic nodular goiter, unspecified type, without mention of thyrotoxic crisis or storm	E05.20	Thyrotoxicosis with toxic multinodular goiter without thyrotoxic crisis or storm
242.31	Toxic nodular goiter, unspecified type, with mention of thyrotoxic crisis or storm	E05.21	Thyrotoxicosis with toxic multinodular goiter with thyrotoxic crisis or storm
242.40	Thyrotoxicosis from *ectopic* thyroid nodule without mention of thyrotoxic crisis or storm	E05.30	Thyrotoxicosis from ectopic thyroid tissue without thyrotoxic crisis or storm
242.41	Thyrotoxicosis from ectopic thyroid nodule with mention of thyrotoxic crisis or storm	E05.31	Thyrotoxicosis from ectopic thyroid tissue with thyrotoxic crisis or storm

Hypothyroidism

The most common cause of congenital hypothyroidism is absence of a thyroid gland at birth. This requires lifelong hormone therapy since thyroxine regulates metabolism and growth. Untreated, congenital hypothyroidism causes serious problems in the central nervous system, developmental delay, and problems with somatic growth. By providing replacement thyroid hormones, almost all of the complications of congenital hypothyroidism are avoidable.

Neurological-type hypothyroidism includes endemic cretinism, which is defined as having impaired physical and mental development with dystrophy of bones and soft tissues. This is due to congenital lack of thyroid secretion. Additionally, patients may have deaf-mutism, spasticity, and motor dysfunction.

A diffuse goiter, which is nontoxic, is a diffuse or nodular enlargement of the thyroid that is not associated with abnormal thyroid function and does not result from an inflammatory or neoplastic process.

An endemic goiter, also called a colloid goiter, is a thyroid enlargement that occurs in groups of people who live in areas with iodine-poor soil.

A myxedematous type-goiter is marked by dry skin and swellings around the lips and nose, in addition to abnormal deposits of mucin in the skin and other tissues.

In the ICD-10-CM code set, an additional code (F70–F79) should be used if applicable, to identify associated mental retardation.

Coding for Congenital Hypothyroidism

ICD-9-CM		ICD-10-CM	
243	Congenital hypothyroidism	E00.0	Congenital iodine-deficiency syndrome neurological type
		E00.1	Congenital iodine-deficiency syndrome myxedematous type
		E00.2	Congenital iodine-deficiency syndrome mixed type
		E00.9	Congenital iodine-deficiency syndrome unspecified
		E03.0	Congenital hypothyroidism with diffuse goiter
		E03.1	Congenital hypothyroidism without goiter

Acquired Hypothyroidism

Hypothyroidism is a deficiency of thyroid hormone. Primary (acquired) hypothyroidism usually develops in older adults, usually after age 40. There are many causes of this type of hypothyroidism, the most common due to any condition that causes inflammation of the gland. For example, the most frequent cause of hypothyroidism is inflammation of the thyroid gland, which damages the gland's cells. Autoimmune and Hashimoto's *thyroiditis* are good examples of diseases in which the immune system attacks the thyroid gland. *Postpartum* thyroiditis may also develop in some women.

Other causes of hypothyroidism include:

- Certain drugs (such as amiodarone, lithium, methimazole, and propylthiouracil [PTU])
- Iodine, resulting from administration or ingestion of iodine
- Postsurgical/postprocedural, due to removal of partial or total thyroid gland
- Radioactive iodine used to treat an overactive thyroid (hyperthyroidism)
- Viral thyroiditis, which may cause hyperthyroidism and is often followed by temporary or permanent hypothyroidism

Coding for Acquired Hypothyroidism

ICD-9-CM		ICD-10-CM	
244.0	Postsurgical hypothyroidism	E89.0	Postprocedural hypothyroidism
244.1	Other postablative hypothyroidism		
244.2	Iodine hypothyroidism	E03.2	Hypothyroidism due to medicaments and other exogenous substances
244.3	Other *iatrogenic* hypothyroidism		
244.8	Other specified acquired hypothyroidism	E01.8	Other iodine- deficiency related thyroid disorders & allied conditions
		E02	Subclinical iodine-deficiency hypothyroidism
		E03.3	Postinfectious hypothyroidism
		E03.8	Other specified hypothyroidism
244.9	Unspecified hypothyroidism	E03.9	Hypothyroidism, unspecified

DEFINITIONS

iatrogenic. Adversely induced in the patient; caused by medical treatment.

postpartum. Period of time following childbirth.

thyroiditis. Inflammation of the thyroid gland.

Hypoparathyroid Conditions

Hypoparathyroidism is a condition in which one or more of the parathyroid glands secrete an abnormally low amount of the parathyroid hormone (PTH). This condition causes decreased levels of calcium and increased levels of phosphorus in the blood, muscle cramping, increased frequency of urination, and cataracts. The most common cause of hypoparathyroidism is injury to the glands during head and neck surgery. Occasionally, hypoparathyroidism is a side-effect of radioactive iodine treatment.

Coding for Hypoparathyroidism

ICD-9-CM		ICD-10-CM	
252.1	Hypoparathyroidism	E20.0	*Idiopathic* hypoparathyroidism
		E20.8	Other hypoparathyroidism
		E20.9	Hypoparathyroidism, unspecified
		E89.2	Postprocedural hypoparathyroidism

Secondary Diabetes Mellitus

Secondary diabetes mellitus (SDM) presents with the same symptoms as diabetes mellitus (discussed in the subsequent section), manifesting with elevated blood sugar levels and resulting in the inability to successfully metabolize carbohydrates, fats, and proteins. Secondary diabetes develops when defects in insulin production and secretion, or defects in the action of insulin occur, but as a result of another, underlying primary cause. This may be caused, for instance, when the islets of Langerhans, responsible for the production of insulin, are absent or destroyed by events such as chronic disease, trauma, or surgical removal of the pancreas. Secondary diabetes can also result from hormonal disturbances, such as *Cushing's syndrome* (described in more detail later in this chapter in the pituitary section) or excessive growth hormone production that results in *acromegaly*.

Nonketotic hyperglycemic-hyperosmolar coma (NKHHC), also referred to as diabetic hyperglycemic hyperosmolar syndrome (HHS), is a complication of secondary diabetes mellitus that is associated with high mortality. This type of coma generally follows an infection, myocardial infarction, stroke, or acute illness. Sometimes it may occur in patients who have not been diagnosed with diabetes or in patients with uncontrolled diabetes. The patient usually presents with a glucose of 600 mg/dL or greater without the presence of ketones.

Hyperglycemia is abnormally high blood sugar, usually greater than 140 mg/dl in a nonfasting, nondiabetic patient. Hyperglycemia in a diabetic patient is not easily quantified; levels vary from patient to patient.

Hyperosmolarity is the increase in osmolarity or the concentration of ions and chemicals in blood or a solution.

Ketoacidosis is an abnormal increase in the acidity of body fluids and tissues (acidosis) caused by the increased accumulation of ketone bodies, most often seen in Type 1 diabetes or excessive alcohol consumption.

Secondary diabetes mellitus is divided into two separate categories in ICD-10-CM. Codes under category E08 Diabetes mellitus due to underlying condition, and E09 Drug or chemical induced diabetes mellitus, identify complications and/or manifestations associated with secondary diabetes mellitus. Codes should be assigned according to the instructions found in the ICD-10-CM tabular section. For example, in category E08 Diabetes mellitus due to underlying condition, code first the underlying condition. In category

EØ9 Drug or chemical induced diabetes mellitus, code first the drug or chemical (T36–T65).

Note that ICD-9-CM codes 249.30 and 249.31 crosswalk to the same group of ICD-10-CM codes.

Coding for Secondary Diabetes Mellitus

ICD-9-CM		ICD-10-CM	
249.20	Secondary diabetes mellitus with hyperosmolarity not stated as uncontrolled, or unspecified	E08.00	Diabetes mellitus due to underlying condition with hyperosmolarity without nonketotic hyperglycemic-hyperosmolar coma (NKHHC)
		E08.01	Diabetes mellitus due to underlying condition with hyperosmolarity with coma
		E09.00	Drug or chemical induced diabetes mellitus with hyperosmolarity without nonketotic hyperglycemic- hyperosmolar coma (NKHHC)
		E09.01	Drug or chemical induced diabetes mellitus with hyperosmolarity with coma
249.21	Secondary diabetes mellitus with hyperosmolarity uncontrolled	E08.01	Diabetes mellitus due to underlying condition with hyperosmolarity with coma
		E08.65	Diabetes mellitus due to underlying condition with hyperglycemia
		E09.01	Drug or chemical induced diabetes mellitus with hyperosmolarity with coma
249.30	Secondary diabetes mellitus with other coma not stated as uncontrolled, or unspecified	E08.11	Diabetes mellitus due to underlying condition with ketoacidosis with coma
		E08.641	Diabetes mellitus due to underlying condition with hypoglycemia with coma
249.31	Secondary diabetes mellitus with other coma uncontrolled	E09.11	Drug or chemical induced diabetes mellitus with ketoacidosis with coma
		E09.641	Drug or chemical induced diabetes mellitus with hypoglycemia with coma

Secondary diabetes mellitus may be complicated by the presence of nephropathy or chronic kidney disease. Chronic kidney disease is decreased renal efficiencies resulting in the kidney's reduced ability to filter waste. The National Kidney Foundation's classification includes five clinical stages, based on the glomerular filtration rate (GFR). The stages of CKD are as follows: stage 1, some kidney damage with a normal or slightly increased GFR value (> 90); stage 2, mild kidney damage with a GFR value of 60 to 89; stage 3, moderate kidney damage with a GFR value of 30 to 59; stage 4, severe kidney damage and a GFR value of 15 to 29; and stage 5, severe kidney damage that has progressed to a GFR value of less than 15. Dialysis or transplantation is required at stage 5.

Nephropathy is defined as a disease or abnormality of the kidney. Note that ICD-9-CM codes 249.40 and 249.41 crosswalk to the same group of ICD-10-CM codes

Coding for Secondary Diabetes Mellitus with Renal Manifestations

ICD-9-CM		ICD-10-CM	
249.40	Secondary diabetes mellitus w/renal manifestations not stated as uncontrolled, unspecified	E08.21	Diabetes mellitus due to underlying condition with diabetic nephropathy
		E08.22	Diabetes mellitus due to underlying condition with diabetic chronic kidney disease
		E08.29	Diabetes mellitus due to underlying condition with other diabetic kidney complication
		E09.21	Drug or chemical induced diabetes mellitus with diabetic nephropathy
		E09.22	Drug or chemical induced diabetes mellitus with diabetic chronic kidney disease
		E09.29	Drug or chemical induced diabetes mellitus with other diabetic kidney complication

Secondary diabetes mellitus may also have *ophthalmic* complications, including cataracts, retinopathy, and macular edema.

Figure 6.10: Cataract

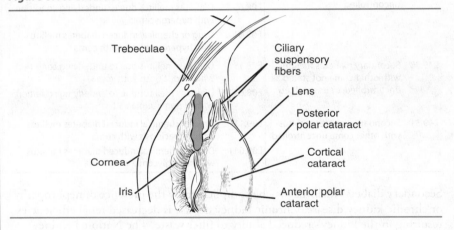

A cataract is a clouding or opacity of the lens that prevents clear images from forming on the *retina*, causing vision impairment or blindness. The classification and coding of cataracts are dependent upon size, shape, location, and etiology.

Diabetic macular edema (DME) occurs when leakage from the blood vessels causes the retina to swell. In DME, the central portion of the retina, the macula, swells and impairs vision. Exudates or plaques may develop in the posterior pole of the retina due to the breakdown of retinal vasculature, which can precipitate vision loss.

Retinopathy usually occurs in diabetes of long duration. It represents a continuum of disease; a progression of pathologic changes in the retina due to microvascular complications inherent in diabetes mellitus. Nonproliferative diabetic retinopathy is indicative of early stage disease. Microaneurysms form, retinal *hemorrhages* occur, and blind spots are characteristic. Increased vessel leakage occurs as the disease progresses, resulting in further vision impairment. The disease progresses from mild to moderate to severe nonproliferative retinopathy and becomes proliferative in its more advanced stage, characterized by new blood vessel formation in the retina due to significant ischemia from the damaged vessels.

DEFINITIONS

hemorrhage. Internal or external bleeding with loss of significant amounts of blood.

ophthalmic. Relating to the eye.

retina. Layer of tissue located at the back of the eye that is sensitive to light similar to film in a camera.

ICD-9-CM codes 249.50 and 249.51 crosswalk to the same group of ICD-10-CM codes. In ICD-9-CM, two or more codes are needed to accurately describe secondary diabetes mellitus with ophthalmic manifestations. However, combination codes have been created in ICD-10-CM. For example, ICD-9-CM codes 249.50, 362.10, and 362.83 are needed to identify secondary diabetes mellitus with retinopathy and macular edema. ICD-10-CM requires only code EØ8.311 or EØ9.311.

Amyotrophy is muscular wasting and weakening that generally occurs in patients with diabetes. It usually affects the thighs and pelvic region.

Autonomic neuropathy describes a disease complication that has affected one or more nerves in the *autonomic nervous system.*

*Mono*neuropathy is a disease process of severe inflammation of one nerve; inflammation of multiple nerves is called *poly*neuropathy.

ICD-9-CM codes 249.60 and 249.61 crosswalk to the same group of ICD-10-CM codes. These codes describe diabetes complications involving the neurological system.

Coding for Secondary Diabetes Mellitus with Neurological Manifestations

ICD-9-CM		ICD-10-CM	
249.6Ø	Secondary diabetes mellitus with neurological manifestations not stated as uncontrolled, or unspecified	EØ8.4Ø	Diabetes mellitus due to underlying condition with diabetic neuropathy
		EØ8.41	Diabetes mellitus due to underlying condition with diabetic mononeuropathy
		EØ8.42	Diabetes mellitus due to underlying condition with diabetic polyneuropathy
		EØ8.43	Diabetes mellitus due to underlying condition with diabetic autonomic (poly)neuropathy
		EØ8.44	Diabetes mellitus due to underlying condition with neurological complications diabetic amyotrophy
		EØ8.49	Diabetes mellitus due to underlying condition with other diabetic neurological complication
		EØ8.61Ø	Diabetes mellitus due to underlying condition with diabetic neuropathic arthropathy
		EØ9.4Ø	Drug or chemical induced diabetes mellitus with neurological complications with diabetic neuropathy, unspecified
		EØ9.41	Drug or chemical induced diabetes mellitus with neurological complications with diabetic mononeuropathy
		EØ9.42	Drug or chemical induced diabetes mellitus with neurological complications with diabetic polyneuropathy
		EØ9.43	Drug or chemical induced diabetes mellitus with neurological complications with diabetic autonomic (poly) neuropathy
		EØ9.44	Drug or chemical induced diabetes mellitus with neurological complications diabetic amyotrophy
		EØ9.49	Drug or chemical induced diabetes mellitus with neurological complications with other diabetic neurological complication
249.61	Secondary diabetes mellitus with neurological manifestations uncontrolled	EØ8.4Ø	Diabetes mellitus due to underlying condition with diabetic neuropathy
		EØ8.65	Diabetes mellitus due to underlying condition with hyperglycemia
		EØ9.4Ø	Drug or chemical induced diabetes mellitus with neurological complications with diabetic neuropathy, unspecified

DEFINITIONS

autonomic nervous system.
Portion of the nervous system that controls involuntary body functions. The fibers of the autonomic nervous system regulate the iris of the eye and the smooth-muscle action of the heart, blood vessels, lungs, glands, stomach, colon, bladder, and other visceral organs that are not under conscious control by the individual. The autonomic nerve fibers exit from the central nervous system and branch out into the sympathetic and parasympathetic nervous systems.

mono-. One or single.

-poly. Much or many.

DEFINITIONS

peripheral. Outside of a structure or organ.

The following section describes complications of secondary diabetes mellitus involving the circulatory system.

Gangrene frequently occurs when a large area of tissue dies, usually resulting from a loss of vascular supply, followed by a bacterial attack or onset of disease.

An angiopathy is any disease of the blood or lymph vessels.

Note that ICD-9-CM codes 249.70 and 249.71 crosswalk to the same group of ICD-10-CM codes.

Coding for Secondary Diabetes Mellitus with Circulatory Manifestations

ICD-9-CM		ICD-10-CM	
249.70	Secondary diabetes mellitus with **peripheral** circulatory disorders, not stated as uncontrolled, or unspecified	E08.51	Diabetes mellitus due to underlying condition with diabetic peripheral angiopathy without gangrene
249.71	Secondary diabetes mellitus with peripheral circulatory disorders, uncontrolled	E08.52	Diabetes mellitus due to underlying condition with diabetic peripheral angiopathy with gangrene
		E09.51	Drug or chemical induced diabetes mellitus with diabetic peripheral angiopathy without gangrene
		E09.52	Drug or chemical induced diabetes mellitus with diabetic peripheral angiopathy with gangrene

The following section describes complications of secondary diabetes mellitus of other specified manifestations, including:

- **Arthropathy:** Joint disease.
- **Dermatitis:** Inflammation of the skin.
- **Ulcer:** Open sore or excavating lesion of skin or the tissue on the surface of an organ from the sloughing of chronically inflamed and necrosing tissue.

Hypoglycemia is abnormally low blood glucose levels. Excessive insulin produced by the pancreas, sometimes associated with tumors, or an overdose of insulin to treat diabetes may be a cause.

Hyperglycemia is just the opposite—abnormally high blood sugar, usually greater than 140 mg/dl in a nonfasting, nondiabetic patient. Hyperglycemia in a diabetic patient is not easily quantified; levels vary from patient to patient.

Note that ICD-9-CM codes 249.80 and 249.81 crosswalk to the same group of ICD-10-CM codes: E08.618–E08.638, E08.649–E08.69, and E09.618–E09.69.

Diabetes Mellitus

Diabetes mellitus (DM) is a complex metabolic disease with multisystem manifestations. It is characterized by high glucose (blood sugar) levels. Normally the hormone insulin controls glucose levels. In patients with diabetes mellitus, insulin is not produced normally or the body has a resistance to it, resulting in elevated blood sugar levels.

Diabetes mellitus has two forms. Diabetes mellitus Type I is caused by inadequate secretion of insulin by the pancreas. Type I, also referred to as type I insulin-dependent diabetes mellitus (IDDM), is classified as an autoimmune disease wherein the patient's immune system incorrectly produces antibodies, resulting in damage to the body's tissues. This type is most often seen at a young age, usually at 6 to 7 years of age, and sometimes in early adulthood as well. The patient requires regular insulin injections due to the autoimmune destruction of pancreatic beta cells, which cease to produce insulin. It is unknown what triggers the autoimmune response.

Diabetes mellitus Type II is caused by the body's inability to respond to insulin, called *insulin resistance.* DM Type II is also referred to as non-insulin-dependent diabetes mellitus (NIDDM) or adult-onset diabetes mellitus (AODM). Type II accounts for 90 to 95 percent of all cases and is usually diagnosed in adulthood as the pancreas gradually loses the ability to produce insulin or the body becomes more resistant to that which is being produced. An increasing number of children are being diagnosed with Type II diabetes due to the increase of childhood obesity. Children are developing Type II DM at an older age than is common with Type I DM, usually around 12 years of age, and they usually have a family history of DM.

The primary factor that distinguishes Type I from Type II is the absence of naturally occurring insulin within the body. Type I diabetics require insulin injections to survive. Type II diabetics may improve their health with insulin injections and may even come to require insulin, but the administration of insulin has no bearing on code selection for diabetes, nor does the age of onset. A patient with Type II diabetes is always coded as having Type II, even when the medical record states the patient requires insulin.

Diabetes can cause a variety of complications, including kidney problems, pain due to nerve damage, blindness, and coronary heart disease.

Many of the terms used in this category to describe complications are the same as those used in secondary diabetes. Please see the definitions in the previous section.

In ICD-10-CM, this category of codes is classified according to Type I or Type II, the body system affected, and the type of complication. The status and the presence of diabetic control are not indicated. Multiple codes within a particular category may be necessary to describe all of the complications of the disease. They should be sequenced based on the reason for a particular encounter.

Coding for Diabetes Mellitus

ICD-9-CM		ICD-10-CM	
250.20	Diabetes with hyperosmolarity, Type II or unspecified type, not stated as uncontrolled	E11.00	Type 2 diabetes mellitus with hyperosmolarity without nonketotic hyperglycemic-hyperosmolar coma (NKHHC)
		E11.01	Type 2 diabetes mellitus with hyperosmolarity with coma
		E13.00	Other specified diabetes mellitus with hyperosmolarity without nonketotic hyperglycemic-hyperosmolar coma (NKHHC)
		E13.01	Other specified diabetes mellitus with hyperosmolarity with coma

Diabetes mellitus may be complicated by the presence of nephropathy or chronic kidney disease. These conditions are described in more detail above in the secondary diabetes section.

Combination codes have been created in ICD-10-CM. For example, in ICD-9-CM, codes 250.41 and 583.81 are needed to accurately identify diabetes mellitus, type 1 with nephropathy. ICD-10-CM requires only code, E10.21.

> **DEFINITIONS**
>
> **insulin resistance syndrome.** Group of health risks that increase the likelihood of developing heart disease, stroke, and diabetes. Diagnosis of insulin resistance syndrome is made if one has three or more of the following: waist measurement of 40 or more inches for men and 35 or more inches for women; blood pressure of 130/85 mm or higher; triglyceride level greater than 150 mg/dl; fasting blood sugar of more than 100 mg/dl; HDL level less than 40 mg/dl in men or less than 50 mg/dl in women.

Coding for Diabetes Mellitus with Renal Manifestations

ICD-9-CM		ICD-10-CM	
250.40	Diabetes with renal manifestations, Type II or unspecified type, not stated as uncontrolled	E11.21	Type 2 diabetes mellitus with diabetic nephropathy
		E11.22	Type 2 diabetes mellitus with diabetic chronic kidney disease
		E11.29	Type 2 diabetes mellitus with other diabetic kidney complication
		E13.21	Other specified diabetes mellitus with diabetic nephropathy
		E13.22	Other specified diabetes mellitus with diabetic chronic kidney disease
		E13.29	Other specified diabetes mellitus with other diabetic kidney complication
250.41	Diabetes with renal manifestations, Type I [juvenile type], not stated as uncontrolled	E10.21	Type 1 diabetes mellitus with diabetic nephropathy
		E10.22	Type 1 diabetes mellitus with diabetic chronic kidney disease
		E10.29	Type 1 diabetes mellitus with other diabetic kidney complication

Like secondary diabetes, diabetes mellitus may also have ophthalmic complications, including cataract, retinopathy, and macular edema. The following table is not a complete mapping of all of the types of ophthalmic manifestations that may occur in diabetes, but gives the coder an idea of what may be seen in ICD-10-CM. For detailed information on ICD-9-CM to ICD-10-CM mapping, see *Ingenix's ICD-10-CM Mappings.*

Coding for Diabetes Mellitus with Ophthalmic Manifestations

ICD-9-CM		ICD-10-CM	
250.50	Diabetes with ophthalmic manifestations, Type II or unspecified type, not stated as uncontrolled	E11.321	Type 2 diabetes mellitus with mild nonproliferative diabetic retinopathy with macular edema
		E11.329	Type 2 diabetes mellitus with mild nonproliferative diabetic retinopathy without macular edema
		E11.331	Type 2 diabetes mellitus with moderate nonproliferative diabetic retinopathy with macular edema
		E11.339	Type 2 diabetes mellitus with moderate nonproliferative diabetic retinopathy without macular edema
		E11.341	Type 2 diabetes mellitus with severe nonproliferative diabetic retinopathy with macular edema
		E11.349	Type 2 diabetes mellitus with severe nonproliferative diabetic retinopathy without macular edema
		E11.351	Type 2 diabetes mellitus with proliferative diabetic retinopathy with macular edema
		E11.359	Type 2 diabetes mellitus with proliferative diabetic retinopathy without macular edema
		E11.36	Type 2 diabetes mellitus with diabetic cataract

ICD-9-CM	ICD-10-CM	
250.51 Diabetes with ophthalmic manifestations, Type I [juvenile type], not stated as uncontrolled	E10.321	Type 1 diabetes mellitus with mild nonproliferative diabetic retinopathy with macular edema
	E10.329	Type 1 diabetes mellitus with mild nonproliferative diabetic retinopathy without macular edema
	E10.331	Type 1 diabetes mellitus with moderate nonproliferative diabetic retinopathy with macular edema
	E10.339	Type 1 diabetes mellitus with moderate nonproliferative diabetic retinopathy without macular edema
	E10.341	Type 1 diabetes mellitus with severe nonproliferative diabetic retinopathy with macular edema
	E10.349	Type 1 diabetes mellitus with severe nonproliferative diabetic retinopathy without macular edema
	E10.351	Type 1 diabetes mellitus with proliferative diabetic retinopathy with macular edema
	E10.359	Type 1 diabetes mellitus with proliferative diabetic retinopathy without macular edema
	E10.36	Type 1 diabetes mellitus with diabetic cataract
	E10.39	Type 1 diabetes mellitus with other diabetic ophthalmic complication

In ICD-9-CM, two or more codes are needed to accurately describe Type 1 diabetes mellitus with neurological manifestations. However, combination codes have been created in ICD-10-CM. For example, ICD-9-CM codes 250.51, 362.01, and 362.07 are needed to identify diabetes mellitus Type 1 with retinopathy and macular edema. ICD-10-CM requires only code, E11.311.

The following codes describe complications involving the neurological system. These conditions are described in more detail in the secondary diabetes section above.

Coding for Diabetes Mellitus with Neurological Manifestations

ICD-9-CM	ICD-10-CM	
250.60 Diabetes with neurological manifestations, Type II or unspecified type, not stated as uncontrolled	E11.40	Type 2 diabetes mellitus with diabetic neuropathy, unspecified
	E11.41	Type 2 diabetes mellitus with diabetic mononeuropathy
	E11.42	Type 2 diabetes mellitus with diabetic polyneuropathy
	E11.43	Type 2 diabetes mellitus with diabetic autonomic (poly) neuropathy
	E11.44	Type 2 diabetes mellitus with diabetic amyotrophy
	E11.49	Type 2 diabetes mellitus with other diabetic neurological complication
	E13.40	Other specified diabetes mellitus with diabetic neuropathy, unspecified
(Continued on next page)	E13.41	Other specified diabetes mellitus with diabetic mononeuropathy

ICD-9-CM	ICD-10-CM	
250.60 Diabetes with neurological manifestations, Type II or unspecified type, not stated as uncontrolled *(Continued)*	E13.42	Other specified diabetes mellitus with diabetic polyneuropathy
	E13.43	Other specified diabetes mellitus with diabetic autonomic (poly) neuropathy
	E13.44	Other specified diabetes mellitus with diabetic amyotrophy
	E13.49	Other specified diabetes mellitus with other diabetic neurological complication
250.61 Diabetes with neurological manifestations, Type I [juvenile type], not stated as uncontrolled	E10.40	Type 1 diabetes mellitus with diabetic neuropathy, unspecified
	E10.41	Type 1 diabetes mellitus with diabetic mononeuropathy
	E10.42	Type 1 diabetes mellitus with diabetic polyneuropathy
	E10.43	Type 1 diabetes mellitus with diabetic autonomic (poly)neuropathy
	E10.44	Type 1 diabetes mellitus with diabetic amyotrophy
	E10.49	Type 1 diabetes mellitus with other diabetic neurological complication

The following codes describe complications involving the circulatory system. Many of the terms used in this category to describe complications are the same as those used in secondary diabetes. Please see the definitions in the previous section.

Coding for Diabetes Mellitus with Circulatory Manifestations

ICD-9-CM	ICD-10-CM	
250.70 Diabetes with peripheral circulatory disorders, Type II or unspecified type, not stated as uncontrolled	E11.51	Type 2 diabetes mellitus with diabetic peripheral angiopathy without gangrene
	E11.52	Type 2 diabetes mellitus with diabetic peripheral angiopathy with gangrene
	E11.59	Type 2 diabetes mellitus with other circulatory complications
	E13.51	Other specified diabetes mellitus with diabetic peripheral angiopathy without gangrene
	E13.52	Other specified diabetes mellitus with diabetic peripheral angiopathy with gangrene
	E13.59	Other specified diabetes mellitus with other circulatory complications
250.71 Diabetes with peripheral circulatory disorders, Type I [juvenile type], not stated as uncontrolled	E10.51	Type 1 diabetes mellitus with diabetic peripheral angiopathy without gangrene
	E10.52	Type 1 diabetes mellitus with diabetic peripheral angiopathy with gangrene
	E10.59	Type 1 diabetes mellitus with other circulatory complications

The following section of diabetes mellitus codes encompasses complications that did not have a category assigned in the other sections previously discussed. Many of the terms used in this category to describe complications are the same as those used in secondary diabetes. Please see the definitions in the previous section.

Coding for Diabetes Mellitus with Other Specified Manifestations

ICD-9-CM		ICD-10-CM	
250.80	Diabetes with other specified manifestations, Type II or unspecified type, not stated as uncontrolled	E11.618	Type 2 diabetes mellitus with other diabetic arthropathy
		E11.620	Type 2 diabetes mellitus with diabetic dermatitis
		E11.621	Type 2 diabetes mellitus with foot ulcer
		E11.622	Type 2 diabetes mellitus with other skin ulcer
		E11.628	Type 2 diabetes mellitus with other skin complications
		E11.630	Type 2 diabetes mellitus with periodontal disease
		E11.638	Type 2 diabetes mellitus with other oral complications
		E11.649	Type 2 diabetes mellitus with hypoglycemia without coma
		E11.65	Type 2 diabetes mellitus with hyperglycemia
		E13.618	Other specified diabetes mellitus with other diabetic arthropathy
		E13.620	Other specified diabetes mellitus with diabetic dermatitis
		E13.621	Other specified diabetes mellitus with foot ulcer
		E13.622	Other specified diabetes mellitus with other skin ulcer
		E13.628	Other specified diabetes mellitus with other skin complications
		E13.630	Other specified diabetes mellitus with *periodontal* disease
		E13.638	Other specified diabetes mellitus with other oral complications
		E13.641	Other specified diabetes mellitus with hypoglycemia with coma
		E13.649	Other specified diabetes mellitus with hypoglycemia without coma
		E13.65	Other specified diabetes mellitus with hyperglycemia
250.81	Diabetes with other specified manifestations, Type I [juvenile type], not stated as uncontrolled	E10.618	Type 1 diabetes mellitus with other diabetic arthropathy
		E10.620	Type 1 diabetes mellitus with diabetic dermatitis
		E10.621	Type 1 diabetes mellitus with foot ulcer
		E10.622	Type 1 diabetes mellitus with other skin ulcer
		E10.628	Type 1 diabetes mellitus with other skin complications
		E10.630	Type 1 diabetes mellitus with periodontal disease
		E10.638	Type 1 diabetes mellitus with other oral complications
		E10.649	Type 1 diabetes mellitus with hypoglycemia without coma
		E10.65	Type 1 diabetes mellitus with hyperglycemia
		E10.69	Type 1 diabetes mellitus with other specified complication

 DEFINITIONS

periodontal. Relating to the tissues that support and surround the teeth.

Pituitary Gland Disorders

Acromegaly and gigantism are caused by a *benign* tumor of the pituitary that stimulates production of excessive growth hormone, causing abnormal growth in particular parts of the body. Acromegaly is a rare, chronic, metabolic disorder and usually develops over many years in adults. Gigantism occurs when excess growth hormone begins to be secreted in childhood.

In ICD-10-CM, code E34.4 Constitutional tall stature is also appropriate for constitutional gigantism.

Coding for Acromegaly and Gigantism

ICD-9-CM		ICD-10-CM	
253.0	Acromegaly and gigantism	E22.0	Acromegaly and pituitary gigantism
		E34.4	Constitutional tall stature

Cushing's syndrome, sometimes called hypercortisolism, is caused when the body is exposed to high levels of the hormone cortisol for a long period of time. This can be the result of glucocorticoid medications or over-secretion of adrenal cortisol. Cushing's syndrome is relatively rare and most commonly affects adults aged 20 to 50. The most common cause of Cushing's syndrome is glucocorticoids. These steroid hormones are chemically similar to naturally produced cortisol and are present in prednisone used for *asthma, rheumatoid arthritis, lupus,* and other inflammatory diseases.

Cushing's syndrome may also be referred to as Cushing's disease. However, the terms are not synonymous. Cushing's disease is specific to one cause of Cushing's syndrome, a benign *tumor* or *hyperplasia* in the pituitary gland that produces large amounts of adrenocorticotropic hormone (ACTH), which subsequently elevates cortisol.

Ectopic *ACTH* syndrome is a condition in which a tumor forms outside the pituitary or adrenal glands and produces ACTH. Such tumors are usually found in the lung, pancreas, thyroid, or thymus gland and can be benign or malignant. The most common forms of these tumors are small-cell lung cancer and *carcinoid tumors.* Other less common types of tumors that can produce ACTH are medullary carcinomas of the thyroid, pancreatic islet cell tumors, and thymomas.

The ICD-10-CM classification code for pituitary-dependent Cushing's disease is appropriate to use for Cushing's disease caused by an overproduction of ATCH by tumors of the pituitary (pituitary-dependent).

Note: Codes have also been introduced in ICD-10-CM to indicate Cushing's syndrome as a result of alcohol or drugs.

Coding for Cushing's Syndrome

ICD-9-CM		ICD-10-CM	
255.0	Cushing's syndrome	E24.0	Pituitary-dependent Cushing's disease
		E24.2	Drug-induced Cushing's syndrome
		E24.3	Ectopic ACTH syndrome
		E24.4	Alcohol-induced pseudo-Cushing's syndrome
		E24.8	Other Cushing's syndrome
		E24.9	Cushing's syndrome, unspecified

DEFINITIONS

ACTH. Adrenocorticotropic hormone. Hormone secreted by the anterior pituitary that acts on the adrenal cortex and its secretion of corticosteroids. ACTH is used in hormone replacement therapy and as a diagnostic aid.

asthma. Narrowing or inflammation of the airway causing obstructed, labored breathing.

benign. Mild or nonmalignant in nature.

carcinoid tumor. Benign or malignant tumor that arises from neuroendocrine cells located throughout the body. The most common sites are the appendix, bronchi, rectum, small intestine, and stomach.

hyperplasia. Abnormal proliferation in the number of normal cells in regular tissue arrangement.

pseudo. Indicates false or imagined.

rheumatoid arthritis. Autoimmune disease causing pain, stiffness, inflammation, and possibly joint destruction.

systemic lupus. Inflammatory connective tissue disease.

tumor. Pathological swelling or enlargement; a neoplastic growth of uncontrolled, abnormal multiplication of cells.

Addison's disease is caused by decreased function of the adrenal cortex as a result of some sort of damage. In this disease, the adrenal glands produce too little cortisol and often insufficient levels of aldosterone. Adrenal cortex damage can result from such things as autoimmune disease, fungal infections, HIV, tuberculosis, tumors, and the use of anticoagulants.

Addisonian crisis occurs when a person with Addison's disease is under extreme physical stress, such as illness, physical shock (e.g., a car accident), or previously undiagnosed Addison's disease.

Coding for Addison's Disease

ICD-9-CM	ICD-10-CM	
255.41 Glucocorticoid deficiency	E27.1	Primary adrenocortical insufficiency
	E27.2	Addisonian crisis
	E27.3	Drug-induced adrenocortical insufficiency
	E89.6	Postprocedural adrenocortical (-medullary) hypofunction

Nutritional Deficiencies

Ingestion of imbalanced amounts of nutrients can disrupt the balance of nutrients required for proper health and endocrine function. One example of this is a goiter, commonly caused by a deficiency of dietary iodine. In the United States, nutritional and vitamin deficiencies are usually the result of poverty, prolonged parenteral feeding, chronic substance abuse, food fads, or extreme diets.

ICD-10-CM has expanded the available categories used to describe nutritional deficiencies. A few will be discussed in the following section.

Kwashiorkor

Kwashiorkor is an African word meaning "first-child, second-child." It refers to the protein-deficit illness that affects the first child when it is weaned to make room for the second child. Instead of protein-rich breast milk, the first child is fed a thin gruel made from sweet potato, banana, or cassava. The gruel is starchy, so there is no energy deficit, but the lack of protein causes edema, lethargy, and impaired growth. Kwashiorkor is considered a third-degree malnutrition disorder.

Marasmic kwashiorkor is a condition in which there is a deficiency of both calories and protein; it is the most severe form of protein-energy malnutrition. It is accompanied by severe tissue wasting, loss of *subcutaneous* fat, and usually *dehydration*.

Coding for Kwashiorkor

ICD-9-CM	ICD-10-CM	
260 Kwashiorkor	E40	Kwashiorkor
	E42	Marasmic kwashiorkor

Thiamine and Niacin Deficiencies

Alcoholism is the main cause of thiamine (vitamin B1) deficiency in the United States. It is also common in people with *malabsorption* problems, which sometimes occur after bariatric surgery. In other countries, it can result from eating a diet of highly polished rice. Infants can develop a thiamine deficiency

DEFINITIONS

dehydration. Condition resulting from an excessive loss of water from the body.

malabsorption. Body's inability to absorb a substance or nutrient, usually occurring in the small intestine.

subcutaneous. Below the skin.

when breast-fed by thiamine-deficient mothers. Thiamine deficiency causes beriberi, with manifestations of *neuritis, edema,* and heart disease.

Wet beriberi describes a thiamine deficiency that involves the cardiovascular system.

Dry beriberi is a thiamine deficiency that also affects the nervous system.

Wernicke's encephalopathy is brain damage in lower parts of the brain called the thalamus and hypothalamus, caused by a lack of thiamine. Symptoms include confusion, *ataxia,* and vision changes.

Niacin deficiency is called pellagra and is characterized by a light-sensitive rash, diarrhea, glossitis, and psychosis. Pellagra is most common in countries in which corn is the main food source and is rare in the United States.

Coding for Beriberi

ICD-9-CM		ICD-10-CM	
265.0	Beriberi	E51.11	Dry beriberi
		E51.12	Wet beriberi
265.1	Other and unspecified manifestations of thiamine deficiency	E51.2	Wernicke's encephalopathy
		E51.8	Other manifestations of thiamine deficiency
		E51.9	Thiamine deficiency, unspecified
265.2	Pellagra	E52	Niacin deficiency [pellagra]

B-group Deficiencies

Ariboflavinosis is riboflavin, or vitamin B2, deficiency that causes inflammation of the lips, tongue fissures, corneal vascularization, and anemia. Ariboflavinosis is associated with milk deficiency, though the disease can also occur secondarily in patients with chronic diseases affecting nutritional absorption.

Pyridoxine, or vitamin B6, is important in blood, the central nervous system, and skin metabolism. It is uncommon to find a primary deficiency of vitamin B6, but secondary deficiency can result in chronic diseases affecting nutritional absorption in patients using oral contraceptives or in alcoholism. Vitamin B6 deficiency causes skin, lip, and tongue disturbances, peripheral neuropathy, and, in infants, convulsions.

Coding for Deficiency of B-complex Components

ICD-9-CM		ICD-10-CM	
266.0	Ariboflavinosis	E53.0	Riboflavin deficiency
266.1	Vitamin B6 deficiency	E53.1	Pyridoxine deficiency
266.2	Other B-complex deficiencies	D81.818	Other biotin-dependent carboxylase deficiency
		D81.819	Biotin-dependent carboxylase deficiency, unspecified
		E53.8	Deficiency of other specified B group vitamins

Ascorbic Acid Deficiency

Vitamin C, or ascorbic acid, is essential for wound healing and connective tissue health, and it facilitates absorption of iron. A deficiency in this vitamin is commonly called scurvy or Cheadle-Moller-Barlow syndrome. Vitamin C is common to many fruits and vegetables. Symptoms of scurvy include bleeding gums, weight loss, myalgias, and slowing of the healing process. The symptoms are reversed with ascorbic acid therapy.

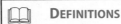

DEFINITIONS

ataxia. Defect in muscular coordination, seen especially when voluntary muscular movements are attempted.

edema. Swelling due to fluid accumulation in the intercellular spaces.

neuritis. Inflammation of a nerve or group of nerves, often manifested by loss of function and reflexes, pain, and numbness or tingling.

ICD-10-CM has further classified vitamin C deficiency with the addition of code E64.2 Sequelae of vitamin C deficiency. When using this code, the condition resulting from the malnutrition or deficiency should be reported first.

Coding for Ascorbic Acid Deficiency

ICD-9-CM		ICD-10-CM	
267	Ascorbic acid deficiency	E54	Ascorbic acid deficiency
		E64.2	Sequelae of vitamin C deficiency

ICD-10-CM has expanded the ICD-9-CM categories used to identify other nutritional deficiencies. Many deficiencies reported as not elsewhere classified or other in ICD-9-CM now have their own code description in ICD-10-CM.

Coding for Other Deficiencies

ICD-9-CM		ICD-10-CM	
269.0	Deficiency of vitamin K	E56.1	Deficiency of vitamin K
269.1	Deficiency of other vitamins	E56.0	Deficiency of vitamin E
		E56.8	Deficiency of other vitamins
269.2	Unspecified vitamin deficiency	E56.9	Vitamin deficiency, unspecified
269.3	Mineral deficiency, not elsewhere classified	E58	Dietary calcium deficiency
		E59	Dietary selenium deficiency
		E60	Dietary zinc deficiency
		E61.0	Copper deficiency
		E61.1	Iron deficiency
		E61.2	Magnesium deficiency
		E61.3	Manganese deficiency
		E61.4	Chromium deficiency
		E61.5	Molybdenum deficiency
		E61.6	Vanadium deficiency
269.8	Other nutritional deficiency	E61.7	Deficiency of multiple nutrient elements
		E61.8	Deficiency of other specified nutrient elements
		E63.0	Essential fatty acid [EFA] deficiency
		E63.1	Imbalance of constituents of food intake
		E63.8	Other specified nutritional deficiencies
		E64.8	Sequelae of other nutritional deficiencies
269.9	Unspecified nutritional deficiency	E61.9	Deficiency of nutrient element, unspecified
		E63.9	Nutritional deficiency, unspecified
		E64.9	Sequelae of unspecified nutritional deficiency

ICD-10-CM has expanded the ICD-9-CM categories used to identify metabolic and immunity disorders. Many disorders reported under one broad category in ICD-9-CM now have their own classification in ICD-10-CM. A few examples follow.

Cystinosis is a genetic metabolic disease that causes the amino acid cystine to accumulate in various organs of the body. The cystine crystallizes and commonly accumulates within the brain, eyes, kidneys, liver, muscles, pancreas, and white blood cells.

Cystinosis is an autosomal recessive genetic disease. In simple terms, both parents are carriers of the abnormal gene. The parents do not show any of the symptoms of cystinosis, but the odds are that one in four of their children will have cystinosis. Cystinosis is a rare disease primarily affecting children, although

DEFINITIONS

albinism. Genetic condition with absence of pigment in skin, hair, and eyes that is often accompanied by astigmatism, photophobia, and nystagmus.

calculus. Abnormal, stone-like concretion of calcium, cholesterol, mineral salts, or other substances that forms in any part of the body.

cataract. Clouding or opacities of the lens that stop clear images from forming on the retina, causing vision impairment or blindness. The classification and coding of cataracts are dependent upon size, shape, location, and etiology.

Fanconi (-de Toni) (-Debré) syndrome. Renal tubular malfunction, including cystinosis and osteomalacia caused by inherited disorders, the result of multiple myeloma, or proximal epithelial growth.

glaucoma. Rise in intraocular pressure, restricting blood flow and decreasing vision.

hypotonia. Diminished muscle tone and stretching resistance.

it can develop in adults. If this condition is left untreated, eventually complete kidney failure will result and other complications, such as *Fanconi syndrome,* may develop.

Cystinuria is a hereditary metabolic disorder characterized by the abnormal transfer of amino acids, such as cystine, lysine, arginine, and ornithine, in the intestines and kidneys. Excessive amounts of cystine in the urine cause the formation of *calculus* in the kidney, bladder, and/or ureter.

Hartnup's disease is an inherited inborn error of metabolism of amino acids in addition to a niacin deficiency. People with this disease are not able to absorb some of the amino acids in their intestines. One of the main amino acids that is not absorbed is tryptophan, which the body uses to make its own form of niacin. Generally individuals with this disease do not have symptoms, but exposure to sunlight, fever, stress, or poor nutrition can cause skin problems, coordination impairment, vision problems, mild mental retardation, gastrointestinal problems, and central nervous system abnormalities. Frequency of attacks usually diminishes with age.

Lowe's syndrome, also referred to as OCRL (oculo-cerebro-renal) syndrome, is a rare genetic condition characterized by anomalies affecting the eye, the nervous system, and the kidney. This disorder occurs almost exclusively in males. Infants with this syndrome are born with congenital *cataracts,* infantile *glaucoma,* neonatal or infantile *hypotonia,* intellectual impairment, and renal tubular dysfunction (Fanconi syndrome).

Phenylketonuria (PKU) is a genetic disorder characterized by an inability to process a part of protein called phenylalanine (Phe). Phe is found in almost all foods. Because of a genetic abnormality, affected individuals lack or have very low levels of an enzyme (phenylalanine hydroxylase or PAH) that converts Phe to other substances the body needs. Extremely elevated Phe levels can cause brain damage and severe mental retardation.

Coding for Disorders of Amino-acid Transport and Metabolism

ICD-9-CM		ICD-10-CM	
270.0	Disturbances of amino-acid transport	E72.00	Disorders of amino-acid transport, unspecified
		E72.01	Cystinuria
		E72.02	Hartnup's disease
		E72.04	Cystinosis
		E72.09	Other disorders of amino-acid transport
270.1	Phenylketonuria (PKU)	E70.0	Classical phenylketonuria
		E70.1	Other hyperphenylalaninemias

Tyrosinemia is a genetic disorder in which the body cannot effectively break down the amino acid tyrosine. Increased levels of tyrosine and its byproducts build up in tissues and organs, leading to serious medical problems such as liver and kidney disturbances and mental retardation. Untreated, tyrosinemia can be fatal.

X-linked ocular albinism (XLOA), which occurs almost exclusively in males, is caused by a gene mutation of the X chromosome. People with XLOA have the developmental and functional vision problems of *albinism.* However, eye, hair, and skin color are usually the same as others in the family or slightly lighter.

Autosomes are the chromosomes that contain genes for general body characteristics. Generally each individual inherits two of these chromosomes: one from the mother and one from the father. In autosomal recessive ocular albinism, albinism is an inherited recessive trait, obvious only when two copies of the gene for that trait are present. In other words, if one parent carries a mutated chromosome and the other does not, the child will not have albinism but instead be a carrier. However, if both parents (that are only carriers) have mutated chromosomes that are passed on, the child will have albinism. In this situation, there is a one in four chance that the child will have albinism.

Tyrosinase negative oculocutaneous albinism type IA (OCA1A) results from a genetic defect in an enzyme called tyrosinase. This enzyme helps the body transform the amino acid tyrosine into pigment. The enzyme is inactive and no melanin is produced; therefore, there is a complete absence of pigment in the skin, hair, and eyes. These individuals also present with *photophobia*, moderate-to-severe reduced *visual acuity*, and *nystagmus*.

In tyrosinase positive oculocutaneous albinism type II (OCA2), the enzyme tyrosinase is present. Generally OCA2 manifests with a minimal-to-moderate amount of pigment remaining in the skin, hair, and eyes. Many patients can develop pigmented freckles, lentigines, and/or *nevi* with age. Individuals with OCA2 have the usual visual anomalies associated with albinism, including decreased acuity and nystagmus. OCA2 is the most prevalent form of oculocutaneous albinism. The occurrence of this disorder is greatly increased in patients with *Willi-Prader* or *Angelman syndrome.*

Chediak-Higashi syndrome is an autosomal recessive immunodeficiency disorder. Individuals with this disorder inherit a defective gene from each parent. This gene affects multiple body areas but has the biggest impact on the immune system. It prevents white blood cells from functioning properly, leaving them unable to fight viruses and bacteria. This disease also manifests symptoms of oculocutaneous albinism (light pigmentation of eyes, hair, and skin, and vision problems), prolonged bleeding times, easy bruisability, and peripheral *neuropathy.*

Hermansky-Pudlak syndrome is an autosomal recessive type of albinism that includes a *coagulation* defect and lung disease. This disease also manifests symptoms of oculocutaneous albinism (light pigmentation of eyes, hair, and skin, and vision problems), in addition to *colitis* and kidney failure.

Coding for Disorders of Aromatic Amino-acid Metabolism

ICD-9-CM		ICD-10-CM	
270.2	Other disturbances of aromatic amino-acid metabolism	E70.20	Disorder of tyrosine metabolism, unspecified
		E70.21	Tyrosinemia
		E70.29	Other disorders of tyrosine metabolism
		E70.30	Albinism, unspecified
		E70.310	X-linked ocular albinism
		E70.311	Autosomal recessive ocular albinism
		E70.318	Other ocular albinism
		E70.319	Ocular albinism, unspecified
		E70.320	Tyrosinase negative oculocutaneous albinism
		E70.321	Tyrosinase positive oculocutaneous albinism
		E70.328	Other oculocutaneous albinism
		E70.329	Oculocutaneous albinism, unspecified
		E70.330	Chediak-Higashi syndrome
		E70.331	Hermansky-Pudlak syndrome
		E70.338	Other albinism with hematologic abnormality
(Continued on next page)		E70.339	Albinism with hematologic abnormality, unspecified

DEFINITIONS

Angelman syndrome. Emergence in early childhood of a pattern of interrupted development, stiff jerky gait, absence or impairment of speech, excessive laughter, and seizures.

coagulation. Clot formation.

colitis. Inflammation of the colon, caused by any number of infections, external influences such as laxatives or radiation, and antibiotics.

neuropathy. Abnormality, disease, or malfunction of the nerves.

nevus. plural of nevi. Benign, pigmented skin lesion that includes congenital lesions of the skin such as birthmarks, telangiectasias (permanent dilations of small blood vessels), vascular spider veins, hemangiomas, and moles.

nystagmus. Rapid, rhythmic, involuntary movements of the eyeball in vertical, horizontal, rotational, or mixed directions that can be congenital, acquired, physiological, neurological, or due to ocular disease.

photophobia. Sensitivity to light.

visual acuity. Clarity of vision.

Willi-Prader syndrome. Typified by rounded face, almond-shaped eyes, strabismus, low forehead, hypogonadism, hypotonia, mental retardation, and an insatiable appetite.

ICD-9-CM	ICD-10-CM
270.2 Other disturbances of aromatic amino-acid metabolism *(Continued)*	E70.39 Other specified albinism E70.5 Disorders of tryptophan metabolism E70.8 Other disorders of aromatic amino-acid metabolism E70.9 Disorder of aromatic amino-acid metabolism, unspecified

Summary

The endocrine system, which is vital to many daily functions, can be affected by numerous conditions. This chapter reviews many of these conditions, and outlines the increased specificity included in the ICD-10-CM code set. In order to be well prepared to transition to ICD-10-CM, it is important to be aware of the basic anatomy and physiology of the endocrine system, as well as the specific disease pathologies that are described in both code sets.

Chapter 7. **Cardiovascular System**

Anatomic Overview

The cardiovascular system houses some of the most important components needed for day-to-day survival. The heart and the approximately 60,000 miles of blood vessels in the circulatory system provide oxygen-rich blood, nutrients such as amino acids and electrolytes, and important hormones to all of the body's cells and carry off carbon dioxide and other waste products of metabolism. In addition, the cardiovascular system stabilizes body temperature and pH. Other body systems work closely with the cardiovascular system to ensure proper functioning and homeostasis, which is the ability of an organism to obtain and maintain internal stability by adjusting its physiological processes. For instance, the digestive system provides needed nutrients to the body by way of the cardiovascular system.

Anatomy of the Heart

The heart, itself, is a small organ, approximately the size of a fist. It is located in the mediastinum, with the majority of it to the left of the body's midline. It is enclosed in a protective, two-layer membrane that positions it in the chest but also allows for expansion as needed for contractions. The outer layer, the fibrous pericardium, is made up of dense connective tissue. The serous pericardium is double layered, with the outermost parietal layer adherent to the fibrous pericardium and the inner visceral layer (epicardium) adherent to the heart's surface. Between these two layers, the pericardial cavity contains lubricating pericardial fluid that decreases friction caused by the beating of the heart.

Figure 7.1: Sections of Heart Muscle

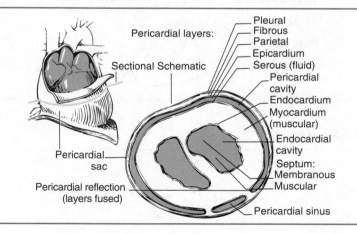

The heart wall comprises three layers: the external epicardium (also called the visceral serous pericardial layer), the middle myocardium, and the endocardium, which is the innermost layer covering the four chambers of the heart, the valves, and the lining of large blood vessels connected to the heart.

The four chambers of the heart include the right and left atria on the upper side and the left and right ventricles on the lower side. The outermost surface of the heart contains channels known as sulci. These sulci, which contain some fat and the coronary blood vessels, delineate the outside margins of the heart chambers.

Each of the four valves of the heart, although located in different areas, function in the same way. The valves open and close in response to pressure differences caused by contraction and relaxation of the heart chambers. This allows blood to flow from areas with higher pressure to those with lower pressure. Valves allow blood to flow in one direction only, preventing backflow when closed.

Between the right atrium and the right ventricle lies the tricuspid valve, through which blood flows. From the right ventricle, blood passes through the pulmonary valve into the pulmonary trunk where it is carried to the lungs for oxygenation. After oxygenation occurs, the blood returns to the left atrium through the four pulmonary veins. It passes from the left atrium through the bicuspid (mitral) valve to the left ventricle. The blood is then passed through the aortic valve into the ascending aorta where some flows into the coronary arteries and the rest passes into the aortic arch and descending aorta where other arteries carry the blood throughout the body.

Collectively, the bicuspid and the tricuspid valves are referred to as the atrioventricular (AV) valves, while the pulmonary and aortic valves are referred to as the semi-lunar (SL) valves.

Figure 7.2: Anatomy

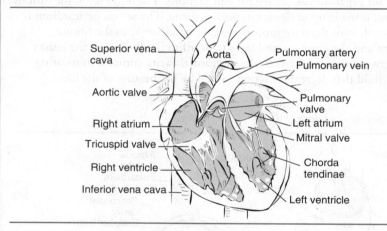

Figure 7.3: Blood Flow

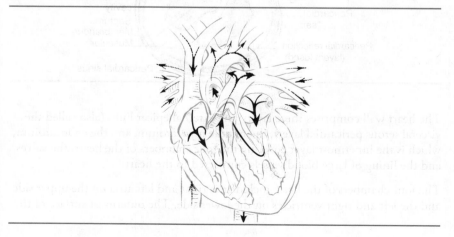

Conduction System of the Heart

Specialized autorhythmic cells in the cardiac muscle not only produce the electrical stimulation that initiates the heartbeat, but also form the conduction system that stimulates the contraction of the heart to make it pump effectively. Inherent in the heart's muscle tissue are the physiological properties of:

- **Automaticity:** Property of a cell to reach a threshold potential and generate an impulse on its own without stimulation from another source.

- **Conductivity:** Ability to transfer an impulse from cell to cell.

- **Contractility:** Property that allows shortening of the muscle when stimulated.

- **Excitability:** Capacity of a cell to respond to a stimulus.

Figure 7.4: Conduction System of the Heart

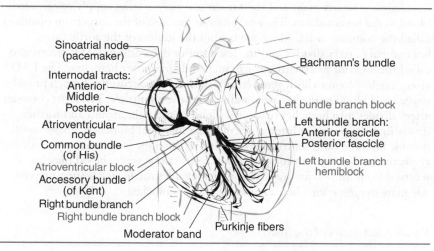

In a normal heart, the muscle is stimulated by impulses that originate in the sinoatrial (SA) node, also referred to as the sinus node and the heart's pacemaker. The impulse goes from the sinus node, through the atria, to the atrioventricular (AV) node, which is positioned between the atria and the ventricles, through the bundle branches, and ends in the Purkinje fibers of the ventricles' walls to initiate systole.

The SA node, under control of the autonomic nervous system, is innervated by parasympathetic nervous system fibers, as well as sympathetic nervous system fibers. Stimulation of the sympathetic nervous system increases the heart rate, raises blood pressure, and increases the force of myocardial contraction. On the other hand, parasympathetic stimulation slows the heart rate, lowers blood pressure, and decreases the force of contraction. The manipulation of the autonomic nervous system by drugs such as beta adrenergic blocking drugs (beta blockers) takes advantage of these effects. Blocking the sympathetic nervous system relieves stress on the heart, causing it to slow down, decreases the force of the heart's contraction, and reduces blood vessel contraction as well. These drugs are useful following myocardial infarction and for treating cardiac dysrhythmias and hypertension.

Cardiac Cycle

A cardiac cycle is the sequence of events that occur during each heartbeat. An impulse from the SA node causes the atria to contract first (atrial systole), while the ventricles relax (ventricular diastole). Atria contraction forces blood through the open AV valves to the ventricles. Since the SL valves are closed, the ventricle is able to fill with approximately 130 cc of blood, a volume referred to as the end-diastolic volume (EDV). When the ventricles contract (ventricular systole), the atria relax (atria diastole). The increased ventricular pressure forces the SL valves open, ejecting blood from the heart. Ventricular ejection is the period of time when the SL valves are open. Each ventricle ejects about 70 cc of blood, leaving approximately 60 cc in the ventricle, referred to as the end systolic volume (ESV). The four chambers of the heart then relax, and the cycle begins again.

Coronary Circulation

The heart has its own system of blood vessels, referred to as coronary or cardiac circulation. The left main and right main coronary arteries supply oxygenated blood to the myocardium. They originate at the base of the aorta from openings called the coronary ostia, which are behind the leaflets of the aortic valve. The left coronary artery divides into the left anterior descending (LAD) artery, also called the anterior interventricular branch and circumflex branches. The LAD artery carries blood to both ventricular walls, and the circumflex branch provides oxygenated blood to the left atrial walls and the left ventricle. The right coronary artery divides into branches that carry blood to the right atrium and further divide into the posterior interventricular and marginal branches. These vessels provide blood to both ventricular walls and to the right ventricular myocardium, respectively. The myocardium has many connections where blood may be received from more than one artery, which enables the heart's tissue to receive adequate oxygen even when a coronary artery is blocked.

Figure 7.5: Arteries of the Heart

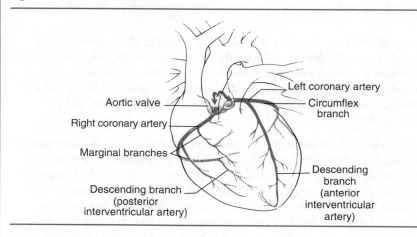

Once the blood has completed its circuit through the arteries, it continues to the capillaries, delivering oxygen and nutrients and collecting CO_2 and any waste product before it drains into the coronary sinus. On the venous side of the coronary circulation are veins that empty deoxygenated blood into the coronary sinus and ultimately into the right atrium, including:

- **Anterior cardiac veins:** Drain the right ventricle.

- **Great cardiac vein:** Drains the left atrium and both ventricles.

- **Middle cardiac vein:** Drains both ventricles.

- **Small cardiac vein:** Drains the right atrium and ventricle.

Circulatory Pathways

The heart and the blood vessels form two distinct, but parallel, circulatory pathways that nourish all of the organs and cells of the body. The systemic circulation includes all of the arteries and arterioles that branch off the aorta as it emerges from the left ventricle to deliver oxygen-rich blood to the body, as well as the veins and venules that eventually drain into the superior and inferior vena cava and the coronary sinus that empties oxygen-poor blood into the right atrium. The blood then goes to the right ventricle, where it is picked up by the pulmonary circulation to be reoxygenated. Blood leaves the right ventricle via the pulmonary trunk, which splits into the right and left pulmonary arteries. These branches further divide, becoming successively smaller until they become pulmonary capillaries surrounding the alveoli in the lungs. The layers of cells that line the alveoli and the surrounding capillaries are very thin and in close proximity to each other. It is here that carbon dioxide is passed from the blood to the alveoli to be exhaled and oxygen from the air is passed from the lungs into the blood, a process known as alveolar capillary exchange. As this cycle continues, the tiny capillaries join together to form venules and ultimately the four (two left, two right) pulmonary veins bring oxygen-rich blood to the left atrium, then the left ventricle, where the oxygenated blood is pumped into the systemic circulation.

Blood Vessel Anatomy: Artery, Veins, Arterioles, Venules, and Capillaries

Although there are variations in the function of each particular blood vessel, the walls of most have the following three layers:

- **Tunica interna:** Innermost layer of the vessel that contains a single layer of endothelium on the inner surface that helps influence blood flow, secretes chemicals that affect capillary permeability, and aids in vessel contraction.

- **Tunica media:** Thick middle layer of mostly smooth muscle cells and extensive elastic fibers. The primary function of this layer is to regulate blood pressure and flow by contraction and dilation.

- **Tunica externa:** Outermost layer of the vessel, its function is to attach the vessel to the surrounding tissue. It is made up of collagen, elastic fibers, and many nerves. In the case of larger vessels, the tunica externa also contains very small vessels that supply blood to the vessel wall.

Arteries transport blood away from the heart to all organs and cells of the body and are divided into two types: elastic and muscular. Elastic, or conducting, arteries have the largest diameter of all arteries in the body and include the aorta, pulmonary trunk, brachiocephalic, common carotid, common iliac, and subclavian arteries. They drive blood forward while the ventricles are relaxed, pushing blood toward smaller arteries. Muscular (distributing) arteries are mid-size arteries that are branches of the elastic arteries. Varying in size from the pencil-sized axillary and femoral arteries to the small, string-size arteries that carry blood to organs, the thick walls of these arteries are able to regulate blood flow with vasoconstriction and vasodilatation. Some examples of muscular arteries include the brachial and radial arteries of the arm. Branching into increasingly smaller arteries, the muscular arteries eventually branch out into the microscopic arterioles that control blood flow into the capillary networks. Changes at this level can impact blood pressure, with arteriole vasodilatation decreasing blood pressure and arteriole vasoconstriction increasing blood pressure.

Upon entering the tissue, arterioles branch off further into capillaries, which are the body's smallest blood vessels. They exchange substances in the blood and interstitial fluid of the body's cells. They are not present in cartilage or in the cornea or lens of the eye, but they are found in abundance in connection with tissues that have high metabolic requirements, such as the nervous system, liver, and muscles.

Figure 7.6: Capillary Bed

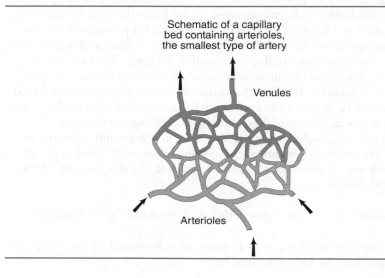

Capillaries function as part of a capillary bed, comprising 10 to 100 capillaries through which blood flows and capillary exchange takes place. Diffusion is the primary mechanism of this process, allowing oxygen, hormones, nutrients, and byproducts of metabolism to cross the capillary walls. Transcytosis may also take place, particularly with larger or lipid-insoluble materials, such as antibodies and proteins. Transcellular transport takes place when the substance becomes enclosed in the wall of the cell and is moved across the cell and expelled through the cell wall on the opposite side.

After capillary exchange takes place, the tiny postcapillary venules continue the exchange of nutrients and waste products, especially for larger molecules. The venules then begin to reunite and become successively larger veins, eventually returning the blood to the right atrium via the inferior and superior vena cava.

DEFINITIONS

anastomosis. Surgically created connection between ducts, blood vessels, or bowel segments to allow flow from one to the other. The majority of tissues in the body can receive blood from more than one artery, which is important when a vessel is blocked or compressed. This other pathway, referred to as collateral circulation, may also occur between arterioles, veins, and venules.

Brain Circulation

The carotid and vertebral arteries supply oxygenated blood to the brain. The carotid arteries are easily palpated under the jaw: one on the left and one on the right. At the top of the neck, the carotids *bifurcate* into the external and internal carotid arteries. The external carotid arteries provide blood and nutrients to the face and scalp, while the internal carotid arteries supply the anterior three-fifths of the cerebrum, with the exception of parts of the temporal and occipital lobes.

The vertebral arteries course along the spinal column, joining together to create the single basilar artery (vertebrobasilar arteries) near the brain stem at the skull base. These arteries nourish the posterior two-fifths of the cerebrum, part of the cerebellum, and the brain stem.

DEFINITIONS

bifurcation. Point of division into two separate branches or structures, such as the site where the trachea divides into the right and left main bronchi or the common carotid artery becomes the external and internal carotid arteries.

Figure 7.7: Cerebrovascular Arteries

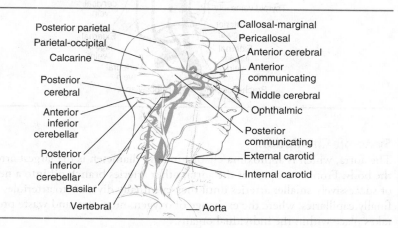

Posterior parietal
Parietal-occipital
Calcarine
Posterior cerebral
Anterior inferior cerebellar
Posterior inferior cerebellar
Basilar
Vertebral

Callosal-marginal
Pericallosal
Anterior cerebral
Anterior communicating
Middle cerebral
Ophthalmic
Posterior communicating
External carotid
Internal carotid
Aorta

The internal-carotid and vertebral arteries converge at the Circle of Willis. It is from the circle of Willis that other arteries—the anterior cerebral artery (ACA), the middle cerebral artery (MCA), and the posterior cerebral artery (PCA)—arise and travel to all parts of the brain. One of the shortcomings of the circle of Willis is that cerebral aneurysms are inclined to develop at the arterial junctions. Deoxygenated blood is removed from the brain via the jugular vein.

Figure 7.8: Head Veins

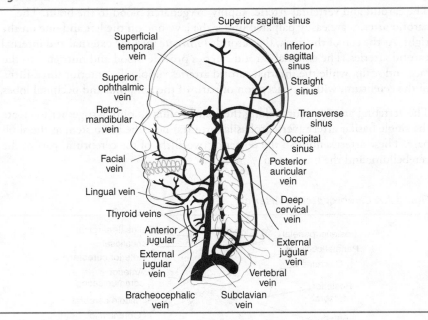

Systemic Circulation

The aorta, which is approximately one inch in diameter, is the largest artery in the body. From every part of the aorta, other arteries branch off into a network of successively smaller arteries until they eventually divide into arterioles and finally capillaries, where the exchange of oxygen, nutrients, and waste products takes place within the individual organs.

The aorta is divided into four segments:

- **Ascending aorta:** Arises from the left ventricle and is the site of the coronary arteries.

- **Aortic arch:** First arching to the left, the aorta descends through the diaphragm. This segment includes arteries that travel to the head, neck, and upper extremities.

- **Thoracic aorta:** Part of the aorta between the arch and the diaphragm that contains arterial branches that supply the bronchi, esophagus, pericardium, mediastinum, intercostal muscles, muscles of the chest, and a portion of the diaphragm.

- **Abdominal aorta:** Portion of the aorta between the diaphragm and the branches of the common iliac arteries that supplies part of the diaphragm, intestines, all of the visceral organs, lower limbs, reproductive organs, bladder, and buttock muscles.

Figure 7.9: Arterial System

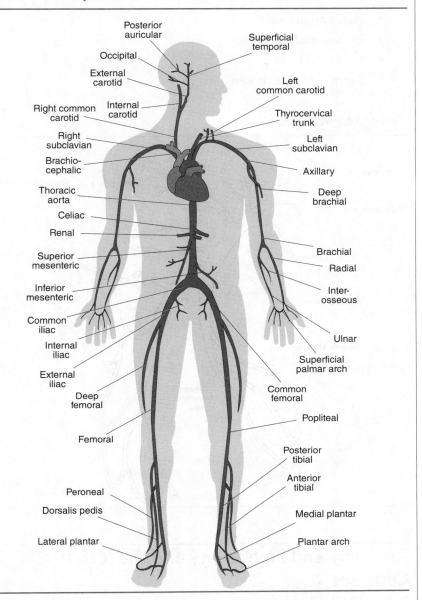

Hepatic Portal System

Simply put, a portal system consists of a network of blood vessels through which blood is transported after passing through one capillary bed to another network of capillaries prior to being returned to systemic circulation. The portal venous system channels blood from parts of the digestive tract, spleen, and pancreas to the liver for processing prior to returning to the heart.

Blood flow to the liver differs from that in the general circulation since the liver receives oxygenated blood, as well as partially deoxygenated blood. Oxygenated blood from the hepatic artery mixes with the nutrient rich blood from the portal vein in the liver sinusoids.

The large veins that make up the portal venous system are:

- Hepatic portal vein
- Inferior mesenteric vein
- Splenic vein
- Superior mesenteric vein

Figure 7.10: Portal System

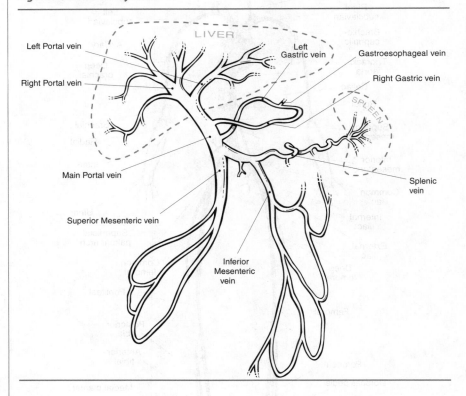

Anatomy and Physiology and the ICD-10-CM Code Set

In ICD-10-CM, diagnosis coding of conditions affecting the cardiovascular system is much more detailed than it is in ICD-9-CM. In many cases, there is one ICD-9-CM code describing a diagnosis, whereas there are several ICD-10-CM codes. Details such as specific anatomical site or the severity of a condition have been incorporated into ICD-10-CM that didn't exist in ICD-9-CM.

For example, ICD-9-CM has one specific code to classify cardiac arrest:

427.5 **Cardiac arrest**

In ICD-10-CM, however, more specific codes are available to classify the cardiac arrest, including:

I46.2 **Cardiac arrest due to underlying cardiac condition**

I46.8 **Cardiac arrest due to other underlying condition**

I46.9 **Cardiac arrest, cause unspecified**

The increased specificity of ICD-10-CM makes it imperative that physicians document more detailed information and that coders are able to determine from documentation the code or codes appropriate for the patient's condition.

Valvular Disorders

Acute rheumatic fever, a complication of strep pharyngitis in children, results in various cardiac conditions in more than a third of patients affected. Depending on the extent of heart inflammation involved, patients with the acute form of the disease may develop heart failure, *pericarditis*, myocarditis, and endocarditis, which is manifested as insufficiency of the mitral (65 to 70 percent of cases) and aortic valves (25 percent of cases).

> 📖 **DEFINITIONS**
>
> **pericarditis.** Inflammation affecting the pericardium.

Figure 7.11: Valvular Function

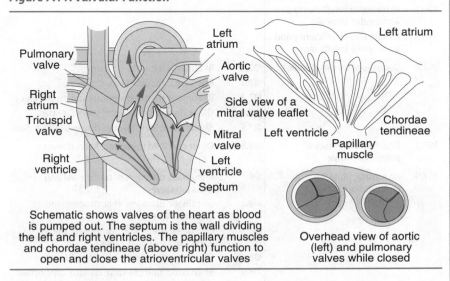

Schematic shows valves of the heart as blood is pumped out. The septum is the wall dividing the left and right ventricles. The papillary muscles and chordae tendineae (above right) function to open and close the atrioventricular valves

Overhead view of aortic (left) and pulmonary valves while closed

Chronic disease may result in arrhythmias, ventricular dysfunction, and dilation of the atria. In adults, acute rheumatic fever is the most common cause of mitral valve stenosis and the leading cause for valvular replacement surgery. Although the mitral valve is most commonly affected, the aortic and tricuspid valves may also be involved.

Chronic manifestations due to protracted disease and continued valve deformity occur in an estimated 9 to 39 percent of adults with previous rheumatic heart disease. Two to 10 years after an acute episode of rheumatic fever, the valve apparatus may fuse, with resulting stenosis or stenosis with insufficiency. Each recurrent episode can extend the valvular damage.

For acute rheumatic heart conditions, there is a one-to-one mapping of the appropriate ICD-9-CM code to the appropriate ICD-10-CM code. For instance, ICD-9-CM code 391.0 for acute rheumatic pericarditis directly correlates to code IØ1.1 in ICD-10-CM. This is also true for some valvular diseases resulting from rheumatic fever. Although ICD-9-CM does classify some conditions as rheumatic in nature, ICD-10-CM has distinguished, in large part, specific valvular diseases caused by rheumatic fever versus those not related to the disease, as well as the specific valve involved as shown in the following table. This differentiation does not always result in additional ICD-10-CM codes, as demonstrated by ICD-9-CM codes 396.0 through 396.8, which map to ICD-10-CM code IØ8.Ø.

Coding for Diseases of the Heart Valves

ICD-9-CM		ICD-10-CM	
Rheumatic			
394.0	Mitral stenosis	I05.0	Rheumatic mitral stenosis
394.2	Mitral stenosis with insufficiency	I05.2	Rheumatic mitral stenosis with insufficiency
394.9	Other and unspecified mitral valve diseases	I05.8	Other rheumatic mitral valve diseases
		I05.9	Rheumatic mitral valve disease, unspecified
396.0	Mitral valve stenosis and aortic valve stenosis	I08.0	Rheumatic disorders of both mitral and aortic valves
396.1	Mitral valve stenosis and aortic valve insufficiency	I08.0	Rheumatic disorders of both mitral and aortic valves
396.2	Mitral valve insufficiency and aortic valve stenosis		
396.3	Mitral valve insufficiency and aortic valve insufficiency		
397.0	Diseases of tricuspid valve	I07.0	Rheumatic tricuspid stenosis
		I07.1	Rheumatic tricuspid insufficiency
		I07.2	Rheumatic tricuspid stenosis and insufficiency
		I07.8	Other rheumatic tricuspid valve diseases
		I07.9	Rheumatic tricuspid valve disease, unspecified
397.1	Rheumatic diseases of pulmonary valve	I09.89	Other specified rheumatic heart diseases
397.9	Rheumatic diseases endocardium valve unspecified	I08.1	Rheumatic disorders of both mitral and tricuspid valves
		I08.2	Rheumatic disorders of both aortic and tricuspid valves
		I08.3	Combined rheumatic disorders of mitral, aortic, and tricuspid valves
		I08.8	Other rheumatic multiple valve diseases
		I08.9	Rheumatic multiple valve disease, unspecified
		I09.1	Rheumatic diseases of endocardium, valve unspecified

There are many differences between the ICD-9-CM and ICD-10-CM terminology used for valvular disorders. Key differences can be as simple as a "disorder" code in ICD-9-CM becoming more specific in ICD-10-CM; however, there are some important terms to be aware of.

Insufficiency is, in general, the inability to perform a function adequately or to the level necessary for the human body. When using the term with regard to valve function, it typically means the valve isn't functioning as well as it should be, allowing blood to flow back into the chamber inappropriately.

Prolapse, specifically mitral valve prolapse, occurs when the cusps of the mitral valve protrude into the left atrium during ventricular systole. It is sometimes referred to as mitral valve prolapse syndrome.

Stenosis means narrowing or contracted. Regarding the valves, it describes a condition in which there has been a narrowing or a stricture caused by a multitude of factors, such as calcification or a congenital malformation.

Understanding these three terms helps when reporting valve disorders in ICD-10-CM. It is not known how payers will handle unspecified codes under the ICD-10-CM code set, so it is important to always code to the highest level of specificity. This may mean querying the provider for additional information.

📖 **DEFINITIONS**

insufficiency. Inadequate closure of the valve, allowing abnormal backward blood flow.

regurgitation. Abnormal backward flow.

stenosis. Narrowing or constriction of a passage.

Coding for Diseases of the Heart Valves

ICD-9-CM		ICD-10-CM	
Nonrheumatic			
424.0	Mitral valve disorders	I34.0	Nonrheumatic mitral (valve) insufficiency
		I34.1	Nonrheumatic mitral (valve) prolapse
		I34.2	Nonrheumatic mitral (valve) stenosis
		I34.8	Other nonrheumatic mitral valve disorders
		I34.9	Nonrheumatic mitral valve disorder unspecified
424.1	Aortic valve disorders	I35.0	Nonrheumatic aortic (valve) stenosis
		I35.1	Nonrheumatic aortic (valve) insufficiency
		I35.2	Nonrheumatic aortic (valve) stenosis with insufficiency
		I35.8	Other nonrheumatic aortic valve disorders
		I35.9	Nonrheumatic aortic valve disorder, unspecified
424.2	Tricuspid valve disorders specified as nonrheumatic	I36.0	Nonrheumatic tricuspid (valve) stenosis
		I36.1	Nonrheumatic tricuspid (valve) insufficiency
		I36.2	Nonrheumatic tricuspid (valve) stenosis with insufficiency
		I36.8	Other nonrheumatic tricuspid valve disorders
		I36.9	Nonrheumatic tricuspid valve disorder, unspecified
424.3	Pulmonary valve disorders	I37.0	Nonrheumatic pulmonary (valve) stenosis
		I37.1	Nonrheumatic pulmonary (valve) insufficiency
		I37.2	Nonrheumatic pulmonary (valve) stenosis with insufficiency
		I37.8	Other nonrheumatic pulmonary valve disorders
		I37.9	Nonrheumatic pulmonary valve disorder, unspecified

Acute Coronary Syndromes

Obstruction of a coronary artery can result in a number of conditions that make up acute coronary syndrome. Depending on the percentage of the artery obstructed, as well as the specific location of the obstruction, the diagnosis may range from unstable angina to non-ST-segment elevation MI (NSTEMI), ST-segment elevation MI (STEMI), or sudden cardiac death. Symptoms for angina and myocardial infarctions (MI) are comparable and include chest discomfort with or without dyspnea, nausea, and diaphoresis. A diagnosis is made by ECG, as well as by the use of specific serologic markers. Treatment may include antiplatelet drugs, anticoagulants, nitrates, and beta-blockers. For STEMI, treatment may also include emergency reperfusion using fibrinolytic drugs, percutaneous intervention, or coronary artery bypass graft surgery.

Myocardial Infarction

Figure 7.12: Acute Myocardial Infarction

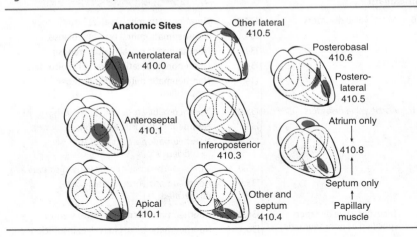

Myocardial infarction, also referred to as a heart attack, may be caused by several conditions but is most frequently attributed to narrowing of the coronary blood vessels due to atheromatous plaques. With rupture of the plaques, thrombi may form in the coronary vessel and vasospasm of the arteries occurs, causing complete or partial vessel occlusion. With the flow of oxygen and nutrients required by the heart blocked, myocardial ischemia begins in the endocardium and extends to the epicardium. Permanent heart damage, most of which occurs in the first two to three hours after infarction, must be quickly reversed to save the heart muscle.

The size and site of the infarction are primary factors in determining death and debility. For instance, anterior infarcts are likely to be larger and have a poorer prognosis than do inferoposterior infarcts. They are most often due to obstruction of the left coronary artery, particularly the anterior descending artery. Inferoposterior infarcts, on the other hand, are indicative of right coronary or dominant left circumflex artery obstruction.

While an MI most often affects the left ventricle, damage may also extend into the right ventricle or the atria. Right ventricular infarction commonly results from obstruction of the right coronary or a dominant left circumflex artery. A right ventricular infarction that complicates a left ventricular infarction represents a grave clinical situation with considerable increase in mortality risk.

Transmural infarcts involve the entire thickness of the myocardium from epicardium to endocardium and are most often distinguished by abnormal Q waves on the patient's ECG. Nontransmural or subendocardial infarcts do not extend through the ventricular wall and result in ST-segment and T-wave (ST-T) abnormalities. The quicker the oxygen supply is restored, the better the chance of saving the heart and minimizing damage. After a period of four to six hours, however, the ischemia caused by an occlusion can cause necrosis to the heart that cannot be reversed.

Other causes of myocardial infarction include:

- Acute anemia due to hemorrhage
- Anomalies such as aneurysms of the coronary arteries

- Aortic dissection, with retrograde involvement of the coronary arteries
- Arteritis
- Chest trauma
- Drugs such as amphetamines, cocaine, and ephedrine
- Emboli of the coronary arteries, due to air, cholesterol, sepsis, and heart valve infection
- Hypoxia secondary to acute pulmonary conditions or carbon monoxide poisoning
- Pediatric coronary artery disease, such as seen with Marfan syndrome and progeria
- Vasospasm of the coronary arteries
- Ventricular hypertrophy (e.g., left ventricular hypertrophy [LVH], idiopathic hypertrophic subaortic stenosis [IHSS], or underlying valve disease)

The risk factors for the formation of atherosclerotic plaque are well documented and include:

- Age
- Diabetes mellitus
- Family history
- Hypercholesterolemia and hypertriglyceridemia (includes inherited lipoprotein disorders)
- Hypertension
- Male gender
- Smoking
- Sedentary lifestyle
- Type A personality

The increased specificity of ICD-10-CM coding is evident in the classification of MIs. For this reason, it is important to understand the details of the condition.

Symptoms indicative of an MI require rapid emergency intervention to restore blood flow to the heart as quickly as possible. An electrocardiogram (ECG) is performed to evaluate the electrical activity of the heart to determine if blood flow through heart tissue has been compromised. One component of an ECG is the ST segment, which is found on the ECG following the QRS complex and continuing into the T wave. Depression or elevation of the ST segment is characteristic of ischemia or injury to the myocardium. The ST segment differentiates between two types of myocardial infarction: ST segment elevation myocardial infarction (STEMI) and non-ST-segment elevation myocardial infarction (NSTEMI). Although both types indicate damage to the heart's blood flow, patients with STEMI are more likely to be candidates for thrombolytic drug (clot buster) therapy, while those with NSTEMI are not. An elevated ST segment signifies a comparatively large amount of damage to the heart muscle is taking place due to total occlusion of a coronary artery. The milder NSTEMI results in a partly occluded artery, which affects only part of the heart muscle. STEMIs account for 30 to 45 percent of all heart attacks.

The ICD-9-CM code book distinguishes between STEMIs and NSTEMIs using inclusion notes under the MI code descriptors. In ICD-10-CM, the code descriptor itself includes the designation of STEMI or NSTEMI. Although ICD-9-CM and ICD-10-CM have specific codes that identify the area of the heart the MI affected, guidelines for MIs vary quite a bit in how they define an episode of care and in the reporting of subsequent MIs.

For instance, ICD-9-CM defines an acute episode of care as a period of eight weeks or less. In ICD-10-CM, this has been redefined as a period of four weeks. In ICD-9-CM, a fifth-digit subclassification of 1 indicates the first episode of care and is used to report the MI whether or not the patient is transferred to another facility. A fifth digit of 2 indicates a patient was admitted for additional treatment of the cardiac condition at any time during the eight-week period following the initial MI. However, if a patient sustains a second MI during the admission for treatment of the initial MI, a fifth digit of 1 is still reported.

ICD-10-CM guidelines indicate that a code from category I21 should be reported when a patient has an initial MI. However, if the patient has another MI within the four-week period of the initial MI, a code from category I22 is reported as well. In this type of scenario, the sequencing of codes indicates the reason for the encounter or admission. For instance, a patient has an MI and is admitted to the hospital, where he suffers a second MI on day five of the hospitalization. In this case, a code from category I21 is sequenced first, and code I22 is sequenced as the secondary diagnosis.

However, if a patient has an MI, is treated, and is discharged home, a code from category I21 is reported. If the same patient has a second MI, a code from category I22 is sequenced first, with a code from category I21 listed as a secondary code to demonstrate the patient is within the four-week time period from the original MI.

In the following table, ICD-10-CM designates each MI as STEMI or NSTEMI, as well as initial or subsequent.

Coding for Myocardial Infarctions

ICD-9-CM		ICD-10-CM	
410.01	AMI of anterolateral wall, initial episode of care	I21.09	ST elevation (STEMI) MI involving other coronary artery of anterior wall
		I22.0	Subsequent ST elevation (STEMI) MI of anterior wall
410.11	AMI of other anterior wall, initial episode of care	I21.01	ST elevation (STEMI) MI involving left main coronary artery
		I21.02	ST elevation (STEMI) MI involving left anterior descending coronary artery
		I21.09	ST elevation (STEMI) MI involving other coronary artery of anterior wall
		I22.0	Subsequent ST elevation (STEMI) MI of anterior wall
410.21	AMI of inferolateral wall, initial episode of care	I21.19	ST elevation (STEMI) MI involving other coronary artery of inferior wall
		I22.1	Subsequent ST elevation (STEMI) MI of inferior wall
410.31	AMI of inferoposterior wall, initial episode of care	I21.11	ST elevation (STEMI) MI involving right coronary artery
		I22.1	Subsequent ST elevation (STEMI) MI of inferior wall
410.41	AMI of other inferior wall, initial episode of care	I21.19	ST elevation (STEMI) MI involving other coronary artery of inferior wall
		I22.1	Subsequent ST elevation (STEMI) MI of inferior wall
410.51	AMI of other lateral wall, initial episode of care	I21.29	ST elevation (STEMI) MI involving other sites
		I22.8	Subsequent ST elevation (STEMI) MI of other sites
410.61	AMI, true posterior wall infarction, initial episode of care	I21.29	ST elevation (STEMI) MI involving other sites
		I22.8	Subsequent ST elevation (STEMI) MI of other sites
410.71	AMI, subendocardial infarction, initial episode of care	I21.4	Non-ST elevation (NSTEMI) MI
		I22.2	Subsequent non-ST elevation (NSTEMI) MI
410.81	AMI of other specified sites, initial episode of care	I21.21	ST elevation (STEMI) MI involving left circumflex coronary artery
		I21.29	ST elevation (STEMI) MI involving other sites
		I22.8	Subsequent ST elevation (STEMI) MI of other sites
410.91	AMI, unspecified site, initial episode of care	I21.3	ST elevation (STEMI) MI of unspecified site
		I22.9	Subsequent ST elevation (STEMI) MI of unspecified site

Atherosclerosis

Arteriosclerosis, also referred to as "hardening of the arteries," occurs when the arteries become narrowed due to *atherosclerosis* and then become hardened by fibrous tissue and calcification. As this process continues, it results in a decrease in blood and oxygen supply to the affected organ. Eventually, the plaque may cause severe or complete obstruction of the artery, causing tissue necrosis. Although this process is often associated with the heart, it may occur in any of the organs, including the brain, kidneys, intestines, eyes, and limbs. Chronic hypertension may also cause arteriosclerosis, with the elevated blood pressure contributing to the thickening of the muscular arterial walls.

 DEFINITIONS

arteriosclerosis. Condition causing thickening of the artery walls.

atherosclerosis. Buildup of yellowish plaques composed of cholesterol and lipoid material within the arteries.

In the heart, atherosclerosis may lead to coronary artery disease, while in the brain, it may lead to a stroke. In the lower extremities, arterial constriction results in pain, numbness, and the sensation of cold legs or feet. Peripheral artery disease (PAD) limits physical movement due to pain, and severe complications such as nonhealing ulcers and gangrene may occur resulting in limb amputation.

Angina

As a general definition, angina is chest pain that occurs due to inadequate blood flow to the heart. In stable angina, rest and mild activity fail to elicit symptoms. However, an increase in activity that puts stress on the heart and increases oxygen demand does cause pain. This occurs because partial blockage of a coronary artery restricts blood flow to the myocardium. The term "stable" is attributed to this type of angina since the pattern or pain is predictable in the sense that it occurs only when the heart is under stress. While plaque is present and causing diminished blood flow, plaque growth is slow and collateral circulation may occur.

"Unstable" angina shares many of the characteristics of myocardial infarction and is included in the range of acute coronary syndromes. It is most commonly caused by atherosclerotic coronary artery disease. In this condition, there is rupture or disruption of the plaque, thrombosis, and vasoconstriction. It often precedes an MI, cardiac arrhythmias, or, in some cases, sudden death. Other names for this condition include acute coronary insufficiency, preinfarction angina, and intermediate syndrome.

Prinzmetal's (variant) angina is a rare form caused by vasospasm. Pain, which occurs most often at rest, may be intense but is treatable with medications.

Microvascular angina causes chest pain in patients seemingly without occlusions of a coronary artery. Pain results when the tiny blood vessels nourishing the heart, as well as the limbs, do not function property. This type of angina is also treated with medications.

In ICD-9-CM, unstable angina is classified to code 411.1 but only when the underlying cause is not identified and when surgery is not performed. If a patient is admitted for bypass surgery or angioplasty to avoid the progression of unstable angina to an infarction, an appropriate code reporting the underlying coronary atherosclerosis is reported first, with unstable angina reported as a secondary code. ICD-10-CM, however, has two subcategories that specifically classify atherosclerosis with angina using combination codes, making the assumption about a causal relationship between the two conditions. These codes are further classified according to whether the condition involves native coronary artery disease, a bypass graft, or a transplanted heart. In addition, ICD-10-CM specifies whether a spasm is documented, a factor not addressed in ICD-9-CM. The following table compares the coding of unstable angina with and without atherosclerotic heart disease in ICD-9-CM and ICD-10-CM.

The following table is not a complete mapping of all of the types of unstable angina and coronary atherosclerosis, but gives the coder an idea of what may be seen in ICD-10-CM. For detailed information on ICD-9-CM to ICD-10-CM mapping, see *Ingenix's ICD-10-CM Mappings*.

Coding for Unstable Angina and Coronary Atherosclerosis

ICD-9-CM		ICD-10-CM	
411.1	Intermediate coronary syndrome	I20.0	Unstable angina
		I25.110	Atherosclerotic heart disease of native coronary artery with unstable angina pectoris
		I25.710	Atherosclerosis of autologous vein coronary artery bypass graft(s) with unstable angina pectoris
		I25.720	Atherosclerosis of autologous artery coronary artery bypass graft(s) with unstable angina pectoris
		I25.730	Atherosclerosis of nonautologous biological coronary artery bypass graft(s) with unstable angina pectoris
		I25.750	Atherosclerosis of native coronary artery of transplanted heart with unstable angina
413.9	Other and unspecified angina pectoris	I20.8	Other forms of angina pectoris
		I20.9	Angina pectoris, unspecified
		I25.111	Atherosclerotic heart disease of native coronary artery with angina pectoris with documented spasm
		I25.118	Atherosclerotic heart disease of native coronary artery with other forms of angina pectoris
		I25.119	Atherosclerotic heart disease of native coronary artery with unspecified angina pectoris
		I25.701	Atherosclerosis of coronary artery bypass graft(s), unspecified, with angina pectoris with documented spasm
		I25.708	Atherosclerosis of coronary artery bypass graft(s), unspecified, with other forms of angina pectoris
414.01	Coronary atherosclerosis native coronary artery	I25.10	Atherosclerotic heart disease of native coronary artery without angina pectoris
		I25.110	Atherosclerotic heart disease of native coronary artery with unstable angina pectoris
		I25.111	Atherosclerotic heart disease of native coronary artery with angina pectoris with documented spasm
		I25.118	Atherosclerotic heart disease of native coronary artery with other forms of angina pectoris
		I25.119	Atherosclerotic heart disease of native coronary artery with unspecified angina pectoris
414.02	Coronary atherosclerosis autologous vein bypass graft	I25.710	Atherosclerosis of autologous vein coronary artery bypass graft(s) with unstable angina pectoris
		I25.711	Atherosclerosis of autologous vein coronary artery bypass graft(s) with angina pectoris with documented spasm
		I25.718	Atherosclerosis of autologous vein coronary artery bypass graft(s) with other forms of angina pectoris
		I25.719	Atherosclerosis of autologous vein coronary artery bypass graft(s) with unspecified angina pectoris

Atherosclerosis of Extremity Arteries

The primary cause of arterial disease of the lower extremities is atherosclerosis. Once the plaque begins to build up in the artery, not only is blood flow reduced, but the arterial walls become stiffer and unable to dilate. This means the leg muscles don't receive adequate blood and oxygen when demand is increased, such as by walking and exercising. Symptoms include pain, fatigue, aching, burning, and discomfort of the calves, feet, or thighs, which subside with rest. If the condition progresses, symptoms begin to appear sooner and during less strenuous activity. Pain and ulceration often limit physical activity. If the condition continues to progress, there is an inadequate supply of blood and oxygen at rest and symptoms do not resolve. Complications most often include unhealed ulcer, gangrene, and amputation of the affected limb.

As the disease progresses, patients may experience:

- Arterial bruits
- Atrophy of calf muscles
- Diminished blood pressure in the affected limb
- Hair loss on feet or legs
- Impotence
- Limb pulses that are weak or absent altogether
- Non-healing ulcers
- Pain and cramps in the legs at night
- Pain or tingling in the feet/toes so severe that the weight of clothes or bed sheets is painful
- Increased pain with leg elevation that improves when the leg is dangled
- Cyanotic or pale, shiny, or tight skin of the feet or toes
- Thickened toenails

Peripheral artery disease (PAD) is a common disorder that primarily affects men older than age 50. A history of any of the following conditions puts the individual at higher risk:

- Abnormal cholesterol level
- Cerebrovascular disease (stroke)
- Coronary artery disease
- Diabetes
- Heart disease (coronary artery disease)
- Hypertension
- Kidney disease with hemodialysis
- Smoking

Growth of an atherosclerotic lesion occurs in three stages. In the first stage, a fatty streak develops with no impediment to blood flow in the vessel. In the second stage, fibrous plaques form. Often located at arterial bifurcations, the lesion can, at this stage, impede blood flow. In the third stage, a complicated lesion develops where the plaque is distorted by calcification, hemorrhage, and mural thrombus. This can lead to embolism and is the underlying cause of vessel obstruction.

Coding atherosclerosis of the extremities is similar in ICD-9-CM and ICD-10-CM. Both systems specify the symptoms of:

- Intermittent *claudication*
- Pain at rest
- Ulceration
- Gangrene

Both classification systems also differentiate between atherosclerosis of a native artery, an autologous bypass graft, or a nonautologous biological bypass graft. However, ICD-10-CM requires the coder to indicate the affected leg (right or left), as well as the specific site of an ulcer (e.g., heel and midfoot or calf). ICD-10-CM also has specific codes to indicate bilateral disease. The following table compares ICD-9-CM and ICD-10-CM coding of atherosclerosis of a native artery of the extremities with an ulcer.

Coding for Atherosclerosis of Native Arteries of the Extremities

ICD-9-CM		ICD-10-CM	
440.23	Atherosclerosis of the extremities with ulceration	I70.231	Atherosclerosis of native arteries of right leg with ulceration of thigh
		I70.232	Atherosclerosis of native arteries of right leg with ulceration of calf
		I70.233	Atherosclerosis of native arteries of right leg with ulceration of ankle
		I70.234	Atherosclerosis of native arteries of right leg with ulceration of heel and midfoot
		I70.235	Atherosclerosis of native arteries of right leg with ulceration of other part of foot
		I70.238	Atherosclerosis of native arteries of right leg with ulceration of other part of lower right leg
		I70.239	Atherosclerosis of native arteries of right leg with ulceration of unspecified site
		I70.241	Atherosclerosis of native arteries of left leg with ulceration of thigh
		I70.242	Atherosclerosis of native arteries of left leg with ulceration of calf
		I70.243	Atherosclerosis of native arteries of left leg with ulceration of ankle
		I70.244	Atherosclerosis of native arteries of left leg with ulceration of heel and midfoot
		I70.245	Atherosclerosis of native arteries of left leg with ulceration of other part of foot
		I70.248	Atherosclerosis of native arteries of left leg with ulceration of other part of lower left leg
		I70.249	Atherosclerosis of native arteries of left leg with ulceration of unspecified site
		I70.25	Atherosclerosis of native arteries of other extremities with ulceration

Diseases of the Aorta

Like other arteries, the aorta and its major branches may also be affected by arteriosclerosis. In fact, the most common cause of thoracic aortic aneurysms, particularly in the descending part, is arteriosclerosis. Although this condition can be an expected part of the aging process, the condition is highly variable. In some patients, the loss of elasticity in the tissue results in dilation, which causes the aorta to become tortuous. On the other hand, advanced dilation may result in a ruptured aneurysm that leads to certain death.

DEFINITIONS

claudication. Lameness, pain, and weakness occurring in the arms or legs during exercise due to muscles not receiving the needed oxygen and nutrients.

INTERESTING A & P FACT

Peripheral emboli are atheroemboli that result from small abdominal aortic aneurysms (AAA), which produce livedo reticularis of the feet, or blue toe syndrome.

Figure 7.13: Thoracic and Abdominal Aortic Aneurysm

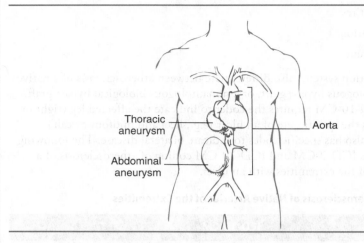

Arteriosclerosis may diminish blood flow to the aortic branches as well and result in a range of conditions due to insufficient blood flow to a given area. For instance, if the renal vessels are involved, the kidneys may become ischemic and possibly lead to renal failure.

Calcium deposits in the aorta also occur due to arteriosclerosis or other conditions. Treatment and outcome of arteriosclerosis vary.

Aortic Dissection

A dissecting aneurysm occurs when the middle arterial layer (media) deteriorates (medial necrosis). Hypertension and arteriosclerosis play a role in this process, causing further damage until a rupture occurs in the innermost arterial layer, which allows blood to fill the wall of the aorta, causing separation of the layers. When the rupture extends through the outermost wall, fatal hemorrhage occurs.

Aortic dissections are seen in individuals with hypertension or arteriosclerosis, or with a family history of aortic (or thoracic) dissection. Less often, it is seen in patients with congenital diseases such as Marfan's syndrome, Ehlers-Danlos syndrome, and congenital valvular disorders. Other conditions that may cause aortic dissection include Takayasu disease, giant cell arteritis, tertiary syphilis, relapsing polychondritis, fungal infections from heart valve surgeries, immunodeficiency, and intravenous drug abuse.

ICD-9-CM and ICD-10-CM classify aortic aneurysms and aortic dissection in much the same way: according to the specific site and whether a rupture or a dissection has occurred.

Venous Phlebitis and Thrombophlebitis

Venous thrombosis may occur in surface veins (superficial thrombophlebitis) or in the deeper veins (deep venous thrombosis, or DVT). When there is an injury to the most inner layer of the vein, hypercoagulability occurs, and a clot may form. The combination of these three conditions is referred to as the Virchow triad. Thrombophlebitis refers to a thrombus that causes vein inflammation (phlebitis) at the site of the injury, reducing venous flow (venous stasis). This condition may be chronic or acute in nature.

 CLINICAL NOTE

Two types of aortic dissections are recognized:

- **Type A:** Dissection to the ascending aorta; may be treated medically for a period of time with interventional catheterization or using open surgical techniques.
- **Type B:** Dissection of the descending aorta; may be treated medically with regular monitoring and medications that include antihypertensive and cholesterol lowering agents.

 CLINICAL NOTE

The terms thrombosis and thrombitis are often used interchangeably.

Figure 7.14: Venous System

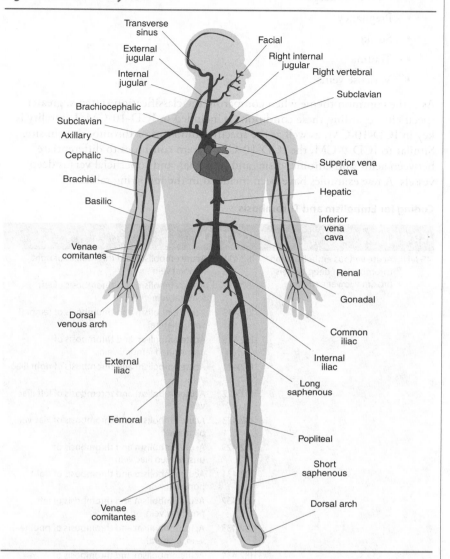

Embolism refers to a condition whereby a *thrombus* or a piece of one breaks off from where it has formed in the vein and migrates through the bloodstream. Emboli seldom develop with superficial thrombophlebitis. However, emboli that occur with DVT, most often found in the veins of the legs, is of utmost concern since they may travel to the lungs (pulmonary embolus), which demands emergent medical treatment to prevent death.

Although the greatest single risk factor for superficial venous thrombosis and DVT is a past medical history of these conditions, other risk factors include:

- Aging
- Abdominal cancer
- Blood coagulation disorders
- Extended bed rest or sitting (e.g., such as on an airplane)
- Heart failure
- Intravenous (IV) catheter usage/use of irritating medications in the IV

 DEFINITIONS

thrombus. Stationary blood clot inside a blood vessel.

- Oral contraceptives
- Pregnancy
- Stroke
- Trauma
- Varicose veins

As is the common theme when comparing the classification systems, greater specificity regarding these conditions is included in ICD-10-CM. Laterality is key in ICD-10-CM, as well as the specific embolism or thrombosis vein site. Similar to ICD-9-CM, the ICD-10-CM system continues to differentiate between acute and chronic, distal and proximal, and superficial versus deep vessels. A few examples have been included in the following tables.

Coding for Embolism and Thrombosis

ICD-9-CM		ICD-10-CM	
453.41	Acute venous embolism and thrombosis of deep vessels proximal lower extremity	I82.411	Acute embolism and thrombosis of right femoral vein
		I82.412	Acute embolism and thrombosis of left femoral vein
		I82.413	Acute embolism and thrombosis of femoral vein, bilateral
		I82.419	Acute embolism and thrombosis of unspecified femoral vein
		I82.421	Acute embolism and thrombosis of right iliac vein
		I82.422	Acute embolism and thrombosis of left iliac vein
		I82.423	Acute embolism and thrombosis of iliac vein, bilateral
		I82.429	Acute embolism and thrombosis of unspecified iliac vein
		I82.431	Acute embolism and thrombosis of right popliteal vein
		I82.432	Acute embolism and thrombosis of left popliteal vein
		I82.433	Acute embolism and thrombosis of popliteal vein, bilateral
		I82.439	Acute embolism and thrombosis of unspecified popliteal vein

Coding for Acute Venous Embolism and Thrombosis of Axillary Veins

ICD-9-CM		ICD-10-CM	
453.84	Acute Venous Embolism & Thrombosis Axillary veins	I82.a11	Acute embolism and thrombosis of right axillary vein
		I82.a12	Acute embolism and thrombosis of left axillary vein
		I82.a13	Acute embolism and thrombosis of axillary vein, bilateral
		I82.a19	Acute embolism and thrombosis of unspecified axillary vein

Varicose Veins

Varicose veins are abnormal, permanently distended, or stretched veins. Once the vein becomes thickened and tortuous, the affected parts of the veins are referred to as varicosities. Most often found in the legs, they may occur in any area of the body, such as hemorrhoids and esophageal varices.

Figure 7.15: Map of Major Veins

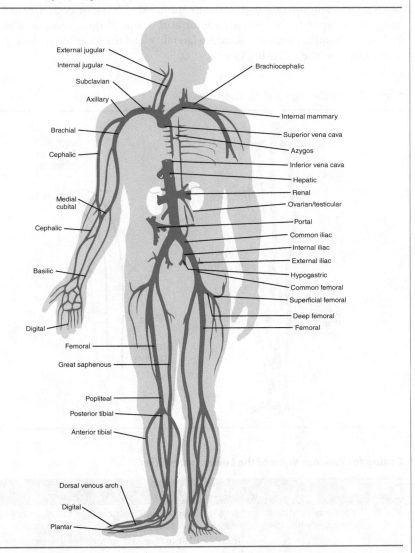

The superficial veins closest to the surface of the skin are the ones that most often develop varicosities. The largest superficial vein is the greater saphenous vein running from the ankle to the thigh on the medial aspect of the leg. Varicosities can also originate from the communicating veins that join the superficial veins to the deep veins.

Although there is much speculation as to why varicosities occur, it is thought to be due to damaged or defective valves in the veins. There are many factors associated with this condition, including:

- Age
- Obesity
- Pregnancy
- Previous leg surgery or trauma
- Spending too much time on one's feet

Although varicose veins of the lower extremities may be asymptomatic, they are often seen in conjunction with inflammation, skin ulcers, or both. Correct code assignment depends on the existence (or not) of one of these complications. ICD-10-CM adds detail by including laterality and the location of the leg ulcer, as is evident in the following table.

Figure 7.16: Veins of Lower Extremities

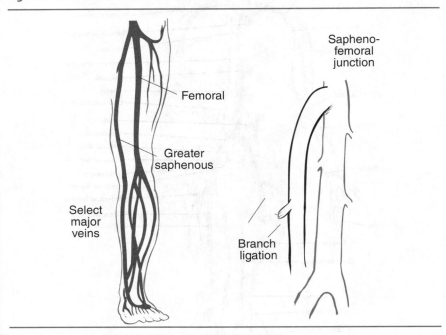

Coding for Varicose Veins of the Lower Extremities

ICD-9-CM		ICD-10-CM	
454.0	Varicose veins of lower extremities with ulcer	I83.001	Varicose veins of unspecified lower extremity with ulcer of thigh
		I83.002	Varicose veins of unspecified lower extremity with ulcer of calf
		I83.003	Varicose veins of unspecified lower extremity with ulcer of ankle
		I83.004	Varicose veins of unspecified lower extremity with ulcer of heel and midfoot
		I83.005	Varicose veins of unspecified lower extremity with ulcer other part of foot
		I83.008	Varicose veins of unspecified lower extremity with ulcer other part of lower leg
		I83.009	Varicose veins of unspecified lower extremity with ulcer of unspecified site
		I83.011	Varicose veins of right lower extremity with ulcer of thigh
		I83.012	Varicose veins of right lower extremity with ulcer of calf
	(Continued on next page)	I83.013	Varicose veins of right lower extremity with ulcer of ankle

ICD-9-CM	ICD-10-CM	
454.0 Varicose veins of lower extremities with ulcer *(Continued)*	I83.013	Varicose veins of right lower extremity with ulcer of ankle
	I83.014	Varicose veins of right lower extremity with ulcer of heel and midfoot
	I83.015	Varicose veins of right lower extremity with ulcer other part of foot
	I83.018	Varicose veins of right lower extremity with ulcer other part of lower leg
	I83.019	Varicose veins of right lower extremity with ulcer of unspecified site
	I83.021	Varicose veins of left lower extremity with ulcer of thigh
	I83.022	Varicose veins of left lower extremity with ulcer of calf
	I83.023	Varicose veins of left lower extremity with ulcer of ankle
	I83.024	Varicose veins of left lower extremity with ulcer of heel and midfoot
	I83.025	Varicose veins of left lower extremity with ulcer other part of foot
	I83.028	Varicose veins of left lower extremity with ulcer other part of lower leg
	I83.029	Varicose veins of left lower extremity with ulcer of unspecified site

Hypertension

Blood pressure is the measurement of the force exerted against the arterial walls produced by the left ventricle during contraction (systole), and pressure that remains in the arteries when the ventricle relaxes (diastole). Blood pressure readings are measured in millimeters of mercury (mmHg) and expressed as two numbers (e.g., 120/80). Either one or both of these numbers may be too high (hypertension). The difference between the two pressures, the systolic and the diastolic, is referred to as the pulse pressure. Normal pulse pressure is 40 mmHg, and if this is increased it provides valuable information about the health of the cardiovascular system. Atherosclerosis is one of the conditions that causes increased pulse pressure. Hypertension is often associated with arterial disease, as well as an increased risk of stroke, heart attack, and heart failure.

Systolic pressure is considered:

- High if over 140 mmHg for the majority of the time
- Normal if below 120 mmHg for the majority of the time

Diastolic pressure is considered:

- High if over 90 mmHg for the majority of the time
- Normal if below 80 mmHg for the majority of the time

Prehypertension may be a concern when:

- Systolic pressure is between 120 and 139 for the majority of the time
- Diastolic blood pressure is between 80 and 89 for the majority of the time

The most common type of hypertension is primary hypertension, previously referred to as "essential" hypertension. Primary hypertension is identified in 85 to 95 percent of all cases, and has no known cause. Although genetics may predispose an individual to this condition, the exact process is not known.

Environmental factors such as obesity, dietary sodium, and stress appear to affect only those individuals with genetic predisposition.

Benign hypertension is defined as a mild to moderate elevation of blood pressure for a protracted period but with no damage to target organs (kidneys, retina, heart).

Risk factors include:

- African American heritage
- Diabetes
- Family history
- High levels of stress or anxiety
- Obesity
- High dietary sodium intake
- Smoking

Hypertension with an identified cause (secondary hypertension) is usually due to a renal disorder. Usually no symptoms develop unless hypertension is severe or long-standing. Diagnosis is by sphygmomanometry. Tests may be done to determine cause, assess damage, and identify other cardiovascular risk factors. Treatment involves lifestyle changes and medication.

High blood pressure resulting from another medical condition or due to a medication is secondary hypertension. This condition may be attributed to conditions such as:

- Atherosclerosis
- Autoimmune diseases
- Chronic kidney disease
- Coarctation of the aorta
- Cocaine use
- Connective tissue disease
- Diabetes with kidney damage
- Endocrine disorders (e.g., adrenal tumors [pheochromocytoma, aldosteronism],Cushing syndrome, thyroid disease)
- Excessive alcohol use
- Medications:
  - appetite suppressants
  - cold medications
  - corticosteroids
  - migraine medications
  - oral contraceptives
- Polycystic kidney disease
- Polynephritis
- Renovascular disease
- Stenosis of renal artery

Examining the dilated retina is integral to assessing damage from hypertension. Examination of the retinal microvascular allows a view of the inner arterial and venous systems and can detect the onset of systemic diseases before symptoms appear. Manifestations of arteriosclerosis include narrowing of the arterioles and sclerosis of the vessels. Cotton wool spots and flame-shaped hemorrhages are often found in hypertensive retinopathy. Edema of the disc indicates malignant hypertension. In many instances, the retinal examination provides the first clue the patient has hypertension.

A hypertensive emergency exists when blood pressure is high enough to damage target organs, such as the cardiovascular system, kidneys, and the central nervous system. A diagnosis of malignant hypertension includes the presence of *papilledema*, with swelling of the optic disc in the eye, caused by an increase in intracranial pressure. Treatment is directed at lowering the patient's blood pressure as quickly as possible. Blood pressure is usually in the 250/150 range.

Accelerated hypertension is a recent major increase over the patient's baseline blood pressure, not associated with target organ damage. Fundoscopic examination often reveals flame-shaped hemorrhages or soft exudates, but without papilledema. Blood pressure is usually in the 220/120 range.

Over a period of time, hypertension damages the brain, cardiovascular system, and the kidneys, increasing the risk of coronary artery disease (CAD), myocardial infarction (MI), renal failure, and cerebrovascular accidents, particularly the hemorrhagic type. As generalized arteriolosclerosis develops, atheromatous plaques form more rapidly in the arteries. Arteriolosclerosis, typified by medial hypertrophy, hyperplasia, and hyalinization, is most readily evident in small arterioles, particularly in the eyes and kidneys. In the kidneys, as these changes continue to constrict the arterial flow, total peripheral vascular resistance increases, and hypertension worsens.

Left ventricular hypertrophy may occur, with resulting diastolic dysfunction. Ultimately, the ventricle dilates, causing dilated cardiomyopathy and heart failure secondary to systolic dysfunction. Nearly all patients with abdominal aortic aneurysms also have hypertension, and thoracic aortic dissection is often an effect of hypertension.

Other complications may include:

- Blood vessel damage (arteriosclerosis)
- Brain damage
- Congestive heart failure
- Chronic kidney disease
- Heart attack
- Hypertensive heart disease
- Loss of vision
- Peripheral artery disease
- Pregnancy complications

Fortunately, in the majority of cases, hypertension can be controlled with medications and lifestyle changes.

There are a wide variety of causes, types, and conditions associated with hypertension, which can make hypertension a challenge from the coding perspective. At first glance, there seems to be a direct, one-to-one correlation between ICD-9-CM codes for hypertension and the equivalent codes in ICD-10-CM. However, comparing the terminology in the codes reveals several important differences. In ICD-9-CM, several categories are available to report "benign" and "malignant" hypertension, such as:

 DEFINITIONS

papilledema. Swelling of the optic disc that is caused by intracranial pressure.

401.0	Essential hypertension, malignant
401.1	Essential hypertension, benign
402.00	Hypertensive heart disease, malignant, without heart failure
402.01	Hypertensive heart disease, malignant, with heart failure
402.10	Hypertensive heart disease, benign, without heart failure
402.11	Hypertensive heart disease, benign, with heart failure
403.00	Hypertensive chronic kidney disease, malignant, with chronic kidney disease stage I—stage IV, or unspecified
403.01	Hypertensive chronic kidney disease, malignant, with chronic kidney disease stage V or end stage renal disease
403.10	Hypertensive chronic kidney disease, benign, with chronic kidney disease stage I—stage IV, or unspecified
403.11	Hypertensive chronic kidney disease, benign, with chronic kidney disease stage V or end-stage renal disease
404.00	Hypertensive heart and chronic kidney disease, benign, without heart failure and with chronic kidney disease stage I through stage IV, or unspecified
404.01	Hypertensive heart and chronic kidney disease, malignant, without heart failure and with chronic kidney disease stage I through stage IV, or unspecified
404.02	Hypertensive heart and chronic kidney disease, malignant, without heart failure and with chronic kidney disease stage I through stage IV, or unspecified
404.03	Hypertensive heart and chronic kidney disease, malignant, without heart failure and with chronic kidney disease stage I through stage IV, or unspecified
404.10	Hypertensive heart and chronic kidney disease, benign, without heart failure and with chronic kidney disease stage I through stage IV, or unspecified
404.11	Hypertensive heart and chronic kidney disease, benign, with heart failure and with chronic kidney disease stage I through stage IV, or unspecified
404.12	Hypertensive heart and chronic kidney disease, benign, without heart failure and with chronic kidney disease stage V, or end stage renal disease
404.13	Hypertensive heart and chronic kidney disease, benign, with heart failure and with chronic kidney disease stage V, or end stage renal disease

The ICD-10-CM classification system, however, has streamlined the hypertension classification and related comorbid conditions. Rather than having separate subcategories for "benign" and "malignant" hypertension, these terms have been integrated into an inclusion note under category I10 Essential hypertension. The following table demonstrates how some of these same codes appear in ICD-10-CM.

Coding for Hypertension

ICD-9-CM		ICD-10-CM	
401.0	Essential hypertension, malignant	I10	Essential primary hypertension
401.1	Essential hypertension, benign		
401.9	Essential hypertension, unspecified		
402.01	Hypertensive heart disease, malignant, with heart failure	I11.0	Hypertensive heart disease with heart failure
402.11	Hypertensive heart disease, benign, with heart failure		
402.91	Hypertensive heart disease, unspecified, with heart failure		
402.00	Hypertensive heart disease, malignant, without heart failure	I11.9	Hypertensive heart disease without heart failure
402.10	Hypertensive heart disease, benign, without heart failure		
402.90	Unspecified hypertensive heart disease without heart failure		
403.01	Hypertensive chronic kidney disease, malignant, with chronic kidney disease stage V or end stage renal disease	I12.0	Hypertensive heart and chronic kidney disease with stage 5 chronic kidney disease or end-stage renal disease.
403.11	Hypertensive chronic kidney disease, benign, with chronic kidney disease stage V or end-stage renal disease		
403.91	Hypertensive chronic kidney disease, unspecified, with chronic kidney disease stage V or end-stage renal disease		

Cerebrovascular Disease

Atherosclerosis of the Precerebral and Cerebral Arteries

The precerebral arteries include the basilar, carotid, and vertebral arteries. The carotid emerges from the aorta as the common carotid artery and bifurcates into the internal and external carotid arteries. This bifurcation is a common site for atherosclerosis, which causes 90 percent of all extracranial carotid lesions. Atherosclerosis may result in narrowing of the common or internal artery. It may become a source of embolization where some of the plaque breaks off and travels to smaller blood vessels in the brain. Once lodged in the small vessel, it can inhibit the flow of blood to the brain temporarily (e.g., transient ischemic attack, or TIA) or permanently (e.g., stroke).

Additional causes of carotid lesions include:

- Aneurysms
- Arteritis
- Bends and twists of the vessel
- Carotid dissection
- Fibromuscular dysplasia
- Radiation
- Vasospasm

ICD-9-CM classifies occlusion and stenosis of the precerebral arteries to category 433, with a fourth digit designating the specific artery involved and a fifth digit indicating if a cerebral infarction occurred.

DEFINITIONS

atheroma. Also referred to as plaque, atherosclerotic plaque, and arterial plaque, it is the buildup of fatty deposit in the innermost lining (intima) of an artery, caused by atherosclerosis.

embolism. Obstruction of a blood vessel resulting from an embolus traveling through the bloodstream. Types of emboli include air, gas, and fat.

thrombosis. Condition arising from the presence or formation of blood clots within a blood vessel that may cause vascular obstruction and insufficient oxygenation.

ICD-10-CM breaks this down even more to indicate if the stenosis or occlusion occurs in the artery on the left side or the right side, and even the specific portion of the artery involved (e.g., left anterior cerebral artery, right middle cerebral artery). It also specifies the arteries involved when pathology is present in bilateral arteries.

When discussing these types of infarcts, it is important to understand the terminology that describes the different mechanisms of vessel blockage. *Thrombosis* occurs when a blood clot forms within a vessel. An *embolism* occurs when an embolus travels through the bloodstream and becomes lodged in a blood vessel, blocking blood flow. Some types of embolism include air emboli, gas emboli, or fat emboli.

ICD-9-CM classifies infarction due to occlusion of one of the precerebral arteries by a thrombosis or embolism to category 433, with includes notes guiding the right code choice. In ICD-10-CM, however, codes differentiate between an infarction of a specific artery due to one of these conditions, as demonstrated in the following table.

Coding for Infarction of the Carotid Artery

ICD-9-CM		ICD-10-CM	
433.11	Occlusion and stenosis of carotid artery with infarction	I63.031	Cerebral infarction due to thrombosis of right carotid artery
		I63.032	Cerebral infarction due to thrombosis of left carotid artery
		I63.039	Cerebral infarction due to thrombosis of unspecified carotid artery
		I63.131	Cerebral infarction due to embolism of right carotid artery
		I63.132	Cerebral infarction due to embolism of left carotid artery
		I63.139	Cerebral infarction due to embolism of unspecified carotid artery
		I63.231	Cerebral infarction due to unspecified occlusion or stenosis of right carotid arteries
		I63.232	Cerebral infarction due to unspecified occlusion or stenosis of left carotid arteries
		I63.239	Cerebral infarction due to unspecified occlusion or stenosis of unspecified carotid arteries

Intracranial Hemorrhage

An intracranial hemorrhage, which may occur at any age and can be due to a wide variety of conditions, is always a medical emergency that requires quick resolution to minimize severe disability due to brain damage or death. The specific location of the bleed and the underlying cause determine the patient's symptoms, the severity of the brain damage, and resulting debility, if any.

Most often due to abnormal arteries found at the base of the brain (cerebral aneurysms), subarachnoid hemorrhage refers to bleeding that occurs due to the rupture of a blood vessel just on the outside of the brain tissue itself and within the skull. Symptoms include a sudden headache, very intense neck pain, and nausea and vomiting. The headache is frequently described as the worst headache of one's life or a thunderclap headache. The rising pressure can quickly result in coma or death. The underlying cause of the hemorrhaging may be traumatic or nontraumatic, with the nontraumatic type being the less common of the two.

ICD-9-CM classifies subarachnoid hemorrhage, nontraumatic, to category 430 and traumatic subarachnoid hemorrhage to category 852. ICD-10-CM, however, goes beyond the traumatic versus nontraumatic classification by identifying the specific vessel that ruptures, as seen in the following table.

Coding for Subarachnoid Hemorrhage

ICD-9-CM		ICD-10-CM	
430	Subarachnoid hemorrhage	I60.00	Nontraumatic subarachnoid hemorrhage from unspecified carotid siphon and bifurcation
		I60.01	Nontraumatic subarachnoid hemorrhage from right carotid siphon and bifurcation
		I60.02	Nontraumatic subarachnoid hemorrhage from left carotid siphon and bifurcation
		I60.10	Nontraumatic subarachnoid hemorrhage from unspecified middle cerebral artery
		I60.11	Nontraumatic subarachnoid hemorrhage from right middle cerebral artery
		I60.12	Nontraumatic subarachnoid hemorrhage from left middle cerebral artery
		I60.20	Nontraumatic subarachnoid hemorrhage from unspecified anterior communicating artery
		I60.21	Nontraumatic subarachnoid hemorrhage from right anterior communicating artery
		I60.22	Nontraumatic subarachnoid hemorrhage from left anterior communicating artery
		I60.30	Nontraumatic subarachnoid hemorrhage from unspecified posterior communicating artery
		I60.31	Nontraumatic subarachnoid hemorrhage from right posterior communicating artery
		I60.32	Nontraumatic subarachnoid hemorrhage from left posterior communicating artery
		I60.50	Nontraumatic subarachnoid hemorrhage from unspecified vertebral artery
		I60.51	Nontraumatic subarachnoid hemorrhage from right vertebral artery
		I60.52	Nontraumatic subarachnoid hemorrhage from left vertebral artery
		I60.6	Nontraumatic subarachnoid hemorrhage from other intracranial arteries
		I60.7	Nontraumatic subarachnoid hemorrhage from unspecified intracranial artery
		I60.8	Other nontraumatic subarachnoid hemorrhage
		I60.9	Nontraumatic subarachnoid hemorrhage, unspecified

An intracerebral hemorrhage, also referred to as an intraparenchymal hemorrhage, intracranial hematoma, or simply ICH, occurs when a blood vessel that is weak or diseased erupts in the brain. The resulting pressure from the blood damages brain cells, and coma or death may occur. This happens most often in the *basal ganglia, brainstem, cerebellum,* or *cortex.* Although this condition is most frequently caused by hypertension, other causes include:

- Aberrant blood vessels, such as arteriovenous malformations (AVM)

- Blood-clotting deficiencies

- Infection

- Traumatic injury

- Tumors

 DEFINITIONS

basal ganglia. Area found at the base of the brain comprising clusters of neurons (nerve cells) that control movement and coordination.

brainstem. Area of the brain that connects the spinal cord to the forebrain and cerebrum; comprises the medulla oblongata, pons Varolii, and midbrain.

cerebellum. Portion of the brain in the rear cranial fossa behind the brainstem responsible for movement coordination.

cerebral cortex. Outermost layer of gray matter of the brain, made up of a collection of nerve cell bodies responsible for higher functions of the brain, such as sensation, thought, reasoning, and memory, and the movement of voluntary muscle.

cerebrum. Primary portion of the brain in the upper part of the cranium that is the largest part of the central nervous system. It is divided into two hemispheres connected by the corpus callosum, with the hemispheres divided into the frontal, parietal, temporal, occipital, and insular lobes. The cerebrum is responsible for intelligence, personality, motor function, planning and organization, and interpretation of sensory input.

parenchymal. Specific fundamental tissue of an organ as distinguished from its connective or supporting tissue.

DEFINITIONS

aphasia. Partial or total loss of the ability to comprehend language or communicate through speaking, the written word, or sign language. Aphasia may result from stroke, injury, Alzheimer's disease, or other disorder. Common types of aphasia include expressive, receptive, anomic, global, and conduction.

apraxia. Impaired sequencing of motor skills. Apraxia can be used to describe a variety of symptoms, from an awkward gait to anomalous speech.

ataxia. Defect in muscular coordination, seen especially when voluntary muscular movements are attempted.

cognitive. Having to do with being aware by drawing from knowledge, such as judgment, reason, perception, and memory.

cortical. Pertaining to the cortex, which is the outer portion of an organ. In the brain it refers to the outer part of the *cerebrum*.

dysarthria. Difficulty pronouncing words.

dysphagia. Difficulty and pain upon swallowing. Common causes of dysphagia are esophagitis, Barrett's esophagus, or late effect of a stroke.

hemianopsia. Loss of partial vision or complete blindness in half of the visual field of one (unilateral hemianopsia) or both (bilateral hemianopsia) eyes.

hemiplegia. Paralysis of one side of the body.

monoplegia. Loss or impairment of motor function in one arm or one leg.

subcortical. Pertaining to the part of the brain below the *cebral cortex*.

Intracerebral hemorrhage accounts for 10 to 15 percent of all strokes. This type of stroke is associated with a much higher rate of mortality than that of the more common acute ischemic stroke, caused by thrombosis or embolism.

Intracerebral hemorrhages (nontraumatic) are classified to category 430 in ICD-9-CM, and traumatic hemorrhages are classified to category 851, regardless of where the bleeding occurs in the brain. ICD-10-CM classifies intracerebral hemorrhages according to whether the bleed was traumatic or nontraumatic, but also designates the specific part of the brain in which the bleed occurred for nontraumatic bleeds.

Coding for Intracerebral Hemorrhage

ICD-9-CM		ICD-10-CM	
431	Intracerebral hemorrhage	I61.0	Nontraumatic intracerebral hemorrhage in hemisphere, *subcortical*
		I61.1	Nontraumatic intracerebral hemorrhage in hemisphere, *cortical*
		I61.2	Nontraumatic intracerebral hemorrhage in hemisphere, unspecified
		I61.3	Nontraumatic intracerebral hemorrhage in brain stem
		I61.4	Nontraumatic intracerebral hemorrhage in cerebellum
		I61.5	Nontraumatic intracerebral hemorrhage, intraventricular
		I61.6	Nontraumatic intracerebral hemorrhage, multiple localized
		I61.8	Other nontraumatic intracerebral hemorrhage
		I61.9	Nontraumatic intracerebral hemorrhage, unspecified

Residual Effects of Cerebrovascular Disease

When a brain injury occurs due to a stroke or other type of cerebrovascular disease or due to a traumatic injury to the brain, residual effects can occur according to the severity and the site of the brain injury. This includes paralysis; speech and language problems, such as *aphasia, dysarthria,* and *dysphasia;* and *cognitive* defects. For both coding classification systems, these residual neurological deficits are reported in addition to the underlying brain injury code regardless of when the deficit occurs. Once again, ICD-10-CM classifies these conditions with greater specificity, including *hemiplegia* and *monoplegia* for which ICD-10-CM indicates if the left or right side or limb is dominant. ICD-9-CM simply refers to the dominant side, with no distinction between right and left. Speech deficits are also classified in much more detail in ICD-10-CM, specifying the underlying cause of the condition, as indicated in the following table.

Coding for Speech and Language Deficits

ICD-9-CM	ICD-10-CM	
438.13 Dysarthria	I69.Ø22	Dysarthria following nontraumatic subarachnoid hemorrhage
	I69.122	Dysarthria following nontraumatic intracerebral hemorrhage
	I69.222	Dysarthria following other nontraumatic intracranial hemorrhage
	I69.322	Dysarthria following cerebral infarction
	I69 822	Dysarthria following other cerebrovascular disease
	I69 922	Dysarthria following unspecified cerebrovascular disease
438.14 *Fluency disorder*	I69.Ø23	Fluency disorder following nontraumatic subarachnoid hemorrhage
	I69.123	Fluency disorder following nontraumatic intracerebral hemorrhage
	I69.223	Fluency disorder following other nontraumatic intracranial hemorrhage
	I69.323	Fluency disorder following cerebral infarction
	I69.823	Fluency disorder following other cerebrovascular disease
	I69.923	Fluency disorder following unspecified cerebrovascular disease

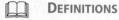 **DEFINITIONS**

fluency disorder. Interruption in the flow of speech, including stuttering due to CVA that impedes communication. Fluency is typified by repetitious sounds and syllables, and anomalous protraction of sounds of speech.

Summary

The cardiovascular system houses some of the most important components needed for day-to-day survival. The heart and blood vessels in the circulatory system provide oxygen-rich blood, nutrients such as amino acids and electrolytes, and important hormones to all of the body's cells and carry off carbon dioxide and other waste products of metabolism. In addition, the cardiovascular system stabilizes body temperature and pH. It makes sense that a system so important to day-to-day survival would be complex, and it is critical that coders understand the function of various parts of the circulatory system in order to code efficiently and effectively under the ICD-10-CM classification system.

Chapter 8

Blood and Blood-Forming Organs

Anatomic Overview

Blood is a *viscous* liquid that the heart pumps through the blood vessels as described in the cardiovascular chapter. It is unique in that it is the only fluid-type tissue in the human body. Its many purposes can be divided into three main functions:

- Transportation
- Regulation
- Protection

The blood travels throughout the body and serves as the transport mechanism for the distribution of oxygen, nutrients, and hormones to the cells and tissues of the entire body. It also carries away the metabolic waste from these structures to the appropriate organ or system for disposal. By doing this, the blood regulates the pH and fluid volumes of the body. Moving throughout the body constantly, it also helps to maintain the body's temperature. There are also multiple types of individual cells within the blood that provide protective functions, such as fighting infection and *hemostasis*.

Due to its many functions, blood has many unique parts. There are formed elements, consisting of red blood cells, white blood cells, and platelets, and plasma, in which the formed elements "float." The formed elements all originate from stem cells in the bone marrow. These stem cells, or hemocytoblasts, can grow into a variety of specialized cell types. Two types of hemocytoblasts that evolve into blood cells: myeloid and lymphoid. Myeloid stem cells eventually form into red blood cells, platelets, and some white blood cells. Lymphoid stem cells become a highly-specialized type of white blood cell known as a lymphocyte, which is discussed in further detail later in this chapter. It is important to note that most blood cells do not divide but are destroyed and replaced by new cells that are formed in the bone marrow.

The composition of blood is obvious in a sample that is left sitting—clotting is prevented as the blood separates, leaving the red blood cells at the bottom, the white bloods cells and platelets in the middle, also called the buffy coat, and the plasma on top. For laboratory blood work, this separation is performed much quicker via *centrifuge*. Being able to separate blood is important in detecting disease and overall health, as each of these blood constituents is unique in structure, function, and life cycle, and a variance in any of these can reveal a disease or disorder. Recognizing and understanding the functions of each of the blood constituents is important to the proper coding of abnormalities that affect the blood and associated organs.

Red Blood Cells

Red blood cells (RBC), or erythrocytes, make up more than 99 percent of the formed elements. These cells travel throughout the body delivering oxygen and removing some of the carbon dioxide cells release. Normal RBCs are dish-shaped—round with a concave depression in the center. Because of its

DEFINITIONS

centrifuge. Machine used to simulate gravitational effects or centrifugal force to separate substances of different densities.

hemostasis. Interruption of blood flow or the cessation or arrest of bleeding.

viscous. Pertaining to something thick, sticky, or glutinous.

INTERESTING A & P FACT

Bone marrow produces an average of an ounce of blood every day, which is approximately 100 billion new cells every day.

dome shape, RBCs can squeeze into even the smallest capillary to perform its function. The depression serves two functions: it increases the surface area in which the diffusion of gases can take place and places the surface closer to the protein molecules that carry oxygen. The protein molecules, known as *hemoglobin*, are responsible for the blood's color. When the RBCs are carrying oxygen, the blood appears bright red; when the hemoglobin is de-oxygenated, the blood appears blue when viewed through blood vessel walls.

Figure 8.1: Red Blood Cells

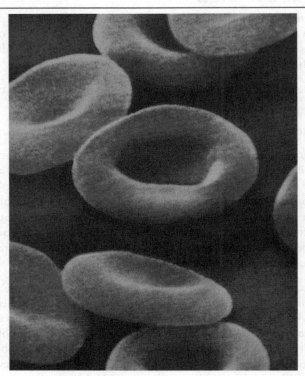

©Bill Longcore/Photo Researchers, Inc.

After about 100 to 120 days in circulation, a red blood cell begins to break down. The cell becomes fragile and brittle, and the hemoglobin becomes less effective. As they move throughout the smaller vessels, the cells begin to fragment. This happens most often in the extremely small vessels of the spleen, which is why the spleen is sometimes referred to as the "red blood cell graveyard." The fragments and ruptured RBCs are then destroyed by *macrophages*. Hemoglobin goes through multiple decomposition phases, resulting in iron that is transported back to the liver for storage and to the bone marrow for later use in producing new hemoglobin. Other byproducts are eventually converted into bilirubin.

RBCs also have surface molecules called antigens and antibodies. Two of these molecules are Rh group and blood type group. These are important in medicine today as they are responsible for determining blood compatibility. If blood is not compatible during a transfusion, the blood could clump, causing *agglutination*.

📖 **DEFINITIONS**

agglutination. Clumping together of cells due to the binding of agglutinin (a protein) molecules on the surface of each cell.

hemoglobin. Oxygen-carrying component of the red blood cell.

macrophage. Type of white blood cell.

The blood type group is determined by identifying up to two antigens on the surface of an erythrocyte. These antigens are known as antigen A and antigen B. The absence or presence of these determine the four blood types:

- **A:** Antigen A is present.
- **B:** Antigen B is present.
- **AB:** Both antigens are present.
- **O:** Neither antigen is present.

Figure 8.2: Blood Types

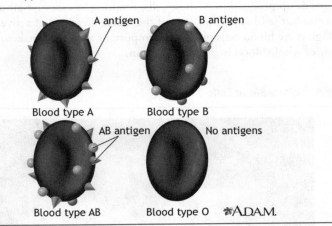

Babies are born without any of these antigens, but two to eight months after birth, the body develops its blood type and, in response, also develops antibodies that float in the plasma that correspond with the antigen. These antibodies attack whichever antigen the body did *not* produce. If the patient develops antigen A, antibody or anti-B is formed; if antigen B is developed, anti-A is formed. When antigens A and B are present, no antibodies are produced. When neither antigen is present, both anti-A and anti-B are formed. These antibodies cause blood to react when an antigen comes into contact with an antibody of the same type (e.g., anti-A attacks antigen A-covered RBCs). These combinations allow only certain blood types to be transfused to other blood types, as is demonstrated in the following table.

Blood Type	Acceptable Blood Type for Transfusion
A	A, O
B	B, O
AB	A, B, AB, O
O	O

> **CLINICAL NOTE**
>
> Blood type O is a universal donor because it is accepted by any blood type. Blood type AB is a universal recipient as it can accept any type of blood.

Rh factor is not as straightforward as blood type. There are many types of Rh antigens attached to the erythrocyte and if any of these are present, the blood is considered Rh-positive. If none are present, it is considered Rh-negative. The main difference between these types of antigens and the blood type is that Rh-negative blood does not automatically develop Rh antibodies (anti-Rh). An Rh-negative patient develops anti-Rh only when exposed to Rh-positive blood, therefore making a reaction unlikely the first time the patient is exposed. However, once the body develops the anti-Rh, the blood reacts if exposed again. An example of this occurs during pregnancy. If an Rh-negative mother carries an

Rh-positive baby, the mother's body develops anti-Rh. This may not impact the first pregnancy, but if the Rh-negative mother carries a second Rh-positive baby, the mother's anti-Rh attacks the Rh-positive red blood cells of the fetus.

White Blood Cells

Unlike red blood cells, there is more than one type of white blood cell (WBC), but they all share the same basic function, to fight infection. Also known as leukocytes, most of their work is performed outside of the bloodstream via *diapedesis*, but they are transported in the blood. Leukocytes are drawn together en masse by chemicals released by damaged tissue or other WBCs, to destroy foreign bodies such as infectious organisms, toxins, or tumor cells. The body then speeds up production of these cells, resulting in excessive amounts of leukocytes in the bloodstream, one of the first indications of active infections. Although these blood cells play a very important role, they make up less than 1 percent of whole blood in a healthy person.

Figure 8.3: White Blood Cells

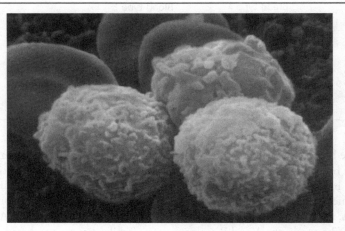

©Dr. Amar/Photo Researchers, Inc.

DEFINITIONS

cytoplasm. All of the substances of a cell except the nucleus.

diapedesis. Passage of blood cells through the walls of blood vessels without damage to the cell or vessel.

granular. Microscopically appearing to have particles resembling sand on its surface.

phagocytosis. Engulfing and ingesting bacteria or other foreign bodies.

There are five types of WBCs that are first classified by the nature of the cell's *cytoplasm*. Some cells have a *granular* cytoplasm and are known as granulocytes. These cells are usually spherical and twice the size of a red blood cell. They have a short lifespan of approximately 12 hours. There are three types of granulocytes: neutrophils, eosinophils, and basophils.

Neutrophils are the "bacteria slayers," being able to ingest and destroy many types of bacteria and some fungi. These types of cells are chemically attracted to inflammation and are usually the first of the leukocytes to arrive at an infection site. Note that immature neutrophils are commonly found in a blood sample, known as *bands*. Bands increase in number during an active infection as the body is producing and releasing as many WBCs as it can to fight off the infection. When the number of aggregate WBCs, neutrophils, and bands all increase significantly, it is known as a "shift to the left" and is highly indicative of an active infection.

Eosinophils make up only 1 to 3 percent of circulating white blood cells. These cells are responsible for moderating allergic reactions by deactivating inflammatory chemicals released and decreasing the immune response by *phagocytosis* of antigen-antibody reactions. They defend against parasites that are too large for phagocytosis. They surround and chemically attack these organisms, dissolving them.

The least type of granulocyte is called a basophil. This type of cell is actively involved in the inflammatory process. Basophils gather at sites of damaged tissues where they release histamine, a chemical that opens the blood vessels to promote blood flow and attract other leukocytes. They also excrete heparin, a naturally occurring chemical that inhibits blood clotting.

Cells that do not have a visibly granular cytoplasm are called agranulocytes. Lymphocytes and monocytes are the two classifications of agranulocytes. Although similar in structure, their functions are completely different.

Lymphocytes are the second most numerous type of leukocyte in the body; however, most of them are not found in the bloodstream. These cells can live for years in the body's lymphoid tissue (e.g., lymph nodes, spleen, etc.), hence the name lymphocyte. There are two types: T-cells and B-cells. T-cells specifically target virus-infected and tumor cells. B-cells eventually become plasma cells, which produce antibodies. More information on lymphocytes can be found in the lymphatic system chapter.

Monocytes are the largest of the blood cells. They are extremely active in the phagocytosis of bacteria, dead cells, and other foreign bodies. When a monocyte leaves the bloodstream, it becomes known as a *macrophage*.

When infectious organisms, dead cells, and leukocytes gather together at an inflamed area, a white viscous fluid, called pus, results. The pus remains while the organisms are present and is eventually absorbed into surrounding tissues if not expelled otherwise.

Platelets

Platelets, also known as thrombocytes, are different from the other formed elements found in the blood in that they are not cells in the strict sense, as they lack a nucleus. A platelet is a fragment of cytoplasm that has chipped off a large cell, called a megakaryocyte, found in the red bone marrow. The fragments that are too large to be considered platelets are diminished in size when they pass through the blood vessels of the lungs. When a blood vessel is damaged, platelets stick to the compromised area, forming a temporary barrier, and release serotonin, a vasoconstrictor that contracts the blood vessel and reduces blood flow to the area.

Figure 8.4: Platelets

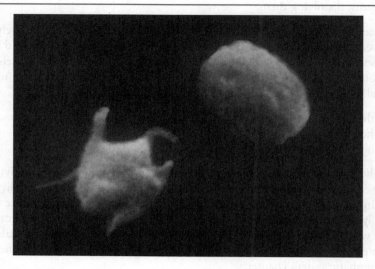

© Kenneth Ewards/Photo Researchers, Inc.

Plasma

Plasma is a straw-colored fluid in which the formed elements are suspended. The plasma carries the formed elements throughout the body. The liquid consists of electrolytes, water, wastes, nutrients, vitamins, hormones, gases, and proteins. The constant adjusting of the different components of the plasma maintains an acceptable pH of blood. The organs secrete and absorb the different substances. For example, the plasma picks up glucose at the small intestine and drops it off at the liver, where it is stored or converted to fat.

Hemostasis

As discussed in the introduction, an important function of blood is hemostasis. This process is a complex reaction to damage to or a break in a blood vessel. There are three mechanisms that occur in quick succession to stop bleeding as quickly as possible. First, the vessel induces a local spasm of its smooth-muscle lining, constricting the flow of blood to the area to allow more time for the other two responses to occur. At this point, platelets flood the area and form a platelet plug, temporarily sealing it. To form the plug, the normally smooth platelet cells begin to swell and grow spike-like processes to stick to other platelets and the exposed collagen fibers of the endothelial lining of the vessel. The last step, referred to as coagulation, takes more than 30 substances, called factors, to complete. During this stage, the liquid blood forms a gel covering the wound, otherwise known as a clot. Clot-forming factors are known as procoagulants. These are numbered I–XIII (i.e., factor VIII, factor X) in the order they were discovered. Factors that inhibit clotting are known as anticoagulants. The formation of a clot and healing of a wound depend on a delicate balance between these two types of factors. As the chemical reactions progress, fibrin strands are produced that form a web to catch the platelets and trap the other formed elements to form a clot.

Figure 8.5: Blood Coagulation

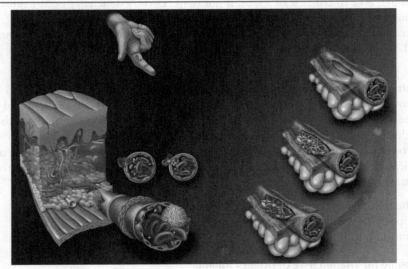

©BSIP/Photo Researchers, Inc.

Once a clot is established and the blood flow is stopped, the clot begins to retract, pulling the edges of the wound together. As the wound is being closed by this process, the platelets involved release a substance that stimulates regrowth of the surrounding original tissue. Because a blood clot is a temporary fix, the body also begins to dissolve it via a process called fibrinolysis. Eventually, the clot is completely absorbed and the wound is closed permanently by new tissue.

Anatomy and Physiology and the ICD-10-CM Code Set

Due to the overall diversity in the composition of the blood and its interaction with other organs and systems, there are many diseases that can affect the blood. Each of the formed blood elements has its own structure and function; each type of blood cell also has its own diseases and abnormalities. In many cases, ICD-9-CM and ICD-10-CM are similar to each other in the blood and blood forming organs chapters. In fact, there is a 69 percent one-to-one equivalent mapping between the synonymous chapters of the two classification systems.

Diseases of the Red Blood Cells

The major differences between the two classification systems regarding diseases of the red blood cells arise with the coding of *anemia*. There are many underlying causes of anemia, and ICD-9-CM effectively categorizes most general forms of anemia. There are, however, categories in which the underlying disease specified by ICD-9-CM is just another manifestation of a bigger underlying issue. For example, because vitamin B12 is used in red blood cell creation, if there is a deficiency in the vitamin, there is a decrease in the RBCs that can be produced. ICD-9-CM groups all B12 deficiency anemias together regardless of etiology, whereas ICD-10-CM takes the selection a step further by identifying the underlying cause of the B12 deficiency.

The most common underlying causes of B12 deficiency are nutritional deficiency and digestive malabsorption. Nutritional deficiency occurs from the

📖 **DEFINITIONS**

anemia. Deficiency in the blood whether in red blood cells, hemoglobin, or total blood count.

lack of B12 in a person's diet but is actually quite rare because the body stores enough B12 to last at least a year, if not years. Dietary deficiency occurs most commonly in chronic alcoholics and elderly on a "tea and toast" diet; occasionally, this impacts people with strict vegan diets as the majority of dietary B12 comes from ingesting meat, poultry, and dairy products.

Digestive malabsorption can come from multiple sources. Vitamin B12 is extracted from ingested proteins once in the stomach. There it attaches to a protein called intrinsic factor (IF). The IF transports the B12 to the terminal ileum of the small intestine where it is absorbed into the bloodstream with the help of a molecule called transcobalamin II (TC II). Any disruption of this process can result in B12 deficiency. Frequent causes are HIV/AIDS, failure to release B12 from protein, IF deficiency, chronic pancreatic disease, competitive parasites, or lack of TC II.

The underlying cause of the B12 deficiency and subsequent anemia is an important piece of documentation needed when assigning codes for this condition in ICD-10-CM.

Coding for Vitamin B-12 Deficiency Anemia

ICD-9-CM		ICD-10-CM	
281.1	Other vitamin B12 deficiency anemia	D51.1	Vitamin B12 deficiency due to selective vitamin B12 malabsorption with proteinuria
		D51.2	Transcobalamin II deficiency
		D51.3	Other dietary vitamin B12 deficiency anemia
		D51.8	Other vitamin B12 deficiency anemias
		D51.9	Vitamin B12 deficiency anemia, unspecified

Closely related to vitamin B12 deficiency is folate deficiency, which also causes anemia. Folate, or folic acid, is an enzyme that works with vitamin B12 in red blood cell production. Folate deficiency is commonly seen during pregnancy, infancy, and periods of stress. It is also frequently caused by pharmaceuticals, such as sulfa-based antibiotics and methotrexate. ICD-10-CM takes all of this into consideration within the folate deficiency anemia category.

Coding for Folate Deficiency Anemia

ICD-9-CM		ICD-10-CM	
281.2	Folate-deficiency anemia	D52.0	Dietary folate deficiency anemia
		D52.1	Drug-induced folate deficiency anemia
		D52.8	Other folate deficiency anemias
		D52.9	Folate deficiency anemia, unspecified

Genetic anemias are also not uncommon in the American population. The two most significant types are sickle cell anemia and thalassemia. Sickle cell anemia and thalassemia are both inherited conditions that impact the red blood cells, but they are significantly different.

Thalassemia is a condition in which the body does not produce enough normal hemoglobin, resulting in severe anemia. An in-depth understanding of the genetic composition of the red blood cell is needed to distinguish between the different types of thalassemia. Hemoglobin is formed by two inherited proteins from both parents. These proteins are known as alpha globin and beta globin. There are four alpha (two from each parent) and two beta (one from each parent) globins that make up hemoglobin. When one or more of the globins are missing or deformed, the incomplete hemoglobin causes misshapen and fragile red blood cells. Due to their frail nature, the affected RBCs break apart and die quickly, resulting in a type of anemia specifically known as thalassemia.

Figure 8.6: Thalassemia

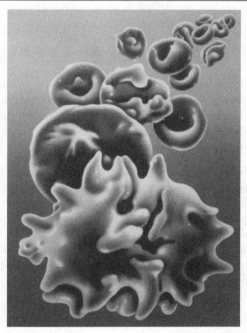

© John Bavosi/Photo Researchers, Inc

The different types of thalassemia are divided by the type and number of missing or deformed globins. The major categories are:

- **Alpha thalassemia:** Also called silent carrier, one alpha globin is missing.
- **Alpha thalassemia minor:** Also called alpha thalassemia trait, two alpha globins are missing.
- **Hemoglobin H disease:** Three alpha globins are missing.
- **Alpha thalassemia major:** Also called hydrops fetalis, four alpha globins are missing.
- **Beta thalassemia minor:** Also called beta thalassemia trait, there is one abnormal and one normal beta globin.
- **Beta thalassemia major:** Also called Cooley's anemia, both beta globins are abnormal.
- **Delta-Beta thalassemia**

ICD-10-CM requires documentation of the specific type of thalassemia in order to code correctly.

 CLINICAL NOTE

Delta-beta thalassemia. About 3 percent of adult hemoglobin is made of alpha and delta globins rather than alpha and beta.

Coding for Thalassemia

ICD-9-CM	ICD-10-CM	
282.49 Other thalassemia	D56.0	Alpha thalassemia
	D56.1	Beta thalassemia
	D56.2	Delta-beta thalassemia
	D56.3	Thalassemia minor
	D56.8	Other thalassemias
	D56.9	Thalassemia, unspecified

It is important to note that any type of thalassemia that is considered minor or as a trait only is reported to D56.3 to properly reflect the severity of the disease. Another type of thalassemia not discussed above involves another red blood cell disorder called sickle cell disease or anemia. Sickle cell can occur with or without thalassemia, depending on the patient's genetics.

Sickle cell disease is characterized (and named) for the crescent or sickle-shaped deformity of the red blood cells caused by defective hemoglobin. The hemoglobin is abnormal due to an abnormal alpha globin, referred to as sickle globin. Because a person gets one alpha globin from each parent, both parents must carry sickle globin for sickle cell disease to occur; both alpha globins must be absent and replaced by sickle globins. If only one parent passes the genetic disposition to create sickle globin, the patient is considered to have sickle cell trait, an asymptomatic carrier status.

Figure 8.7: Normal and Sickle Red Blood Cells

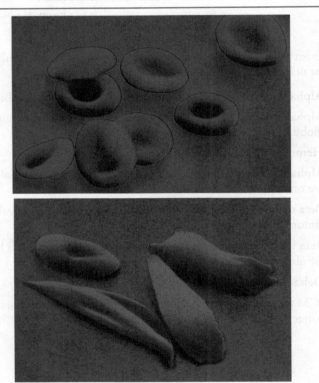

© Omikron/Photo Researchers, Inc

There are three main types of sickle cell disease:

- **Hemoglobin SS (Hb-SS):** Hemoglobin S gene is inherited from both parents.

- **Hemoglobin SC (Hb-C):** Hemoglobin S is inherited from one parent and hemoglobin C is inherited from the other parent.

- **Sickle beta thalassemia (thalassemia Hb-S):** Hemoglobin S is inherited from one parent, and the beta thalassemia gene is inherited from the other parent.

In sickle cell anemia, the hook-shape of the red blood cells not only makes the cells more fragile but also leads them to get trapped in blood vessels, causing blocked vessels. When this occurs, the blood flow is stopped, possibly leading to pain and tissue damage. Usually when a blockage episode occurs, the affected area is extremely painful. This is called a *crisis*. A sickle cell crisis can manifest in many ways but is commonly classified as vaso-occlusive pain in the bones, abdomen, or major joints; acute chest syndrome, in which blood is trapped in the small vessels of the lungs; and splenic sequestration, when blood cells clog the spleen, causing it to enlarge.

ICD-9-CM does distinguish between the main types of sickle cell disease and also provides codes for with and without crisis. However, the type of crisis is coded elsewhere. ICD-10-CM eliminates the need, in some cases, for an additional code to be reported as the categories are further expanded to include this information.

Coding for Sickle Cell Disease

ICD-9-CM		ICD-10-CM	
282.42	Sickle cell thalassemia with crisis	D57.411	Sickle-cell thalassemia with acute chest syndrome
		D57.412	Sickle-cell thalassemia with splenic sequestration
		D57.419	Sickle-cell thalassemia with crisis unspecified
282.62	Hb-SS disease with crisis	D57.01	Hb-SS disease with acute chest syndrome
		D57.02	Hb-SS disease with splenic sequestration
		D57.00	Hb-SS disease with crisis unspecified
282.64	Sickle-cell/Hb-C disease with crisis	D57.211	Sickle-cell/Hb-C disease with acute chest syndrome
		D57.212	Sickle-cell/Hb-C disease with splenic sequestration
		D57.219	Sickle-cell/Hb-C with crisis unspecified

Diseases of White Blood Cells

As discussed in the anatomic overview of this chapter, all of the formed elements of the blood arise from myeloid or lymphoid stem cells in the red bone marrow. In some instances, the blood and bone marrow develop cancer and the stem cells produce abnormal, immature, and excessive white blood cells. This is known as leukemia, a generalized term that encompasses a variety of disease processes. Most leukemias can be classified as myeloid or lymphoid, depending on the malfunctioning stem cell producing the abnormal cells. Lymphocytic leukemia evolves from the lymphoid stem cells and myeloid leukemia the myeloid cells. These can be further divided into acute and chronic types—acute developing suddenly and chronic developing over a period of time. Knowing these generalizations is the most important piece of information needed to assign a code in ICD-9-CM or ICD-10-CM. However, ICD-10-CM further differentiates specific types of leukemia that fall under broader "other specified" categories in ICD-9-CM. The more specific types of lymphocytic leukemia featured in ICD-10-CM include:

- **Prolymphocytic leukemia of B-cell type:** Aggressive form of chronic lymphocytic leukemia involving mature B-cells.

- **Prolymphocytic leukemia of T-cell type:** Very rare form of chronic lymphoid leukemia involving mature T cells.

- **Mature B-cell leukemia, Burkitt type:** Form of acute lymphoid leukemia.

There is one additional type of lymphocytic leukemia that ICD-10-CM identifies. Occasionally leukemia is caused by a virus called the human T-lymphotropic virus (HTLV). In this type of disorder, the virus infects healthy T-cells and replicates within them.

Another important factor in choosing a code for any type of leukemia in either classification system is whether the cancer is active, in remission, or in relapse. The disease is considered active when it is first discovered and is current and causing signs and symptoms. Once treatment is rendered, usually in the form of chemotherapy or induction therapy, the abnormal blood cells disappear from the blood and the disease disappears. When this occurs, the patient is considered in remission. A relapse is when the disease returns after the patient has achieved remission. A patient can relapse multiple times.

Applying all of the above knowledge is the best way to assign the most appropriate code in ICD-9-CM or ICD-10-CM, but some additional understanding of the cell types is required for the new classification system.

Coding for Lymphocytic Leukemia

ICD-9-CM		ICD-10-CM	
204.80	Other lymphoid leukemia without achieved remission	C91.30	Prolymphocytic leukemia of B-cell type not having achieved remission
		C91.50	Adult T-cell lymphoma/leukemia (HTLV-1-associated) not having achieved remission
		C91.60	Prolymphocytic leukemia of T-cell type not having achieved remission
		C91.a0	Mature B-cell leukemia Burkitt-type not having achieved remission
		C91.z0	Other lymphoid leukemia not having achieved remission
204.81	Other lymphoid leukemia in remission	C91.31	Prolymphocytic leukemia of B-cell type in remission
		C91.51	Adult T-cell lymphoma/leukemia (HTLV-1-associated) in remission
		C91.61	Prolymphocytic leukemia of T-cell type in remission
		C91.a1	Mature B-cell leukemia Burkitt-type in remission
		C91.z1	Other lymphoid leukemia in remission
204.82	Other lymphoid leukemia in relapse	C91.32	Prolymphocytic leukemia of B-cell type in relapse
		C91.52	Adult T-cell lymphoma/leukemia (HTLV-1-associated) in relapse
		C91.62	Prolymphocytic leukemia of T-cell type in relapse
		C91.a2	Mature B-cell leukemia Burkitt-type in relapse
		C91.z2	Other lymphoid leukemia in relapse

Myeloid leukemia follows the same basic concepts as lymphocytic. But again, ICD-10-CM categorizes the more common types of specific acute myeloid leukemia. Those that are featured in the new classification system are:

- **Acute myeloblastic leukemia (AML):** Hemocytoblasts that form the myeloid stem cells are abnormal, causing immature and abnormal blood cells.

- **Acute promyelocytic leukemia (APL):** Blood cells are abnormal and there are excess promyelocytes or unevolved granulocytes found in the bloodstream.

- **Acute myelomonocytic leukemia (AMML):** Monocytes, as well as myeloid cells, are impacted.

- **Acute myeloid leukemia with 11q23-abnormality:** AML with a chromosomal abnormality.

- **Acute myeloid leukemia with multilineage dysplasia:** AML in patients who have previously been diagnosed with *myelodysplastic syndrome* or *myeloproliferative disease*.

Coding for Acute Myeloid Leukemia

ICD-9-CM		ICD-10-CM	
205.00	Acute myeloid leukemia without achieved remission	C92.0[0,1,2]	Acute myeloblastic leukemia
		C92.4[0,1,2]	Acute promyelocytic leukemia
		C92.5[0,1,2]	Acute myelomonocytic leukemia
		C92.6[0,1,2]	Acute myeloid leukemia with 11q23-abnormality
		C92.a[0,1,2]	Acute myeloid leukemia with multilineage dysplasia
		5th Character meanings for codes as indicated *0 not having achieved remission* *1 in remission* *2 in relapse*	

Although there are many other types of diseases that impact the white blood cells, reporting for most of them is considerably similar between the two coding systems and does not require any additional knowledge.

Plasma Disorders

Most plasma disorders have a one-to-one crosswalk between ICD-9-CM and ICD-10-CM. However, because many plasma abnormalities can indicate other more serious diseases, specific classifications have been added to the newer coding system that identify abnormal findings in the plasma. Knowing the most commonly discussed plasma proteins is crucial to understanding the ICD-10-CM codes. The three protein abnormalities ICD-10-CM tracks are albumin, globulin, and alphafetoprotein. The differences are highlighted below.

Coding for Plasma Abnormalities

ICD-9-CM		ICD-10-CM	
790.99	Other nonspecific findings on examination of blood	R70.1	Abnormal plasma viscosity
		R77.0	Abnormality of albumin
		R77.1	Abnormality of globulin
		R77.2	Abnormality of alphafetoprotein
		R77.8	Other specified abnormalities of plasma proteins
		R77.9	Abnormality of plasma protein, unspecified

Abnormal Laboratory Blood Tests

Because blood transports substances to and from the organs and body systems, many abnormalities and diseases of different types can be diagnosed via a simple blood test that analyzes the constituents—not just the formed elements, but the electrolytes, chemicals, and variety of other substances. There are times when medical documentation specifies only that there was an abnormal blood test result. When using ICD-9-CM, these types of lab results were mostly classified as "other" abnormal chemistry.

ICD-10-CM has expanded this general code to capture a few more specific and common findings that can increase reporting capabilities for blood tests. The following table highlights a few of these new codes.

Coding for Abnormal Blood Chemistry

ICD-9-CM		ICD-10-CM	
790.6	Other abnormal blood chemistry	E79.0	Hyperuricemia without signs of inflammatory arthritis and tophaceous disease
		R78.71	Abnormal lead level in blood
		R78.79	Finding of abnormal level of heavy metals in the blood
		R78.89	Finding of other specified substances, not normally found in blood
		R79.0	Abnormal level of blood mineral

Summary

The blood and blood-forming organs chapters for both ICD-9-CM and ICD-10-CM are relatively small and concise. Most of the codes applicable to diseases of these tissues are covered well in both classification systems; however, ICD-10-CM has expanded some ICD-9-CM code descriptions. These expansions require more knowledge of the anatomy and physiology of the blood and blood cells as discussed throughout this chapter.

Chapter 9. **Lymphatic System**

Anatomic Overview

The lymphatic system plays a key role in the movement and drainage of fluid in the tissues and the transporting of lipids, and is integral to the body's fight against infection and disease.

The lymphatic system comprises *lymphatic capillaries, lymphatic vessels,* and lymph nodes, as well as *lymph fluid* and lymphatic tissues such as the thymus, spleen, and lymphatic nodules.

This complex system begins at the cellular level. Lymphatic capillaries lie among the cells and are one-way structures that allow *interstitial fluid* to flow into but not out of the capillary. Once the interstitial fluid is in the lymphatic capillary, it is called lymph. The capillaries combine to become lymphatic vessels. Lymphatic nodes are found along the lymphatic vessels. These nodes are bean-shaped and contain masses of B and T-cells. Lymph fluid flows through nodes as it traverses the lymphatic system. In key areas of the lymphatic system there are a series, or "chain," of lymph nodes.

Figure 9.1: Lymphatic Capillaries

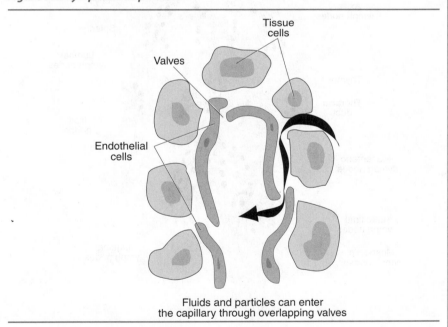

Fluids and particles can enter
the capillary through overlapping valves

The subcutaneous lymphatic vessels generally follow the same route as blood veins, and the visceral lymphatic vessels generally follow the same route as arteries. Avascular tissues, such as cartilage, epidermis, and corneal tissue, do not have lymphatic vessels.

Eventually the lymphatic vessels combine into lymph trunks. The trunks and the areas they drain include:

DEFINITIONS

interstitial fluid. Extracellular fluid filtered through capillaries and drained as lymph that surrounds most tissue outside of blood or lymph vessels.

lymphatic capillary. Small tubular structure in the tissue that collects interstitial fluid using a one-way design; capillaries then combine into lymphatic vessels.

lymphatic fluid. Clear, sometimes yellow fluid that flows through the tissues in the body, through the lymphatic system, and into the bloodstream.

lymphatic vessel. Vessels with interspersed lymph nodes that transport lymph from the lymphatic capillaries to the lymph trunks.

- **Lumbar trunk:** Abdominal wall, lower limbs, pelvis, kidneys, and adrenal glands
- **Intestinal trunk:** Intestines, stomach, pancreas, spleen, and liver
- **Bronchomediastinal trunk:** Heart, lung, and thoracic wall
- **Subclavian trunk:** Upper limbs
- **Jugular trunk:** Head and neck

The lymph flows from the *lymphatic trunk* into the *thoracic duct* or the *right lymphatic duct.* The entire left side of the body, lower abdomen and pelvic area, and lower extremities are drained by the thoracic duct. Only the right side of the head, right upper extremity, and right thoracic area are drained by the right lymphatic duct. The lymph from the thoracic duct is returned to the bloodstream.

Figure 9.2: Lymphatic System

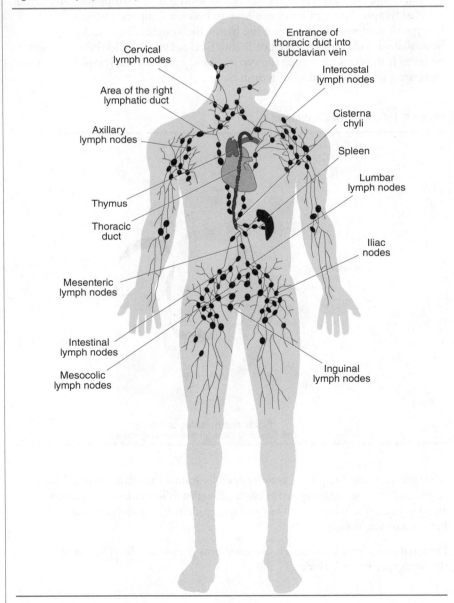

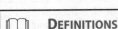

DEFINITIONS

lymphatic trunk. Large vessel created when multiple lymphatic vessels combine.

right lymphatic duct. Large vessel that drains lymph from the lymphatic vessels and trunks of the head, right upper extremity, and right thoracic area.

thoracic duct. Large vessel that drains lymph from the lymphatic vessels and trunks of the left side of the body, lower abdomen and pelvic area, and lower extremities.

Immune response occurs primarily in the secondary lymphatic organs and tissues, lymph nodes, spleen, and lymphatic nodes. The primary lymphatic organs and tissues include red bone marrow production areas and the thymus.

Lymphatic Structures

Thymus

The thymus is located in the upper part of the chest, right beneath the sternum. The thymus contains large numbers of *T-cells* and is larger in infancy and childhood than in adulthood. Immature T-cells move from the red bone marrow to the thymus, where they multiply and mature. Epithelial cells in the thymus help the T-cells learn to differentiate between the body's cells and foreign matter. Mature T-cells can be found in the lymph nodes, spleen, and lymphatic tissue. *Dendritic cells,* also contained in the thymus, are important to immune response. *Microphages* within the thymus help to remove dead and dying cells.

Figure 9.3: Thyroid Gland

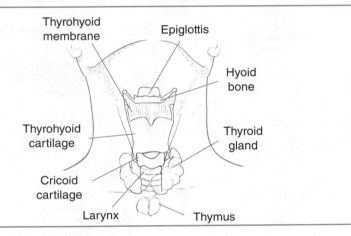

Thyrohyoid membrane
Epiglottis
Hyoid bone
Thyrohyoid cartilage
Thyroid gland
Cricoid cartilage
Larynx
Thymus

Lymph Nodes

There are approximately 600 lymph nodes in the body with greater groupings occurring in the axillae, near the mammary glands, and groin. It is important to realize that lymph nodes may be superficial or deep and that the lymph fluid flows one way only through the node. Foreign substances are trapped as they enter the lymph node. Macrocytes destroy some of the foreign material, and lymphocytes destroy other material through the immune response. Multiple lymphatic vessels may feed into a single lymph node that may terminate in one or more vessels.

INTERESTING A & P FACT

The thymus is quite large in infancy and childhood; however, after puberty the thymus begins to shrink.

DEFINITIONS

B-cells. Type of lymphocyte produced and maturing within the bone marrow to fight foreign matter, such as bacteria and viruses, and trigger an immune response.

dendritic cells. Antigen-presenting cells (APC) that activate T-cells, capture antigens, and help to create immunological memory with B-cells.

microphage. Small phagocyte that ingests foreign matter and other small things like dead tissue and cells.

T-cells. Type of lymphocyte that matures in the thymus and aids in adaptive immunity by destroying infected cells or activating an immune response. T-cell levels are an indicator of health for HIV/AIDS, some types of leukemia, and other diseases.

Figure 9.4: Lymph Node

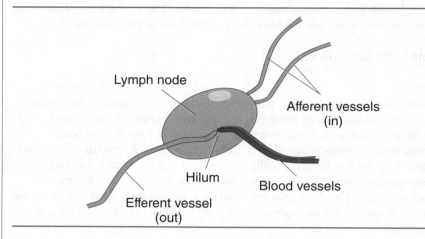

Figure 9.5: Axllary Lymph Nodes

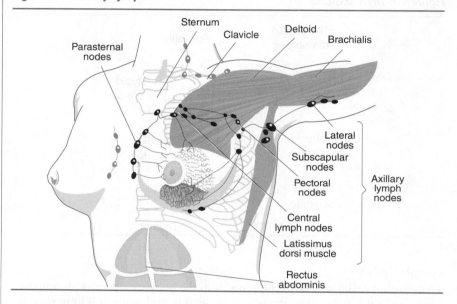

Spleen

The spleen is made up of lymphatic tissue, the splenic artery, the splenic vein, and efferent lymphatic vessels. The lymphatic tissue contains lymphocytes and microphages called white pulp. The white pulp surrounds central arteries that branch off the splenic artery. The spleen also contains areas termed red pulp, which is made up of splenic cords or tissue that contains microphages, lymphocytes, red blood cells, plasma cells, and granulocytes. Red pulp also has venous sinuses that are filled with blood.

Blood enters the venous sinuses via the splenic artery, where the surrounding white pulp contains the B and T-cells that provide the immune response and microphages that eradicate pathogens. The red pulp stores up to a third of the body's platelet supply and eliminates worn-out or bad cells and platelets by microphages.

Figure 9.6: Lymph Nodes of Trunk

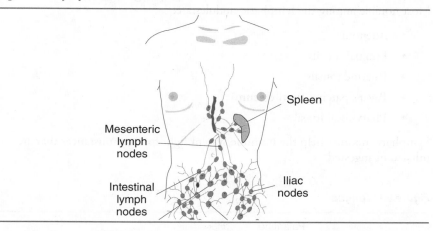

Lymphatic Nodules

Lymph nodes are encapsulated, whereas nodules are not encapsulated. Lymphatic nodules are found in connective tissue such as:

- Gastrointestinal lining
- Reproductive tract
- Respiratory airway
- Urinary tract

In the gastrointestinal lining, lymphatic nodules begin the process of transporting dietary lipids within the lymphatic system. These lipids are transported to the venous blood system.

Figure 9.7: Lymphatic Drainage

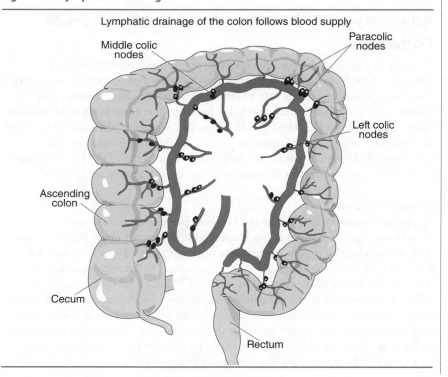

Lymphatic drainage of the colon follows blood supply

Lymphatic nodules may be solitary or they may be larger masses of nodules. Most notable among the lymphatic nodules are:

- Adenoids
- Lingual tonsils
- Palatine tonsils
- Peyer's patches (in the ileum)
- Pharyngeal tonsil

Lymphatic nodules help the immune system fight foreign substances that are inhaled or ingested.

Figure 9.8: Tongue

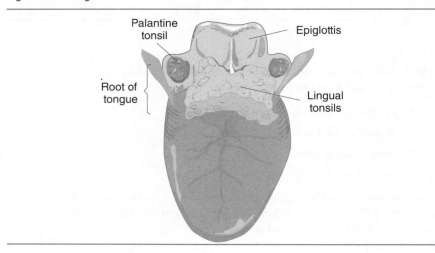

Anatomy and Physiology and the ICD-10-CM Code Set

The primary goals of the lymphatic system are to move interstitial fluid throughout the body to help maintain fluid balance, and to provide immunity from foreign matter that may try to enter the body and cause damage and disease. The lymphatic system also helps prevent some cancers. In the transition from ICD-9-CM to ICD-10-CM, coders must understand the pathophysiology of conditions affecting the lymphatic system, as well as the anatomy and pathology of the system itself. This section discusses some of the key differences between the two code sets and points out important items to be aware of.

Lymphatic Cancer

Lymphatic cancer is categorized as *Hodgkin's lymphoma* and all other *lymphomas*. Reticulosarcoma, lymphosarcoma, Burkitt's tumor, marginal zone lymphoma, mantle cell, and large cell lymphoma have a direct crosswalk to ICD-10-CM codes, although some descriptors use different terminology to describe the disease than was used in ICD-9-CM. ICD-10-CM tends to use the cell type, as opposed to the "disease name," to describe the malignancy. Primary central nervous system, anaplastic large cell, and other variants of lymphoma may require additional information in the medical record, as well as require the coder to understand additional information about the patient's disease process, to appropriately report these services under ICD-10-CM.

To code primary central nervous system lymphomas in ICD-10-CM, the lymphoma must be specified as diffuse large B-cell or nonfollicular lymphoma.

Hodgkin's lymphoma is a malignancy of the lymphatic system that may initially present with localized swelling of the lymph nodes. As the disease progresses, the swelling may become more generalized, spread to the spleen, and even involve the liver. Hodgkin's lymphoma is differentiated by the presence of a specific cell type, Reed-Sternberg. Hodgkin's lymphoma is further divided into lymphocyte-rich classical and nodular lymphocyte predominant types, as is demonstrated in the table below. Code selection is based upon the site and type of lymphatic cells.

Coding for Hodgkin's Disease

ICD-9-CM		ICD-10-CM	
201.40	Hodgkin's disease, lymphocytic-histiocytic predominance, unspecified site, extranodal and solid organ sites	C81.00	Nodular lymphocyte predominant Hodgkin lymphoma, unspecified site
		C81.09	Nodular lymphocyte predominant Hodgkin lymphoma, extranodal and solid organ sites
		C81.40	Lymphocyte-rich classical Hodgkin lymphoma, unspecified site
		C81.49	Lymphocyte-rich classical Hodgkin lymphoma, extranodal and solid organ sites
201.41	Hodgkin's disease, lymphocytic-histiocytic predominance of lymph nodes of head, face, and neck	C81.01	Nodular lymphocyte predominant Hodgkin lymphoma, lymph nodes of head, face, and neck
		C81.41	Lymphocyte-rich classical Hodgkin lymphoma, lymph nodes of head, face, and neck
201.42	Hodgkin's disease, lymphocytic-histiocytic predominance of intrathoracic lymph nodes	C81.02	Nodular lymphocyte predominant Hodgkin lymphoma, intrathoracic lymph nodes
		C81.42	Lymphocyte-rich classical Hodgkin lymphoma, intrathoracic lymph nodes
201.43	Hodgkin's disease, lymphocytic-histiocytic predominance of intra-abdominal lymph nodes	C81.03	Nodular lymphocyte predominant Hodgkin lymphoma, intra-abdominal lymph nodes
		C81.43	Lymphocyte-rich classical Hodgkin lymphoma, intra-abdominal lymph nodes
201.44	Hodgkin's disease, lymphocytic-histiocytic predominance of lymph nodes of axilla and upper limb	C81.04	Nodular lymphocyte predominant Hodgkin lymphoma, lymph nodes of axilla and upper limb
		C81.44	Lymphocyte-rich classical Hodgkin lymphoma, lymph nodes of axilla and upper limb
201.45	Hodgkin's disease, lymphocytic-histiocytic predominance of lymph nodes of inguinal region and lower limb	C81.05	Nodular lymphocyte predominant Hodgkin lymphoma, lymph nodes of inguinal region and lower limb
		C81.45	Lymphocyte-rich classical Hodgkin lymphoma, lymph nodes of inguinal region and lower limb
201.46	Hodgkin's disease, lymphocytic-histiocytic predominance of intrapelvic lymph nodes	C81.06	Nodular lymphocyte predominant Hodgkin lymphoma, intrapelvic lymph nodes
		C81.46	Lymphocyte-rich classical Hodgkin lymphoma, intrapelvic lymph nodes
201.47	Hodgkin's disease, lymphocytic-histiocytic predominance of spleen	C81.07	Nodular lymphocyte predominant Hodgkin lymphoma, spleen
		C81.47	Lymphocyte-rich classical Hodgkin lymphoma, spleen

CODING AXIOM

As with other neoplasms, the correct diagnosis code for all lymphomas depends on the affected sites.

ICD-9-CM		ICD-10-CM	
201.48	Hodgkin's disease, lymphocytic-histiocytic predominance of lymph nodes of multiple sites	C81.08	Nodular lymphocyte predominant Hodgkin lymphoma, lymph nodes of multiple sites
		C81.48	Lymphocyte-rich classical Hodgkin lymphoma, lymph nodes of multiple sites

As previously discussed, lymphoma is reported as Hodgkin's lymphoma or all other lymphomas. In ICD-10-CM, many of the lymphoma codes require additional information for reporting. However, there are exceptions, such as classical Hodgkin's lymphoma. These codes are separated in ICD-9-CM and reported according to the Hodgkin's lymphoma type: paragranuloma, granuloma, or sarcoma. In ICD-10-CM, they are grouped together as "classical Hodgkin's lymphoma" and are reported by site. Below is an example of this collapse of ICD-9-CM codes into a single ICD-10-CM code occurring in the head, face, and neck area.

Coding for Hodgkin's Paragranuloma

ICD-9-CM		ICD-10-CM	
201.01	Hodgkin's paragranuloma of lymph nodes of head, face, and neck	C81.71	Other classical Hodgkin lymphoma, lymph nodes of head, face, and neck
201.11	Hodgkin's granuloma of lymph nodes of head, face, and neck		
201.21	Hodgkin's sarcoma of lymph nodes of head, face, and neck		

Lymphoma codes are selected based on the site of the affected cells and by cell type: large B-cell and other nonfollicular cell. Diffuse large B-cell lymphoma is one of the most common of the lymphomas and is quite aggressive. Standard therapy for this type of lymphoma includes one of several types of chemotherapy treatments.

Coding for Primary Central Nervous System Lymphoma

ICD-9-CM		ICD-10-CM	
200.50	Primary central nervous system lymphoma, unspecified site, extranodal and solid organ sites	C83.39	Diffuse large B-cell lymphoma, extranodal and solid organ sites
		C83.80	Other nonfollicular lymphoma, unspecified site
		C83.89	Other nonfollicular lymphoma, extranodal and solid organ sites
200.51	Primary central nervous system lymphoma, lymph nodes of head, face, and neck	C83.31	Diffuse large B-cell lymphoma, lymph nodes of head, face, and neck
		C83.81	Other nonfollicular lymphoma, lymph nodes of head, face, and neck
200.52	Primary central nervous system lymphoma, intrathoracic lymph nodes	C83.32	Diffuse large B-cell lymphoma, intrathoracic lymph nodes
		C83.82	Other nonfollicular lymphoma, intrathoracic lymph nodes
200.53	Primary central nervous system lymphoma, intra-abdominal lymph nodes	C83.33	Diffuse large B-cell lymphoma, intra-abdominal lymph nodes
		C83.83	Other nonfollicular lymphoma, intra-abdominal lymph nodes
200.54	Primary central nervous system lymphoma, lymph nodes of axilla and upper limb	C83.34	Diffuse large B-cell lymphoma, lymph nodes of axilla and upper limb
		C83.84	Other nonfollicular lymphoma, lymph nodes of axilla and upper limb

ICD-9-CM		ICD-10-CM	
200.55	Primary central nervous system lymphoma, lymph nodes of inguinal region and lower limb	C83.35	Diffuse large B-cell lymphoma, lymph nodes of inguinal region and lower limb
		C83.85	Other nonfollicular lymphoma, lymph nodes of inguinal region and lower limb
200.56	Primary central nervous system lymphoma, intrapelvic lymph nodes	C83.36	Diffuse large B-cell lymphoma, intrapelvic lymph nodes
		C83.86	Other nonfollicular lymphoma, intrapelvic lymph nodes
200.57	Primary central nervous system lymphoma, spleen	C83.37	Diffuse large B-cell lymphoma, spleen
		C83.87	Other nonfollicular lymphoma, spleen
200.58	Primary central nervous system lymphoma, lymph nodes of multiple sites	C83.38	Diffuse large B-cell lymphoma, lymph nodes of multiple sites
		C83.88	Other nonfollicular lymphoma, lymph nodes of multiple sites

When reporting anaplastic large cell lymphoma in ICD-10-CM, it is necessary to identify whether the cells are anaplastic lymphoma kinase (ALK) positive or ALK negative. Those identified as ALK positive are believed to have a more positive prognosis, although treatment for both is similar. ALK is an enzyme, but the ALK gene is shown to be an "oncogene," having a direct link to many large cell lymphomas. ALK-positive patients are positive for this specific oncogene, whereas ALK-negative patients do not have this specific gene but still have the anaplastic large cell lymphoma.

Coding for Anaplastic Large Cell Lymphoma

ICD-9-CM		ICD-10-CM	
200.60	Anaplastic large cell lymphoma, unspecified site, extranodal and solid organ sites	C84.60	Anaplastic large cell lymphoma, ALK-positive, unspecified site
		C84.69	Anaplastic large cell lymphoma, ALK-positive, extranodal and solid organ sites
		C84.70	Anaplastic large cell lymphoma, ALK-negative, unspecified site
		C84.79	Anaplastic large cell lymphoma, ALK-negative, extranodal and solid organ sites
200.61	Anaplastic large cell lymphoma, lymph nodes of head, face, and neck	C84.61	Anaplastic large cell lymphoma, ALK-positive, lymph nodes of head, face, and neck
		C84.71	Anaplastic large cell lymphoma, ALK-negative, lymph nodes of head, face, and neck
200.62	Anaplastic large cell lymphoma, intrathoracic lymph nodes	C84.62	Anaplastic large cell lymphoma, ALK-positive, intrathoracic lymph nodes
		C84.72	Anaplastic large cell lymphoma, ALK-negative, intrathoracic lymph nodes
200.63	Anaplastic large cell lymphoma, intra-abdominal lymph nodes	C84.63	Anaplastic large cell lymphoma, ALK-positive, intra-abdominal lymph nodes
		C84.73	Anaplastic large cell lymphoma, ALK-negative, intra-abdominal lymph nodes
200.64	Anaplastic large cell lymphoma, lymph nodes of axilla and upper limb	C84.64	Anaplastic large cell lymphoma, ALK-positive, lymph nodes of axilla and upper limb
		C84.74	Anaplastic large cell lymphoma, ALK-negative, lymph nodes of axilla and upper limb

Variants of lymphoma and reticulosarcoma of the lymph nodes require further definition in ICD-10-CM. It is important to note if it is small cell, B-cell lymphoma, or other nonfollicular lymphoma. In ICD-9-CM, only the lymphoma or reticulosarcoma site is required. Due to the increased specificity in

ICD-10-CM, there may be a learning curve for providers. Coders can help their providers understand the new levels of specificity in the ICD-10-CM code set. In some instances, a provider query may be needed, especially if the provider is not readily available.

Coding for Other Nonfollicular Lymphoma

ICD-9-CM		ICD-10-CM	
200.80	Other nonfollicular lymphoma, lymph nodes of multiple sites	C83.00	Small cell B-cell lymphoma, unspecified site
		C83.09	Small cell B-cell lymphoma, extranodal and solid organ sites
		C83.80	Other nonfollicular lymphoma, unspecified site
		C83.89	Other nonfollicular lymphoma, extranodal and solid organ sites
		C83.90	Non-follicular lymphoma, unspecified, unspecified site
		C83.99	Nonfollicular lymphoma, unspecified, extranodal, and solid organ sites
		C86.5	Angioimmunoblastic T-cell lymphoma
		C86.6	Primary cutaneous CD30-positive T-cell proliferations
200.81	Other named variants of lymphosarcoma and reticulosarcoma of lymph nodes of head, face, and neck	C83.01	Small cell B-cell lymphoma, lymph nodes of head, face, and neck
		C83.81	Other nonfollicular lymphoma, lymph nodes of head, face, and neck
		C83.91	Nonfollicular lymphoma, unspecified, lymph nodes of head, face, and neck
200.82	Other named variants of lymphosarcoma and reticulosarcoma of intrathoracic lymph nodes	C83.02	Small cell B-cell lymphoma, intrathoracic lymph nodes
		C83.82	Other nonfollicular lymphoma, intrathoracic lymph nodes
		C83.92	Nonfollicular lymphoma, unspecified, intrathoracic lymph nodes
200.83	Other named variants of lymphosarcoma and reticulosarcoma of intra-abdominal lymph nodes	C83.03	Small cell B-cell lymphoma, intra-abdominal lymph nodes
		C83.83	Other nonfollicular lymphoma, intra-abdominal lymph nodes
		C83.93	lymphoma, unspecified, intra-abdominal lymph nodes
200.84	Other named variants of lymphosarcoma and reticulosarcoma of lymph nodes of axilla and upper limb	C83.04	Small cell B-cell lymphoma, lymph nodes of axilla and upper limb
		C83.84	Other nonfollicular lymphoma, lymph nodes of axilla and upper limb
		C83.94	Nonfollicular lymphoma, unspecified, lymph nodes of axilla and upper limb
200.85	Other named variants of lymphosarcoma and reticulosarcoma of lymph nodes of inguinal region and lower limb	C83.05	Small cell B-cell lymphoma, lymph nodes of inguinal region and lower limb
		C83.85	Other nonfollicular lymphoma, lymph nodes of inguinal region and lower limb
		C83.95	Nonfollicular lymphoma, unspecified, lymph nodes of inguinal region and lower limb
200.86	Other named variants of lymphosarcoma and reticulosarcoma of intrapelvic lymph nodes	C83.06	Small cell B-cell lymphoma, intrapelvic lymph nodes
		C83.86	Other nonfollicular lymphoma, intrapelvic lymph nodes
		C83.96	Nonfollicular lymphoma, unspecified, intrapelvic lymph nodes

ICD-9-CM		ICD-10-CM	
200.87	Other named variants of lymphosarcoma and reticulosarcoma of spleen	C83.07	Small cell B-cell lymphoma, spleen
		C83.87	Other nonfollicular lymphoma, spleen
		C83.97	Nonfollicular lymphoma, unspecified, spleen
200.88	Other named variants of lymphosarcoma and reticulosarcoma of lymph nodes of multiple sites	C83.08	Small cell B-cell lymphoma, lymph nodes of multiple sites
		C83.88	Other nonfollicular lymphoma, lymph nodes of multiple sites
		C83.98	Nonfollicular lymphoma, unspecified, lymph nodes of multiple sites

Follicular lymphoma is a form of non-Hodgkin's lymphoma characterized by specific types of tumors. These tumors are made up of follicles that contain cells called centroblasts and centrocytes. In ICD-10-CM, nodular lymphoma is specified by lymphoma type. Codes specify the grade of follicular lymphoma (I, II, III, IIIa, IIIb) and whether it is diffuse follicle, cutaneous follicle, other types of follicular lymphoma, or unspecified follicular lymphoma. Note that the term nodular is not included in these codes. Although there is some controversy over the grading system, the World Health Organization recommends the following:

- Grade I: < 5 centroblasts per high power field
- Grade II: 6–15 centroblasts per high power field
- Grade III: > 15 centroblasts per high power field
  - grade IIIa: centrocytes are still present
  - grade IIIb: follicles consist almost entirely of centroblasts

The following table illustrates how these codes are reported in ICD-10-CM. This table is not all-inclusive of the nodular lymphoma codes but gives the coder an idea of what to expect.

Coding for Nodular Lymphoma

ICD-9-CM		ICD-10-CM	
202.00	Nodular lymphoma, unspecified site, extranodal and solid organ sites	C82.00	Follicular lymphoma grade I, unspecified site
		C82.09	Follicular lymphoma grade I, extranodal and solid organ sites
		C82.10	Follicular lymphoma grade II, unspecified site
		C82.19	Follicular lymphoma grade II, extranodal and solid organ sites
		C82.20	Follicular lymphoma grade III, unspecified, unspecified site
		C82.29	Follicular lymphoma grade III, unspecified, extranodal and solid organ sites
		C82.30	Follicular lymphoma grade IIIa, unspecified site
		C82.39	Follicular lymphoma grade IIIa, extranodal and solid organ sites
		C82.40	Follicular lymphoma grade IIIb, unspecified site
		C82.49	Follicular lymphoma grade IIIb, extranodal and solid organ sites
		C82.60	Cutaneous follicle center lymphoma, unspecified site
		C82.69	Cutaneous follicle center lymphoma, extranodal and solid organ sites
(Continued on next page)			

ICD-9-CM		ICD-10-CM	
202.00	Nodular lymphoma, unspecified site, extranodal and solid organ sites *(Continued)*	C82.80	Other types of follicular lymphoma, unspecified site
		C82.89	Other types of follicular lymphoma, extranodal and solid organ sites
		C82.90	Follicular lymphoma, unspecified, unspecified site
		C82.99	Follicular lymphoma, unspecified, extranodal and solid organ sites

Other malignant lymphomas are reported only by site in ICD-9-CM. However, in ICD-10-CM, the type of lymphoma needs to be indicated—B-cell, large B-cell, or non-Hodgkin's lymphoma—and the lymphoma site must be identified to select a final diagnosis code. The following table contains an example of a "generic" ICD-9-CM code that links to more specific ICD-10-CM codes. These types of examples are found throughout the ICD-10-CM manual.

Blastic NK-cell lymphoma is a very rare and aggressive form of lymphoma that affects the natural killer cells of the immune system. In the early stages, patients often present with skin lesions and lymphadenopathy, and this disease typically affects elderly patients. Unfortunately, the condition is resistant to most of the common lymphoma treatments: chemotherapy, radiation therapy, and bone marrow transplantation. Prognosis tends to be poor for most patients diagnosed with blastic NK-cell lymphoma.

Coding for Other Malignant Lymphomas

ICD-9-CM		ICD-10-CM	
202.80	Other malignant lymphomas, unspecified site, extranodal and solid organ sites	C85.10	Unspecified B-cell lymphoma, unspecified site
		C85.19	Unspecified B-cell lymphoma, extranodal and solid organ sites
		C85.20	Mediastinal (thymic) large B-cell lymphoma, unspecified site
		C85.29	Mediastinal (thymic) large B-cell lymphoma, extranodal and solid organ sites
		C85.80	Other specified types of non-Hodgkin lymphoma, unspecified site
		C85.89	Other specified types of non-Hodgkin lymphoma, extranodal and solid organ sites
		C85.90	Other specified types of non-Hodgkin lymphoma, extranodal and solid organ sites
		C85.99	Non-Hodgkin lymphoma, unspecified, extranodal and solid organ sites
		C86.4	Blastic NK-cell lymphoma
202.81	Other malignant lymphomas of lymph nodes of head, face, and neck	C85.11	Unspecified B-cell lymphoma, lymph nodes of head, face, and neck
		C85.21	Mediastinal (thymic) large B-cell lymphoma, lymph nodes of head, face, and neck
		C85.81	Other specified types of non-Hodgkin lymphoma, lymph nodes of head, face, and neck
		C85.91	Non-Hodgkin lymphoma, unspecified, lymph nodes of head, face, and neck
		C86.0	Extranodal NK/T-cell lymphoma, nasal type

ICD-9-CM		ICD-10-CM	
202.82	Other malignant lymphomas of intrathoracic lymph nodes	C82.52	Diffuse follicle center lymphoma, intrathoracic lymph nodes
		C84.92	Mature T/NK-cell lymphomas, unspecified, intrathoracic lymph nodes
		C85.12	Unspecified B-cell lymphoma, intrathoracic lymph nodes
		C85.22	Mediastinal (thymic) large B-cell lymphoma, intrathoracic lymph nodes
		C85.82	Other specified types of non-Hodgkin lymphoma, intrathoracic lymph nodes
		C85.92	Non-Hodgkin lymphoma, unspecified, intrathoracic lymph nodes
202.83	Other malignant lymphomas of intra-abdominal lymph nodes	C85.13	Unspecified B-cell lymphoma, intra-abdominal lymph nodes
		C85.23	Mediastinal (thymic) large B-cell lymphoma, intra-abdominal lymph nodes
		C85.83	Other specified types of non-Hodgkin lymphoma, intra-abdominal lymph nodes
		C85.93	Non-Hodgkin lymphoma, unspecified, intra-abdominal lymph nodes
		C86.2	Enteropathy-type (intestinal) T-cell lymphoma
		C86.3	Subcutaneous panniculitis-like T-cell lymphoma

Lymphatic Disease

Sarcoidosis begins as inflammation and progresses to clusters of cells referred to as granulomas. Granulomas in general are typically a collection of immune cells that have attempted to wall off substances they deem foreign. In sarcoidosis, granulomas typically contain star-shaped structures called Schaumann bodies. The most common sites for sarcoidosis are the lymph nodes of the chest, skin, or lungs; however, it can also be found in the eyes, liver, brain, and heart. Nearly 66 percent of all patients may be termed as in remission within 10 years. Löfgren's syndrome, a frequent symptom of sarcoidosis, is also reported with ICD-9-CM code 135; however, a specific index or tabular reference is not yet available in ICD-10-CM. Sarcoidosis is differentiated according to the specific site.

Coding for Sarcoidosis

ICD-9-CM		ICD-10-CM	
135	Sarcoidosis	D86.1	Sarcoidosis of lymph nodes
		D86.2	Sarcoidosis of lung with sarcoidosis of lymph nodes
		D86.89	Sarcoidosis of other sites
		D86.9	Sarcoidosis, unspecified

Lymphadenitis, inflammation of the lymph nodes, is often localized and changes in the ICD-10-CM code set require that the location be identified. Note that coding only for acute conditions, not chronic lymphadenitis, calls for this additional information. In ICD-9-CM, rubric 289 is used to report chronic disease, and I88.0 through I88.9 is used in ICD-10-CM.

When reporting acute lymphadenitis, the site of the inflamed lymph nodes is used to determine the correct ICD-10-CM code.

Coding for Acute Lymphadenitis

ICD-9-CM		ICD-10-CM	
683	Acute lymphadenitis	L04.0	Acute lymphadenitis of face, head and neck
		L04.1	Acute lymphadenitis of trunk
		L04.2	Acute lymphadenitis of upper limb
		L04.3	Acute lymphadenitis of lower limb
		L04.8	Acute lymphadenitis of other sites
		L04.9	Acute lymphadenitis, unspecified

Enlargement of the lymph nodes without inflammation is reported with ICD-9-CM code 785.6. ICD-10-CM requires additional information about the nature of the enlarged lymph nodes, however. The term lymphadenopathy may also be used in the provider's documentation to describe this condition. Although there is not an "official" standard to follow, commonly "localized" describes the enlargement of lymph nodes in a single area of the body. "Generalized" describes the enlargement of lymph nodes in two or more areas of the body.

Coding for Enlargement of Lymph Nodes

ICD-9-CM		ICD-10-CM	
785.6	Enlargement of lymph nodes	R59.0	Localized enlarged lymph nodes
		R59.1	Generalized enlarged lymph nodes
		R59.9	Enlarged lymph nodes, unspecified

Immunity

The lymphatic system is integral to the body's immunity. The specificity for ICD-10-CM includes more detail to further define the type of immunity deficiency disorders than does ICD-9-CM.

Severe combined immunodeficiency disease (SCID) is characterized by a complete lack of or a significant deficiency of B-cells and T-cells in the body, which results in a lack of humoral and cell-mediated immunity in the body. It is somewhat commonly known as "Bubble boy syndrome," as one of the more famous cases occurred in the 1970s and 1980s involving a young boy who lived for 12 years in a germ-free plastic bubble. This disease is typically diagnosed in the first 3 to 6 months of life, when the patient's susceptibility to infection becomes obvious.

Major histocompatibility complex class I and class II are the two primary classes of human leukocyte antigens in genetic makeup that code proteins to assist in our immune response. Class I antigens are found on the surface of all nucleated cells. Class II antigens are found only on immunocompetent T-cells, such as macrophages and B-cells. A deficiency of this antigen significantly affects our immune response.

Hyperimmunoglobulin E (IgE) syndrome is a rare immunodeficiency disease, characterized by several symptoms, including multiple recurrent skin abscesses, upper respiratory issues such as pneumonia, high serum levels of IgE, issues related to teeth, and various other concerns. It is sometimes called Job syndrome, as originally it was thought that these patients were reminiscent of the biblical character Job, whose body was covered with boils by Satan. Treatment usually involves control of infections, although there is no single treatment for this condition.

Immune reconstitution syndrome is a condition that typically affects patients with immunosuppression or AIDS, whereby the immune system begins to recover and during that recovery responds to some type of a previously acquired infection with an overwhelming inflammatory response, making the infection worse. In some cases, the resulting inflammation can be quite dangerous to the patient and needs treatment. However, in many cases, this response often means that the body has a better chance to fight the infection than it did previously. There is no best treatment known for this condition.

Coding for Immunity Deficiency

ICD-9-CM		ICD-10-CM	
279.2	Combined immunity deficiency	D81.0	Severe combined immunodeficiency [SCID] with reticular dysgenesis
		D81.1	Severe combined immunodeficiency [SCID] with low T- and B-cell numbers
		D81.2	Severe combined immunodeficiency [SCID] with low or normal B-cell numbers
		D81.6	Major histocompatibility complex class I deficiency
		D81.7	Major histocompatibility complex class II deficiency
		D81.89	Other combined immunodeficiencies
		D81.9	Combined immunodeficiency, unspecified
279.8	Other specified disorders involving the immune mechanism	D82.2	Immunodeficiency with short-limbed stature
		D82.3	Immunodeficiency following hereditary defective response to Epstein-Barr virus
		D82.4	Hyperimmunoglobulin E [IgE] syndrome
		D82.8	Immunodeficiency associated with other specified major defects
		D82.9	Immunodeficiency associated with major defect, unspecified
		D84.0	Lymphocyte function antigen-1 [LFA-1] defect
		D84.1	Defects in the complement system
		D89.3	Immune reconstitution syndrome
		D89.89	Other specified disorders involving the immune mechanism, not elsewhere classified

When using ICD-10-CM codes to report mononucleosis, another immune disorder, more information is required from the documentation, including the type of virus causing mononucleosis and the absence or presence of complications. This may require additional information from the laboratory, which may delay coding.

Coding for Infectious Mononucleosis

ICD-9-CM		ICD-10-CM	
075	Infectious mononucleosis	B27.00	Gammaherpesviral mononucleosis without complication
		B27.09	Gammaherpesviral mononucleosis with other complications
		B27.10	Cytomegaloviral mononucleosis without complications
		B27.19	Cytomegaloviral mononucleosis with other complication
(Continued on next page)		B27.80	Other infectious mononucleosis without complication

ICD-9-CM		ICD-10-CM	
Ø75 Infectious mononucleosis *(Continued)*		B27.89	Other infectious mononucleosis with other complication
		B27.9Ø	Infectious mononucleosis, unspecified without complication
		B27.99	Infectious mononucleosis, unspecified with other complication

Spleen

Splenic sequestration and other diseases of the spleen are more detailed in ICD-10-CM than in ICD-9-CM. In ICD-10-CM, splenic sequestration codes depend on the type of sickle cell disorder and other splenic diseases depend on the type of disease.

Splenic sequestration is caused when the red blood cells become trapped in the spleen, which causes a significant decrease in the hemoglobin level in the body. This can cause the patient to go into hypovolemic shock and is a leading cause of death in children with sickle cell disease.

Coding for Splenic Sequestration

ICD-9-CM		ICD-10-CM	
289.52	Splenic sequestration	D57.Ø2	Hb-SS disease with splenic sequestration
		D57.212	Sickle-cell/Hb-C disease with splenic sequestration
		D57.412	Sickle-cell thalassemia with splenic sequestration
		D57.812	Other sickle-cell disorders with splenic sequestration

Hyposplenism describes a reduction in the spleen function. An infarction of the spleen occurs when the oxygen supply to the spleen is interrupted in some way, typically due to the splenic artery's being occluded. This interruption in the oxygen supply causes tissue death in various areas of the spleen.

Coding for Other Diseases of the Spleen

ICD-9-CM		ICD-10-CM	
289.59	Other diseases of spleen	D73.Ø	Hyposplenism
		D73.3	Abscess of spleen
		D73.4	Cyst of spleen
		D73.5	Infarction of spleen
		D73.89	Other diseases of spleen

Summary

The lymphatic system moves interstitial fluid throughout the body to help maintain fluid balance, transport lipids, and help the body fight off disease. The lymphatic system does not have a specific section in the ICD-9-CM or ICD-10-CM manual; codes are spread throughout the various sections. Coders and providers must increase their knowledge of lymphatic system diseases to correctly report the lymphatic conditions described in the ICD-10-CM manual.

Chapter 10. **Respiratory System**

Anatomic Overview

The respiratory system comprises all the organs and structures involved in breathing. Oxygen is inhaled and carbon dioxide is expelled. Any malfunction within this process can lead to cell death within the tissues of the various organs of the body by reducing the amount of oxygen distributed to these organs or causing excess waste within the body's tissues. The *capillary* blood vessels enable the body to balance the fluid within every cell of the body. The respiratory system also helps regulate pH in the blood, as well as playing a vital role in our sense of smell and ability to vocalize sounds.

Function of the Respiratory System

When air enters the body through the nose or mouth, the *diaphragm* tightens, allowing more room within the chest cavity for the lungs to expand and take in the air. The *intercostal muscles* also contract, lifting the rib cage and helping to enlarge the area. The air moves into the lungs and *bronchial tubes,* reaching the *alveoli.* Running by these alveoli are capillaries carrying blood that has traveled through the body and been pumped from the right side of the heart through the pulmonary artery and then into capillaries. The alveoli transport the oxygen to the capillaries where hemoglobin helps it flow into the bloodstream. As the oxygen is absorbed, the carbon dioxide is extracted from the capillaries into the alveoli and is exhaled as a waste gas. The oxygenated blood then travels through the pulmonary vein to the left side of the heart, which pumps it to the rest of the body.

When the diaphragm and intercostal muscles relax, they minimize the space within the chest cavity. This causes air rich in carbon dioxide to leave the body.

The respiratory center in the brain stem sends signals via the spinal cord and nerves to the muscles responsible for breathing, allowing for regular function. This is not to say that a person cannot change his or her own breathing pattern voluntarily, such as during exercise, holding of breath, or when outside emotional factors warrant an increase or decrease in airflow. The body is also built with internal sensors that may adjust breathing as needed. For example, the brain works with the *carotid artery* and *aorta* to determine adequate levels of oxygen and carbon dioxide within the bloodstream. In addition, air passages can detect the presence of foreign matter that can cause problems, thus promoting a cough or sneeze to eliminate the foreign matter.

Functional Anatomy of the Respiratory System

There are two main parts to the respiratory system. The upper respiratory tract, situated above the chest, contains the nose, pharynx, and larynx. The lower respiratory tract, located within the chest, contains the trachea, bronchial tree, and the lungs.

📖 DEFINITIONS

alveoli. Last structure within the lung and the primary spot for gas exchange between the lungs and capillaries.

aorta. Largest artery in the body. It is connected to the left ventricle of the heart and progresses through the thorax, leading to the abdomen, and divides into smaller branches to reach other parts of the body.

bronchial tubes. Part of the respiratory structure connecting the lungs to the trachea, allowing for air exchange within the lungs.

capillary. Tiny, minute blood vessel that connects the arterioles (smallest arteries) and the venules (smallest veins) and acts as a semipermeable membrane between the blood and the tissue fluid.

carotid arteries. Two blood vessels on either side of the neck just below the jaw that supply blood to the brain.

diaphragm. Muscular wall separating the thorax and its structures from the abdomen.

intercostal muscles. Muscles within the rib cage responsible for movement when breathing.

Figure 10.1: Lower Respiratory System

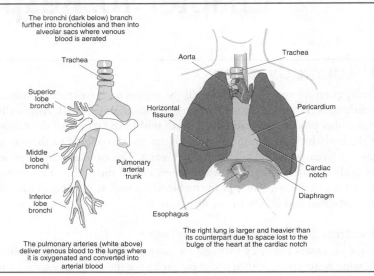

The bronchi (dark below) branch further into bronchioles and then into alveolar sacs where venous blood is aerated

The pulmonary arteries (white above) deliver venous blood to the lungs where it is oxygenated and converted into arterial blood

The right lung is larger and heavier than its counterpart due to space lost to the bulge of the heart at the cardiac notch

DEFINITIONS

cartilage. Nonvascular, fibrous, connective tissue that supports body tissues. Cartilage is less solid than bone.

hyoid bone. Single, U-shaped bone palpable in the neck above the larynx and below the mandible (lower jaw) with various muscles attached but not articulating with any other bone.

lingual tonsils. Tonsils positioned at the base of the tongue that house lymph nodes and become inflamed from bacterial or viral infections.

palatine tonsils. Tonsils seen at the back of the mouth and considered one of the body's primary defenses against infections of the respiratory and digestive systems.

turbinates. Shell-shaped elevations along the wall of the nasal cavity. The inferior turbinate is a separate bone, while the superior and middle turbinates are part of the ethmoid bone.

The nose is made up of bone and *cartilage* covered with skin on the outside and mucous membrane on the inside. Within the nose there are hairs known as cilia that catch germs and other particles inhaled with air. The internal nose comprises the paranasal sinuses and nasolacrimal ducts located over the roof of the mouth separated by the palatine bones. The nasal cavity is split by the septum and opens inside the nostrils, leading to the *turbinate* and then to the pharynx.

The paranasal sinuses are lined with mucous membranes that help produce secretions that drain into the nasal cavity. The sinuses provide a means to produce sound by serving as resonating chambers.

The pharynx, or throat, sends food into the esophagus and air into the larynx. This structure is positioned posterior to the oral cavity and runs between the nasal cavities and larynx. The pharynx is broken down into three parts: nasopharynx, oropharynx, and laryngopharynx. The oropharynx and laryngopharynx are considered part of the respiratory system, as well as the digestive system. The nasopharynx is situated just above the pharynx behind the nasal cavity leading to the soft palate. The soft palate is a moveable muscular structure at the back of the mouth that closes the nasal cavity when swallowing occurs.

There are five structures running off the nasopharynx:

- Two internal nares
- Two openings into auditory canals
- The opening leading to the oropharynx

The back wall of the nasopharynx is where the adenoids are positioned. The oropharynx is the middle portion of the pharynx at the back of the mouth starting at the soft palate and running to the *hyoid bone.* The hyoid bone is a single, u-shaped bone located in the neck just below the jaw but above the larynx. The *palatine* and *lingual tonsils* are positioned within the oropharynx.

The adenoids and tonsils are the first structures to encounter bacteria and viruses that enter the body and are considered the initial step in the body's immune response system. They can also be the site of recurrent bacterial infections and potentially lead to air passage obstructions or swallowing problems due to inflammation from these infections. Various symptoms indicate infection, but the most common are:

- Sore throat
- Difficulty/painful swallowing
- Fever
- White spots at the back of the throat
- Bad breath
- Swollen neck glands

Although typically such conditions are treated with antibiotics, in chronic cases, surgical removal of the adenoids or tonsils may be necessary. Surgery may also be a form of treatment in children with recurrent ear infections that could lead to hearing loss. In adults, tumors or other masses may require tonsil and/or adenoid removal.

The last section of the pharynx is the laryngopharynx that starts at the hyoid bone and connects to the esophagus and larynx. It is considered part of both the respiratory and the digestive systems, as it is both a pathway for air as well as a pathway for the digestive tract.

The larynx, or voice box, is the tubular structure between the laryngopharynx and the trachea and is responsible for speech. At the entrance of the larynx is the epiglottis, which closes when food is swallowed to prevent it from entering the respiratory tract. If foreign material enters the larynx, a reflex cough forces the glottis to open, sending air through the upper respiratory channels and typically expelling the foreign matter.

The larynx houses two pairs of vocal cords: false vocal cords positioned superior to the true vocal cords. Ligaments within the vocal cords stretch into the airway, constricting the glottis. When air hits this area, vibration occurs, producing sound. The pharynx, mouth, nasal cavity, and sinuses provide a type of echo chamber so that understandable speech can be produced.

Figure 10.2: Larynx

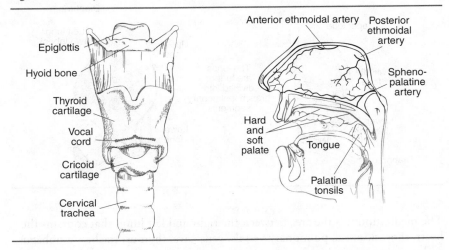

The trachea, or windpipe, begins at the larynx and divides into two branches within the chest: the left and right primary bronchi. The trachea is 12 centimeters in length and 2½ centimeters wide and is made up of C-shaped rings of hyaline cartilage within the *smooth muscle*.

The walls of the trachea are lined with mucous membranes that get more complex structurally as they travel deeper within the bronchial tree. Further within the respiratory tract, the epithelial tissue that lines the trachea begins to contain cilia that help move mucus and any potential foreign matter up and out of the respiratory tract to keep the lungs and respiratory channels clear. An area known as the *carina* is an internal ridge formed by a portion of the last hyaline tracheal cartilage where the trachea divides into the right and left bronchi. The membrane in this area is the most sensitive to foreign matter and is primarily responsible for the reflex to expel any irritants in the respiratory tract.

The right bronchus enters the right lung and is shorter and wider than the left bronchus, which enters the left lung. The bronchi inside the lungs split into secondary bronchi, one for each lobe within the lung. This branching continues to progress into tertiary bronchi, bronchioles, and finally terminal bronchioles. The end result is a structure resembling an upside down tree, referred to as the bronchial tree.

The lungs are situated within the thoracic cavity, separated by the heart and other anatomic structures, and held in place by ligaments. Fissures, or deep grooves, divide each lung into lobes. The left lung contains two lobes while the right lung contains three. This division is further subdivided into bronchopulmonary segments, each supplied by a tertiary bronchus. The left lung contains eight such segments while the right lung contains 10. Disorders or anomalies in these segments can be removed and/or corrected with little upset to the neighboring lung tissues. The bronchopulmonary segments within the lungs include smaller subdivisions referred to as lobules. The lobules are protected by *connective tissue* each made up of a *lymphatic vessel,* an *arteriole,* a *venule,* and a *terminal bronchiole.* The terminal bronchioles divide further to establish very small respiratory bronchioles, which finally branch further to form the alveolar ducts.

Figure 10.3: Lungs

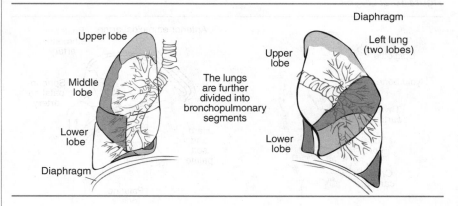

The mediastinum is the area between the right and left lungs that contains the heart, thoracic aorta, pulmonary vessels, vena cava, thymus, trachea, esophagus, and various nerves.

The primary bronchi, pulmonary blood vessels, and pleural tissue are contained within the mediastinum and form the root of the lung, entering through the triangular depression known as the hilum that is above and behind the cardiac impression. Once this network enters the lung, the bronchus and pulmonary veins and arteries divide, making up a vast network of capillaries and alveoli covering an area of 85 square meters. This area is referred to as the respiratory membrane with the primary function of providing gas exchange between air and blood.

The pleura are thin membranes covering the lungs and lining the inside of the chest wall. The pleura surround the lungs and are divided into the visceral and parietal layers. The visceral layer encapsulates the lung surface and the area between the lobes, while the parietal layer covers the inside surface of the chest wall. The area between these layers is the pleural cavity, which contains pleural fluid produced by the membranes. That fluid functions as a lubricant to decrease friction during respiration.

Figure 10.4: Upper Respiratory System

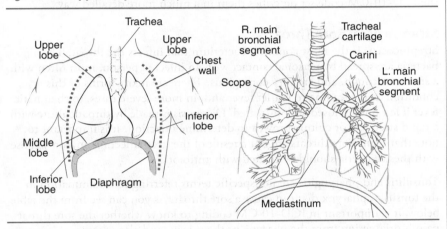

For the respiratory system to function properly, there must be adequate gas exchange within the lungs, as well as within the body's tissues. Gas exchange that takes place within the lungs is referred to as external respiration, and exchange within body tissues is referred to as internal respiration. Internal respiration can occur only via the diffusion process, meaning that gas exchange occurs through membranes, typically from a systemic capillary to the systemic tissue cells. Gases diffuse from an area of higher partial pressure or larger volume area to lower partial pressure or smaller volume area.

External respiration happens through three processes:

- **Ventilation:** Gas exchange within the pulmonary air passages.

- **Pulmonary perfusion:** Blood flow from the right side of the heart to the left side of the heart by way of pulmonary vessels.

- **Diffusion:** As discussed above in internal respiration, gas exchange through membranes where movement occurs from higher partial pressure or larger volume area to lower partial pressure or smaller volume area.

In addition to the breathing functions within the respiratory system, there is an acid-base (pH) balance function. The respiratory system helps regulate pH but not to the extent of the urinary system. When carbon dioxide increases within the body fluids, hydrogen ion levels increase, causing a decrease in blood pH. The respiratory system provides a natural buffer for this process. The rate and depth of breathing can have a major effect on the pH of body fluids, as the amount of carbon dioxide exhaled truly affects the overall acid-base balance in the body.

Anatomy and Physiology and the ICD-10-CM Code Set

The respiratory system can be affected by many disease states, as well as injury and other underlying factors. It is important to remember that breathing requires the use of several muscles within the neck, chest, and abdomen, including the diaphragm, in addition to the nerves that control these movements. An injury to the spinal cord may damage the nerves that signal the brain to control independent breathing. It is important to understand the terminology surrounding many of these disease states and underlying factors as the ICD-10-CM code set describes them in a much more detailed way.

Streptococcal Sore Throat

Streptococcus is the most common bacterium that infects the throat. The bacteria are spread by personal contact with an infected person, most often with a sneeze or cough, and are very contagious. There are many forms of this condition, some leading to scarlet fever and, in more severe cases, to rheumatic fever if left undiagnosed and untreated. Diagnosis is made by throat culture with a rapid strep test or culture growth to determine infection. It is important to note that many sore throats are not a result of the strep infection and only those with these bacteria should be treated with antibiotics.

Tonsillitis and pharyngitis are nonspecific terms referring to inflammation in the tonsils or pharynx that can cause a sore throat. As you can see from the table below, it is important in ICD-10-CM coding to know whether the sore throat pain is originating from the pharynx or the tonsils, and also whether this is a recurrent problem if the patient has a tonsillitis.

Coding for Streptococcal Sore Throat

ICD-9-CM		ICD-10-CM	
Ø34.Ø	Streptococcal sore throat	JØ2.Ø	Streptococcal pharyngitis
		JØ3.ØØ	Acute streptococcal tonsillitis, unspecified
		JØ3.Ø1	Acute recurrent streptococcal tonsillitis

Common symptoms for strep throat include fever, swollen neck glands, and white spots on the tonsils. However, these symptoms do not always indicate strep infection and may accompany several symptoms displayed in tonsillitis and pharyngitis, such as:

- Sore throat
- Headache
- Difficulty swallowing
- Muscle aches
- Weakness

Many symptoms are similar to the common cold or any number of viral infections, and strep throat infection must be determined by lab testing for proper diagnosis and prescription antibiotic treatment.

In order to report strep throat, the diagnosis needs to be documented in the medical record. Lab results may be needed before assigning the streptococcal codes if a rapid strep culture isn't available.

Aspergillosis

Aspergillosis is a fungal infection, growth, or allergic response that typically does not affect people with a normal immune system. This fungus grows in stored grain, compost, and other vegetation during the decay process. This condition presents as pneumonia or a fungal growth in the location of a previous lung disorder, such as tuberculosis or a lung abscess.

Allergic bronchopulmonary aspergillosis is an allergic reaction to this fungus that usually affects people who suffer from asthma or cystic fibrosis. Symptoms common to this form of aspergillosis include:

- Productive cough
- Fever
- Malaise
- Wheezing
- Weight loss
- Repeated airway obstruction

Additional symptoms may be seen that are specific to the body area affected, such as shortness of breath if the reaction is within the lung or sinusitis if the condition involves the nasal passages. Blood tests and a chest x-ray may help diagnose the condition, and in some cases a bronchoscopy may be performed to obtain a tissue sample from the trachea. Allergic bronchopulmonary aspergillosis is normally treated with prednisone to address the symptoms, in conjunction with an antifungal medication to attempt to eradicate the fungus.

Figure 10.5: Bronchoscopy

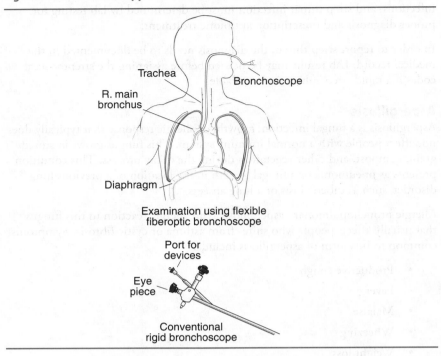

Invasive pulmonary aspergillosis is a more serious condition, as it spreads to other parts of the body and, like the allergic form, it is seen primarily in people with decreased white blood cell counts with disorders such as AIDS, cancer, and leukemia. This condition is treated with antifungal medications; however, significant fungal growth within the lung tissue may require surgical removal.

Aspergilloma is a fungal growth that can invade previously healthy tissue to form an abscess within the lungs. The growth may also spread to the brain, as well as other organs. Symptoms may never develop, and treatment may not be necessary except when coughing produces blood, in which case the bleeding needs to be controlled. Surgical intervention is a last resort due to complexity and high risk but may be necessary when excessive bleeding occurs within the lungs and/or breathing difficulties escalate.

Tonsillar aspergillosis is much like other forms of aspergillosis but occurs specifically within the tonsil region. It is treated much like other forms of aspergillosis—with steroid and antifungal therapies.

Disseminated aspergillosis is seen throughout various areas of the body, indicating a compromised immune system. This condition is often quite difficult to diagnose and can be fatal, to be discovered only at *necropsy.*

Penicilliosis is a fungal pulmonary infection caused by *Penicillium marneffei,* and tends to be an opportunistic infection affecting HIV-positive individuals.

Geotrichosis is an uncommon fungal infection that causes lesions in various areas of the body with the initial attack on the lungs. This condition commonly occurs in immunosuppressed individuals with diabetes. The patients may deal with oral lesions, abdominal pain, diarrhea, rectal bleeding, cough with a thick, bloody sputum, and pulmonary lesions. Each of these symptoms is treated differently, depending on the severity.

 DEFINITIONS

necropsy. Postmortem examination performed to ascertain the cause of death or the changes caused by disease.

Coding for Aspergillosis

ICD-9-CM		ICD-10-CM	
117.3	Aspergillosis	B44.Ø	Invasive pulmonary aspergillosis
		B44.1	Other pulmonary aspergillosis
		B44.2	Tonsillar aspergillosis
		B44.7	Disseminated aspergillosis
		B44.89	Other forms of aspergillosis
		B44.9	Aspergillosis unspecified
		B48.4	Penicillosis
117.9	Other and unspecified *mycoses*	B48.3	Geotrichosis
		B49	Unspecified mycosis

> 📖 **DEFINITIONS**
>
> **mycosis.** Fungal disease in any organ of the body.

Acute Bronchitis and Bronchiolitis

Bronchitis is a common condition that typically results from an upper respiratory infection or virus affecting the respiratory system. This condition affects the bronchial tubes, causing inflammation within the lining. Bronchiolitis is a similar condition, also common, affecting the bronchioles within the lung. Both conditions typically have a rapid onset and short duration in their acute form, typically resolving within a week or two.

Figure 10.6: Bronchioli and Alveoli

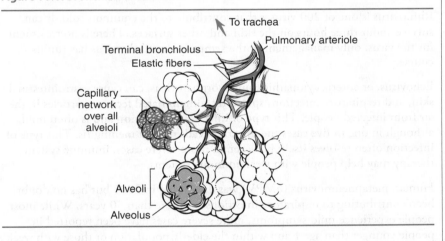

These conditions may be caused by a number of infective agents.

Mycoplasma pneumoniae is a bacterium often acquired when a person is exposed to someone with pneumonia. It typically is a mild form of pneumonia and is often referred to as atypical or walking pneumonia. The condition is characterized by a nine- to 12-day incubation period in most instances, and typically results in symptoms of an upper respiratory infection, dry cough, and fever.

Hemophilus influenzae is a bacterium that can lead to infections within the respiratory tract, which may progress and infect other organs. This bacterium is spread through sneezing, coughing, and touching. The symptoms vary depending on the organ affected and is usually detected by laboratory analysis of body tissue. It is important to note that children are immunized against type B (Hib) to prevent more serious and even deadly infections caused by these bacteria.

Streptococcus is a bacterium, commonly referred to as "strep," that causes infections such as strep throat, pneumonia, and rheumatic and scarlet fevers. It is a gram-positive bacterium, and there are many forms of streptococcal bacteria that grow in humans.

Coxsackie virus appears in the human digestive tract and is spread by unwashed hands and contaminated surfaces. This virus can show signs of mild flu-like symptoms that resolve on their own. However, the virus can also lead to more severe conditions, such as hand, foot, and mouth disease. Due to the transmission method, this virus tends to spread amongst children quickly, especially during warm weather months.

Parainfluenza virus is one of many viruses leading to respiratory infections, most often mild in older children and adults since they have been exposed and the body has built up an immunity to the virus. However, infants and people with a weakened immune system experience more severe symptoms with bronchiolitis caused by parainfluenza.

Respiratory syncytial virus, commonly known as RSV, is a large contributor to respiratory infections among children. Adults may experience this type of infection with mild cold-type symptoms, while children with underlying conditions that affect the lungs and immune systems can experience more serious symptoms and illness. RSV is highly contagious and is spread through contaminated surfaces and coughing, sneezing, and touching.

Rhinovirus is one of 200 viruses that contribute to the common cold. It can survive about three hours on the skin and other surfaces. There is no treatment for the virus, only management of the symptoms until the virus has run its course.

Echovirus, or enteric cytopathic human orphan virus, can cause gastrointestinal, skin, and respiratory infections spread by contaminated feces or particles in the air from infected people. This type of infection is common and is often mild, although in one in five cases the infection leads to viral meningitis. This type of infection often resolves itself; however, in more severe cases, immune system therapy may help people with weak immune systems.

Human metapneumovirus (hMPV) was discovered in 2001 but has no doubt been contributing to respiratory infections for more than 50 years. While most people experience mild symptoms, more severe cases have been reported in people younger than age 1 and within the elderly population or those with weak immune systems. Infection often occurs three to five days after exposure by close contact with an infected person or surface containing the virus. Transplant patients are among those at highest risk for acquiring this type of infection.

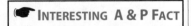
INTERESTING A & P FACT

Rhinovirus causes a cold in adults approximately 30 to 35 percent of the time. There are more than 110 types of rhinoviruses currently identified.

Coding for Acute Bronchitis

ICD-9-CM		ICD-10-CM	
466.0	Acute bronchitis	J20.0	Acute bronchitis due to mycoplasma pneumoniae
		J20.1	Acute bronchitis due to hemophilus influenzae
		J20.2	Acute bronchitis due to streptococcus
		J20.3	Acute bronchitis due to coxsackievirus
		J20.4	Acute bronchitis due to parainfluenza virus
		J20.5	Acute bronchitis due to respiratory syncytial virus
		J20.6	Acute bronchitis due to rhinovirus
		J20.7	Acute bronchitis due to echovirus
		J20.8	Acute bronchitis due to other specified organisms
		J20.9	Acute bronchitis, unspecified

Coding for these types of bronchitis and bronchiolitis will be more complicated under the ICD-10-CM code set due to the new codes established identifying the cause of the infection. In ICD-9-CM, acute bronchitis and bronchiolitis are coded with 466.xx. As illustrated in the tables above and below, understanding the various types of infectious agents is the key to correct code assignment under the ICD-10-CM system.

Coding for Acute Bronchiolitis

ICD-9-CM		ICD-10-CM	
466.19	Acute bronchiolitis due to other infectious organisms	J21.1	Acute bronchiolitis due to human metapneumovirus
		J21.8	Acute bronchiolitis due to other specified organisms
		J21.9	Acute bronchiolitis, unspecified

To code for bronchitis and bronchiolitis under ICD-10-CM, the coder needs to determine from the documentation which organism contributed to the condition—it is not enough to understand whether the patient presents with acute bronchitis or acute bronchiolitis. To code the encounter to the highest level of specificity, the coder may need to query the provider for additional information on the type of infectious agent.

Pneumonia in Whooping Cough and Other Infectious Diseases

Pneumonia is a lung infection caused by bacteria or viruses. When bacteria are the cause, the infection presents quickly with symptoms such as cough, fever, shortness of breath, chills, weakness, and nausea. When a virus is the cause, the infection presents more slowly and, while symptoms are similar, they may not be as easy to identify.

Whooping cough is a common name for a condition sometimes associated with pneumonia called pertussis, named after the bacterium *Bordetella pertussis,* its causative agent. Pertussis is a highly contagious respiratory disease and has been known as whooping cough due to its symptoms: severe coughing, followed by a loud "whooping" inspiration. Children in the United States generally receive vaccines for pertussis.

Parapertussis is similar to whooping cough in etiology and symptoms and can occur at any age, although it primarily affects children ages 3 to 5. Parapertussis

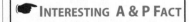

INTERESTING A & P FACT

Prior to widespread vaccination for *Bordetella pertussis,* which began in the 1940s, whooping cough killed 5,000 to 10,000 people in the United States every year. With vaccination, that number has dropped to fewer than 30 per year.

occurs less frequently than pertussis and has a shorter duration as well. Vaccination against whooping cough does not provide immunity to parapertussis, and most people recover completely with extremely rare complications due to this infection.

Ascariasis is an intestinal infection caused by roundworms and is most prevalent in unsanitary or overcrowded populations of the world. The symptoms, though rare in many cases, depend on the volume of worms and the site of infestation. Ascariasis pneumonia is caused by the roundworm larvae that travel through the bloodstream or lymph system into the lungs, causing coughing, shortness of breath, and wheezing lasting about six days before the larvae are expelled through a cough or reingested.

Coding for Pneumonia in Whooping Cough and Other Infectious Diseases

ICD-9-CM		ICD-10-CM	
484.3	Pneumonia in whooping cough	A37.Ø1	Whooping cough due to Bordetella pertussis with pneumonia
		A37.11	Whooping cough due to Bordetella parapertussis with pneumonia
		A37.81	Whooping cough due to other Bordetella species with pneumonia
		A37.91	Whooping cough, unspecified species with pneumonia
484.8	Pneumonia in other infectious diseases classified elsewhere	B77.81	Ascariasis pneumonia
		J17	Pneumonia in diseases classified elsewhere

What was previously reported as pneumonia in whooping cough within the ICD-9-CM code set is broken down even further within ICD-10-CM to allow for specific causal agents to be reported that contribute to the condition. As has been the case with other conditions, it is important to understand how these causal agents relate. Coders need this information at the time of code selection, as it is not yet certain how payers will react to unlisted codes in the ICD-10-CM code set. Using the highest level of specificity at all times will be key to accurate payment for providers.

Emphysematous Bleb and Other Emphysema

Emphysema is a condition of the respiratory system that restricts the air flow during exhalation because the bronchioles and alveoli deteriorate gradually. This causes a loss of lung elasticity, which can result in significant breathing difficulty. As this condition progresses, the spherical air sacs within the lungs become irregular and contain holes, reducing not only the number of air sacs but also the amount of oxygen that can circulate into the blood from the lungs (a decrease in the gas exchange). As the air sacs deteriorate, the openings collapse, trapping air within the lungs. Treatment for this condition can slow down the deterioration; however, once the damage is done, it cannot be reversed or cured. Smoking and air pollution are main contributors to emphysema.

☛ **INTERESTING A & P FACT**

In addition to smoking and air pollution, some patients with emphysema, especially those that are diagnosed early in life, acquire the disease due to a rare genetic deficiency of serum alpha-1 antitrypsin (AAT). AAT protects the elasticity of the lungs and due to deficiency enzymes in the body cause damage resulting in emphysema.

Figure 10.7: Emphysema

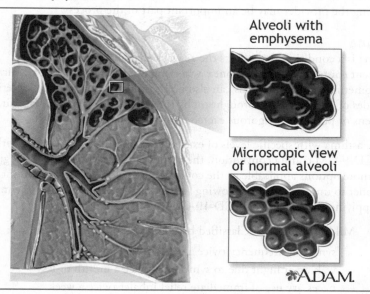

Alveoli with emphysema

Microscopic view of normal alveoli

✤A.D.A.M.

Emphysematous bleb are blisters larger than 1 mm within an emphysematous lung that contain blood or serum. It is a fairly generic term, referring more to a symptom that occurs during emphysema than to a disease process itself.

Macleod's syndrome is a form of emphysema in which one lung becomes somewhat transparent in conjunction with the reduced oxygen and carbon dioxide exchange within the blood. Macleod's syndrome is also known as Swyer James syndrome or SJS.

Panlobular emphysema affects all parts of the lobes within the lungs. The right lung having three lobes and the left lung having two lobes, also further divides into hundreds of smaller lobules each containing a bronchiole and its own group of alveoli. A person with panlobular emphysema has a condition directly affecting all of these areas.

Centrilobular emphysema occurs mainly in the central part of the lobule and is the most common form of emphysema mostly in the upper lobe and more frequently seen in men than women. It is also associated with chronic bronchitis.

Coding for Emphysematous Bleb and other Emphysema

ICD-9-CM		ICD-10-CM	
492.Ø	Emphysematous bleb	J43.9	Emphysema unspecified
492.8	Other emphysema	J43.Ø	Unilateral pulmonary emphysema [Macleod's syndrome]
		J43.1	Panlobular emphysema
		J43.2	Centrilobular emphysema
		J43.8	Other emphysema
		J43.9	Emphysema unspecified

Although the ICD-10-CM code set allows for coding unspecified emphysema, it is clear the expansion of the terms narrows down the exact nature of the condition and tracks the variations of the disease. Keep in mind that unspecified codes may not be acceptable for payment purposes, so using the most specific code available based on the documentation will be important. In some instances, querying the provider may be an important part of the process.

Asthma

Asthma is a condition that affects the airways characterized by typically recurrent episodes of severe dyspnea, wheezing on inspiration and/or expiration, and sometimes coughing. This can also be accompanied by mucous secretions. Episodes of asthma can be brought on by infections, inhalation of cold air, allergens or pollutants, vigorous exercise, or emotional stress.

While asthma with specific levels of exacerbation is currently specified within the ICD-9-CM coding convention, the conversion to ICD-10-CM will give even more options applicable to the condition. It will be vitally important for the coder to understand the following terms when interpreting documentation and applying the appropriate ICD-10-CM codes.

- **Mild intermittent:** Classified based on the following indications:
  - symptom frequency twice a week or less
  - waking at night due to symptoms twice a month or less
  - necessary use of immediate relief inhaler twice a week
  - little or no interference with daily activities
  - normal peak flow readings between symptoms
  - not requiring the use of oral steroids to control or requiring them once per year
- **Mild persistent** Classified based on the following indications:
  - symptom frequency more than two days a week, but not every day
  - waking at night due to symptoms three to four times a month
  - necessary use of immediate relief inhaler more than two times a week
  - minor interference with daily activities
  - peak flow readings equal to 80 percent of personal norm
  - requiring the use of oral steroids twice a year
- **Moderate persistent:** Classified based on the following indications:
  - daily symptoms
  - waking at night due to symptoms more than one time a week
  - necessary use of immediate relief inhaler daily
  - some interference with daily activities
  - peak flow reading from 60 to 80 percent of personal norm
  - requiring the use of oral steroids twice a year
- **Severe persistent:** Classified based on the following indications:
  - frequent symptoms throughout the day
  - waking at night due to symptoms often every night
  - necessary use of immediate relief inhaler several times daily
  - symptoms that severely limit daily activities
  - peak flow readings less than 60 percent of personal norm
  - requiring the use of oral steroids two or more times a year

Currently, asthma is classified into groups: extrinsic and intrinsic. Asthma caused by allergies is known as extrinsic or allergic asthma. This form of asthma is a response to an irritant inhaled or ingested. Intrinsic asthma is typically seen in people aged 30 or older and is typically chronic and persistent rather than episodic in nature. Intrinsic asthma is often related to respiratory infections, inhaled chemicals, and/or pollution.

Coding for Extrinsic Asthma

ICD-9-CM		ICD-10-CM	
493.00	Extrinsic asthma, unspecified	J45.20	Mild intermittent asthma, uncomplicated
		J45.30	Mild persistent asthma, uncomplicated
		J45.40	Moderate persistent asthma, uncomplicated
		J45.50	Severe persistent asthma, uncomplicated
493.01	Extrinsic asthma with status asthmaticus	J45.22	Mild intermittent asthma, with status asthmaticus
		J45.32	Mild persistent asthma, with status asthmaticus
		J45.42	Moderate persistent asthma, with status asthmaticus
		J45.52	Severe persistent asthma, with status asthmaticus
493.02	Extrinsic asthma with exacerbation	J45.21	Mild intermittent asthma, with acute exacerbation
		J45.31	Mild persistent asthma, with acute exacerbation
		J45.41	Moderate persistent asthma, with acute exacerbation
		J45.51	Severe persistent asthma, with acute exacerbation

An exacerbation of a patient's condition is simply an increase in the seriousness of his or her disease, typically marked by a greater intensity of signs and symptoms. In the case of asthma, this often means an asthma attack, prompting the patient to seek medical assistance to receive medication to clear his or her airway to assist in breathing.

Status asthmaticus is classified as an acute and severe asthma attack that does not respond to the typical treatment with bronchodilators and can lead to respiratory failure. Because this type of an attack requires immediate medical intervention, it is important to recognize the early symptoms, such as shortness of breath and difficulty talking in complete sentences.

Coding for Intrinsic Asthma

ICD-9-CM		ICD-10-CM	
493.10	Intrinsic asthma, unspecified	J45.20	Mild intermittent asthma, uncomplicated
		J45.30	Mild persistent asthma, uncomplicated
		J45.40	Moderate persistent asthma, uncomplicated
		J45.50	Severe persistent asthma, uncomplicated
493.11	Intrinsic asthma with status asthmaticus	J45.22	Mild intermittent asthma, with status asthmaticus
		J45.32	Mild persistent asthma, with status asthmaticus
		J45.42	Moderate persistent asthma, with status asthmaticus
		J45.52	Severe persistent asthma, with status asthmaticus

ICD-9-CM		ICD-10-CM	
493.12	Intrinsic asthma with exacerbation	J45.21	Mild intermittent asthma, with acute exacerbation
		J45.31	Mild persistent asthma, with acute exacerbation
		J45.41	Moderate persistent asthma, with acute exacerbation
		J45.51	Severe persistent asthma, with acute exacerbation

Pneumoconiosis Due to Silica and Other Inorganic Dust

Pneumoconiosis is a condition caused by inhaling dust particles, typically associated with occupations that require regular exposure to mineral dusts. This condition is a form of interstitial lung disease that contributes to the inflammation of the air sacs, causing the lung tissue to harden. There is no cure for this disease, and treatment is focused on managing the patient's symptoms.

There are several common forms of pneumoconiosis in the United States:

- Asbestosis
- Silicosis
- Coal worker's pneumoconiosis
- Talc pneumoconiosis
- Kaolin pneumoconiosis
- Siderosis of the lung

Figure 10.8: Alveoli, Asbestoses, Air Sacs

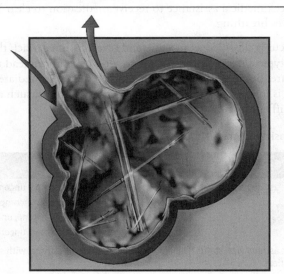

Definitions and Other Classifications of Pneumoconiosis

Asbestosis is a generic term for a group of minerals that cause this form of lung disease. These minerals are taken from underground deposits and have been historically used in insulation, tiles, and automobile parts. People who work in these industries are not the only groups that develop this condition. Those who live or work in structures that contain asbestos products that have begun to break down have also been known to acquire this condition; however, symptoms do not often occur until 20 years or more after exposure. In these patients, chest films often show small linear opacities distributed throughout the lung. This disease tends to be progressive, beginning with shortness of breath, progressing eventually to respiratory failure.

Silicosis is caused by regular exposure to white crystal compounds often associated with sand and quartz as seen in the manufacturing of glass and concrete products. This condition is often characterized by the development of nodular fibrosis in the lungs.

Coal worker's pneumoconiosis affects people who work in mines, manufacturing, or shipping of coal and graphite products with regular inhalation of these particles. It is characterized by the deposit of coal dust in the lungs and the formation of black nodules on the bronchioles, which results in focal emphysema. This condition is often referred to as black lung disease or anthracosis, and the progress can often be halted if further exposure to coal dust is prevented.

Talc pneumoconiosis is caused by regular exposure to talc dust often present in industries such as cosmetics, pharmaceutical, paper, ceramics, and electronics manufacturing. This stage of the disease is considered "simple pneumoconiosis;" continued overexposure leads to fibrosis.

Kaolin, or china clay, pneumoconiosis is named for the mineral that causes it (kaolin), which is used in the manufacturing of ceramics, paper, pharmaceuticals, and cosmetics.

Siderosis, also called welder's or silver polisher's lung, arises from exposure to iron particles or dust. A person with this condition may not display any symptoms, but a chest x-ray will show an abnormality in one or both of the lungs.

Aluminosis may also be referred to as aluminum lung. Typically, this condition afflicts those working in explosive or abrasive aluminum manufacturing, particularly aluminum welders or polishers. Recent studies show a small portion of these workers develops this condition over the course of 25 years or more of exposure.

Bauxite fibrosis of the lung is due to inhalation of bauxite dust, which can be found in combinations of hydrated aluminum oxides that include iron and silicon. Those who work with abrasive materials in spark plugs and furnaces are exposed to this type of dust.

Berylliosis is caused by the light-weight metallic element beryllium, which is used in aerospace, semiconductors, electrical industries, and copper alloy in springs. The most common use of this element is in electric light bulbs and fluorescent tubes. This condition was first recognized in the 1940s as an occupational lung disease. It remains very rare.

Graphite fibrosis of the lung is caused by the dust from graphite, which is one of many mineral forms of carbon with a wide variety of uses. Graphite can be mixed with clay as is done for making pencils and has uses in lubricants, polish, batteries, and nuclear reactor cores.

Stannosis results from overexposure to tin dust (stannic or tin oxide) and can be seen on a chest x-ray presenting as dense masses. These oxides are often used in the production of glass, enamels, and ceramic glazes.

Byssinosis, also referred to as brown lung disease, causes narrowing of air passages, like asthma. The primary cause of this condition is inhalation of cotton, which is frequently used in the textile industry.

Flax-dresser's disease is a form of byssinosis that is caused by inhaling remnants of flax, which is grown for the seed it produces and the oil component of that seed. The oil produced has many industrial, household, and animal uses, such as paint, varnish, ink, and protein meal for livestock. Recently flax seed has been recognized as a beneficial additive to human food due to the fatty acids in the oil.

Cannabinosis is another form of byssinosis specific to the inhalation of hemp and other unprocessed fibers within the textile manufacturing industry. People working in factories that produce yarn, thread, and fabric containing hemp are at increased risk of developing this condition.

As illustrated in the following table, it is important under ICD-10-CM to gather information from providers about the root of the patient's pneumoconiosis. What was previously a simple pneumoconiosis due to a type of inorganic dust is now a berylliosis or a siderosis. Coders must gather the most detailed information they can from the patient's history to code to the highest level of specificity.

Coding for Pneumoconiosis Due to Silica and Other Inorganic Dust

ICD-9-CM		ICD-10-CM	
502	Pneumoconiosis due to other silica or silicates	J62.0	Pneumoconiosis due to talc dust
		J62.8	Pneumoconiosis due to other dust containing silica
503	Pneumoconiosis due to other inorganic dust	J63.0	Aluminosis of lung
		J63.1	Bauxite fibrosis of lung
		J63.2	Berylliosis
		J63.3	Graphite fibrosis of lung
		J63.4	Siderosis
		J63.5	Stannosis
		J63.6	Pneumoconiosis due to other specified inorganic dust
504	Pneumonopathy due to inhalation of other dust	J66.0	Byssinosis
		J66.1	Flax-dresser's disease
		J66.2	Cannabinosis
		J66.8	Airway disease due to other specified organic dust

The pneumoconiosis group of diseases in particular is coded quite differently under the ICD-10-CM code set. It will take practice and physician education to ensure that the documentation specifies the form of the condition being tested for and treated so that ICD-10-CM coding is accurate. Accurate coding, in turn, is needed to determine the medical necessity of tests ordered to confirm diagnosis and determine the appropriate course of treatment, as well as to follow the progression of the disease.

Pleurisy

Pleurisy is a condition that is seen when the membrane lining the chest surrounding the lungs becomes inflamed. This condition may be in conjunction with pleural effusion, when fluid from the vessels or lymphatic system leak into the membrane lining. The typical symptoms associated with pleurisy are chest pain during inhale/exhale phases of breathing, shortness of breath, nonproductive cough, and fevers/chills. Chest pain increases with coughing, sneezing, and deep breathing and may radiate to the shoulder area. If pleurisy is accompanied by effusion, chest pain may subside due to the fluid accumulation that provides lubrication. However, excessive fluid retention adds pressure to the lungs, making it difficult to breathe. When this fluid becomes infected, additional symptoms occur. This condition is then known as empyema.

Pleural plaque is seen within the chest cavity as deposits of fibrous tissue, which may be attributed to asbestos exposure. These deposits often become calcified and can be viewed on a chest x-ray, depending on the density of the calcification. In recent studies, about 10 to 40 percent of these deposits appear on a standard chest radiograph. This plaque is typically benign in nature, and treatment focuses on symptoms, if any are present. Other studies indicate that 80 percent of patients with pleural plaque have been exposed to some form of asbestos. Patients with pleural plaque have an elevated risk of diffuse pleural fibrosis.

Fibrothorax is simply fibrosis within the pleural lining of the lungs. It is commonly seen as a stiff layer surrounding the lung and is attributed to traumatic hemothorax or pleural effusion.

Chylous pleural effusion is fluid within the pleural space that appears opaque and white, but the fluid is no longer opaque when combined with ether. This condition is due to the leaking of lymph contents into the space, usually as a result of thoracic duct damage or injury, as well as mediastinal lymphoma.

Hemothorax occurs when blood accumulates within the pleural cavity. While the most common contributor to this condition is trauma to the chest, it may also be observed in patients with the following conditions:

- Clotting defects
- Necrosis of lung tissue
- Cancer of the lung or within the pleura
- Central venous catheter placement
- Surgery within the chest cavity
- Tuberculosis

Hemothorax symptoms can range from anxiety and chest pain to shortness of breath and increased heart rate. Additionally, the physician may notice absence of breath sounds in the affected area, which requires further testing such as chest x-ray, computed tomography scan, or thoracentesis. Treatment centers on stopping the bleeding via a chest tube that may be left in place over the course of several days. If this is unsuccessful, a *thoracotomy* may be necessary.

 DEFINITIONS

thoracotomy. Surgical procedure during which an incision is made into the chest to puncture the pleural space so that the blood and/or fluid from the area can be drained.

Figure 10.9: Pleural Effusion

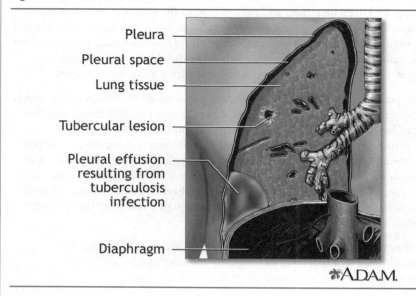

Pleura

Pleural space

Lung tissue

Tubercular lesion

Pleural effusion resulting from tuberculosis infection

Diaphragm

✽A.D.A.M.

Coding for Pleurisy and Related Effusion

ICD-9-CM		ICD-10-CM	
511.0	Pleurisy without mention of effusion or current tuberculosis	J86.9	Pyothorax with fistula
		J92.0	Pleural plaque with presence of asbestos
		J92.9	Pleural plaque without asbestos
		J94.1	Fibrothorax
		J94.8	Other specified pleural conditions
		J94.9	Pleural condition, unspecified
		R09.1	Pleurisy
511.89	Other specified forms of effusion, except tuberculosis	J90	Pleural effusion not elsewhere classified
		J94.0	Chylous effusion
		J94.2	Hemothorax

Understanding the differentiation between the forms of pleurisy is important for coders. Without the appropriate documentation, the coder may need to query the provider for additional information. In some instances, there may not be additional information and a simple diagnosis of pleurisy will be used.

Lung Abscess

An abscess within the lung is a growth often filled with pus and typically due to some kind of infection causing the surrounding tissue to become inflamed. Bacteria normally in the mouth may be inhaled into the lungs, leading to an infection as seen in some cases of periodontal disease. An abscess can also form in people with a weak immune system or airway obstruction. Symptoms that can indicate a lung abscess include productive cough, fever, loss of appetite, and fatigue mirroring pneumonia. A chest x-ray typically shows the presence of a lung abscess. In most cases, symptoms are slow to develop except when the infection is caused by *Staphylococcus aureus,* in which case they appear suddenly and can be fatal if not treated immediately. Most abscesses of the lung are treated with antibiotics. In some rare cases, a bronchoscopy is performed and a tube is inserted to drain the abscess.

Gangrene of the lung can occur when an area is cut off from regular blood supply. The lack of blood supply may be a result of an infection, injury, or disease.

Necrosis is the death of tissue and may occur in addition to gangrene.

Coding for Lung Abscess

ICD-9-CM		ICD-10-CM	
513.0	Abscess of lung	J85.0	Gangrene and necrosis of lung
		J85.1	Abscess of lung with pneumonia
		J85.2	Abscess of lung without pneumonia

There is only one applicable ICD-9-CM code for abscess of the lung; however, ICD-10-CM requires the coder to query the physician for more specific details if the documentation does not indicate gangrene or necrosis, or whether or not the abscess was somehow connected to pneumonia.

Pulmonary Congestion and Hypostasis

Pulmonary congestion is the build-up of fluid within the lungs, often as a result of an infection or congestive heart failure. Hypostasis is the accumulation of deposits of a specific substance in a body area because of lack of activity. With regard to the respiratory system, hypostasis typically occurs in the lungs of elderly and debilitated people because of lack of movement. Both conditions are coded in ICD-9-CM with code 514, but in ICD-10-CM, the specific type of congestion must be specified, as described below.

ICD-10-CM code J18.2 Hypostatic pneumonia, unspecified organism, is specifically associated with a lack of movement over a long period of time. Fluids settle in the patient's lung, causing the pneumonia. This condition often affects elderly, debilitated, or bedridden people. There may be an organism that is causing the pneumonia, but this particular code does not require that the organism be specifically identified.

ICD-10-CM code J18.1 Chronic pulmonary edema, is caused by excessive fluid within the lungs, causing inflammation. This is often a result of congestive heart failure.

Acute Chest Syndrome

Acute chest syndrome is associated with various forms of sickle-cell diseases. Coding for these conditions requires the use of more than one ICD-9-CM code, with acute chest syndrome code 517.3 as the secondary code. ICD-10-CM allows for more specific coding by using one primary code with the option of an additional code to specify any associated fever.

Hb-SS disease, also referred to as sickle cell anemia, is a hereditary deficiency within the red blood cells. This condition causes an irregular shape in the cells that decreases the amount of oxygen that can be carried throughout the body to the various organs. Symptoms, as well as episodes, can vary between patients. Some people have only one episode every few years, while others present with many episodes throughout a given year and still others require hospitalization. Typically symptoms are not seen until the patient is at least 4 months old. Common symptoms include:

- Abdominal pain
- Bone pain

- Developmental delay
- Fatigue
- Fever
- Increased heart rate
- Jaundice
- Chest pain
- Increased thirst
- Increased urination
- Skin ulcers

Ongoing treatment is frequently necessary to manage the condition outside of recurring episodes and may include folic acid supplements, as well as hydration.

Hb-C disease, or hemoglobin C disease, is a genetic blood disorder most often seen in those of African descent. This condition leads to anemia, in which the typical life span of the red blood cells is much shorter than normal. Most people with this condition do not display any symptoms but can develop jaundice, enlargement of the spleen, or gallstones that require treatment. Typically, this condition is managed with a folic acid supplement to assist in the production of normal red blood cells and control the anemia.

Thalassemia is another genetic blood disorder that reduces the number of red blood cells within the body. Mild cases require no treatment; however, more severe cases may require regular blood transfusions. Symptoms depend on the type and severity of the condition and can surface as early as newborn through age 2, while some people may never experience any symptoms.

Coding for Acute Chest Syndrome

ICD-9-CM		ICD-10-CM	
517.3	Acute chest syndrome	D57.01	Hb-SS disease with acute chest syndrome
		D57.211	Sickle-cell/Hb-C disease with acute chest syndrome
		D57.411	Sickle-cell thalassemia with acute chest syndrome
		D57.811	Other sickle-cell disorders with acute chest syndrome

Lung Involvement in Other Diseases

Coding in ICD-9-CM for lung involvement in diseases coded elsewhere obviously requires more than one code, with the secondary code 517.8 and instruction to code first the underlying condition. With ICD-10-CM, there is typically one specific code for the disease manifested within the lung.

Systemic lupus erythematosus (SLE) interferes with the body's normal immune response. This condition causes the body to attack normal, healthy cells, leading to inflammation in various parts of the body and, for this definition, specifically the lungs. It affects nine times more women than men, with symptoms occurring between the ages of 10 and 50. When the lungs are affected by SLE, symptoms include chest pain when breathing deeply, coughing up blood, and shortness of breath. A physician may hear a *pleural friction rub* when the patient is examined, and a chest x-ray may show *pleuritis* or pleurisy. Treatment might include nonsteroidal anti-inflammatory medications to control symptoms.

Dermatopolymyositis is a muscle disorder causing inflammation and weakness, as well as a skin rash. Symptoms of lung involvement reported, as in pulmonary

 DEFINITIONS

pleural friction rub. Low, grating sound heard when pleural surfaces rub against each other. This may be confused with a pericardial rub; cessation of the sound when the patient holds his or her breath indicates a pleural friction rub.

pleuritis. Inflammation of the lining surrounding the lungs and lining the inside of the chest.

fibrosis, are painful respiration and alveolitis and are often treated with corticosteroids.

Polymyositis is a muscle disorder causing inflammation and weakness in the skeletal muscles closest to the trunk of the body. This condition can occur at any age but is most common in adults ages 30 to 50 and is seen more in women than men. Symptoms develop slowly and progress over time, with lung involvement displayed in shortness of breath and speech deterioration. The overall cause cannot be pinpointed even though it is suggested the condition may be brought on by an infection. However, since symptoms at initial onset are slow to develop, it is almost impossible to determine the initial source.

Sicca syndrome, also referred to as Sjögren syndrome, is an autoimmune disease often displayed in conjunction with another condition such as polymyositis. Sicca syndrome is characterized by a significantly decreased fluid production within the body. Specific lung involvement relates to potential respiratory infections and pneumonias due to the dryness.

Coding for Lung Involvement in Other Diseases Classified Elsewhere

ICD-9-CM		ICD-10-CM	
517.8	Lung involvement in other diseases classified elsewhere	J99	Respiratory disorders in diseases classified elsewhere
		M32.13	Lung involvement in systemic lupus erythematosus
		M33.01	Juvenile dermatopolymyositis with respiratory involvement
		M33.11	Other dermatopolymyositis with respiratory involvement
		M33.21	Polymyositis with respiratory involvement
		M33.91	Dermatopolymyositis, unspecified, with respiratory involvement
		M35.02	Sicca syndrome, with lung involvement

Injuries

Many injuries can occur throughout the respiratory system. The ICD-10-CM code set allows the coder to more specifically describe the type and location of the injury, which in turn requires additional documentation and knowledge of terms. Here are some important terms to be aware of in defining injuries under the ICD-10-CM code set:

- **Unilateral:** Affecting one side of the body, or in the case of the lungs, affecting only one lung.

- **Bilateral:** Affecting both sides, or both lungs.

- **Initial encounter:** First visit to treat the injury.

Primary blast is an injury directly related to an explosive and the damage the shock wave's impact has on the body. Body organs that are filled with gas are typically the most affected by such an explosion, with the lungs often being the most severely affected and the most common fatality. The injury should be considered a primary blast if a person is exposed to an explosion and has symptoms of *bradycardia, apnea,* and *hypotension.* While usually present at initial evaluation, symptoms delayed as far out as 48 hours afterward are not uncommon. The effects can be seen on a chest x-ray and, in some cases, a *thoracostomy* may be necessary to avoid complications of anesthesia or air transport to a hospital.

DEFINITIONS

apnea. Absence of breathing.

bradycardia. Slowed heart rate, usually defined as rate less than 60 beats per minute.

hypotension. Decreased blood pressure below the normal rate.

thoracostomy. Creation of an opening in the chest wall for drainage.

A contusion is a superficial injury, often a bruise, as a result of trauma without a break in the skin. However, even this kind of injury can have serious complications when the contusion affects the respiratory system, particularly the lungs.

A laceration is a torn, ragged-edged wound. The initial concern is infection or damage to organs underneath the laceration. Deeper lacerations may require irrigation and/or stitches to close the affected area.

Coding for Injury Related to the Bronchus without Mention of Open Wound in Cavity

ICD-9-CM		ICD-10-CM	
862.21	Bronchus injury without mention of open wound in cavity	S27.401A	Unspecified injury of bronchus, unilateral, initial encounter
		S27.402	Unspecified injury of bronchus, bilateral, initial encounter
		S27.409A	Unspecified injury of bronchus, unspecified, initial encounter
		S27.411A	Primary blast injury of bronchus, unilateral, initial encounter
		S27.412A	Primary blast injury of bronchus, bilateral, initial encounter
		S27.419A	Primary blast injury of bronchus, unspecified, initial encounter
		S27.421A	Contusion of bronchus, unilateral, initial encounter
		S27.422A	Contusion of bronchus, bilateral, initial encounter
		S27.429A	Contusion of bronchus, unspecified, initial encounter
		S27.431A	Laceration of bronchus, unilateral, initial encounter
		S27.432A	Laceration of bronchus, bilateral, initial encounter
		S27.439A	Laceration of bronchus, unspecified, initial encounter
		S27.491A	Other injury of bronchus, unilateral, initial encounter
		S27.492A	Other injury of bronchus, bilateral, initial encounter
		S27.499A	Other injury of bronchus, unspecified, initial encounter

 DEFINITIONS

atelectasis. Collapse of lung tissue, typically alveoli, affecting part or all of one lung, preventing normal oxygen absorption to healthy tissues.

A pulmonary contusion affects the lung tissue itself, leading to fluid and blood accumulation within the alveolar areas of the lung. About 20 percent of cases of blunt chest injuries also reported pulmonary contusions. In some cases, crackling noises known as rales can be heard in the chest through a stethoscope. If the contusion is left undiagnosed, complications such as *atelectasis,* pneumonia, and respiratory failure may occur. Once diagnosed, most lung contusions resolve in less than a week with fluid restriction and careful observation. Larger contusions may require more extensive treatment like oxygen or mechanical ventilation.

Coding for Injury of Other Specified Intrathoracic Organ without Open Wound in Cavity

ICD-9-CM		ICD-10-CM	
862.29	Injury to other specified intrathoracic organs without mention of open wound into cavity	S27.50xA	Unspecified injury of thoracic trachea, initial encounter
		S27.51xA	Primary blast injury of thoracic trachea, initial encounter
		S27.52xA	Contusion of thoracic trachea, initial encounter
		S27.53xA	Laceration of thoracic trachea, initial encounter
		S27.59xA	Other injury of thoracic trachea, initial encounter
		S27.60xA	Unspecified injury of pleura, initial encounter
		S27.63xA	Laceration of pleura, initial encounter
		S27.69xA	Other injury of pleura, initial encounter
		S27.892A	Contusion of other specified intrathoracic organs, initial encounter
		S27.893A	Laceration of other specified intrathoracic organs, initial encounter
		S27.898A	Other injury of other specified intrathoracic organs, initial encounter
		S27.899A	Unspecified injury of other specified intrathoracic organs, initial encounter

Multiple and Unspecified Injuries to Intrathoracic Organs, with Open Wound into Cavity

Multiple injuries within the thoracic cavity have additional codes to capture various circumstances not covered elsewhere and when more than one injury, complication, or area might be affected.

Figure 10.10: Firearm Injury, X-ray

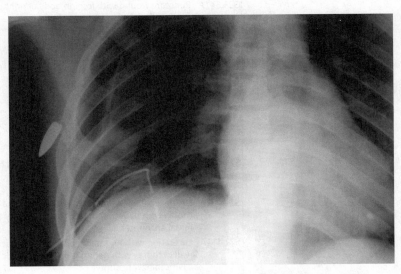

© Mauro Fermariello/Photo Researchers, Inc.

A penetrating wound is one that pierces the skin and enters the body, possibly affecting underlying structures and organs.

A puncture is any injury that creates a hole in the skin and/or internal tissues or organs.

An open bite is a wound caused by teeth, human or animal.

A foreign body is an object or substance found in an organ or tissue that does not belong there under normal circumstances. The following table is an example of some of the many ICD-10-CM codes that ICD-9-CM code 862.9 maps to. For detailed information on ICD-9-CM to ICD-10-CM mapping, see *Ingenix's ICD-10-CM Mappings.*

Coding for Multiple and Unspecified Injuries to the Intrathoracic Organs, with Open Wound into Cavity

ICD-9-CM		ICD-10-CM	
862.9	Injury to multiple and unspecified intrathoracic organs with open wound into cavity	S27.9xxA	Injury of unspecified intrathoracic organ, initial encounter
		AND	
		S21.311A	Laceration without foreign body of right front wall of thorax with penetration into thoracic cavity, initial encounter
		S21.312A	Laceration without foreign body of left front wall of thorax with penetration into thoracic cavity, initial encounter
		S21.321A	Laceration with foreign body of right front wall of thorax with penetration into thoracic cavity, initial encounter
		S21.322A	Laceration with foreign body of front wall of thorax with penetration into thoracic cavity, initial encounter
		S21.331A	Puncture wound without foreign body of right front wall of thorax with penetration into thoracic cavity, initial encounter
		S21.332A	Puncture wound without foreign body of left front wall of thorax with penetration into thoracic cavity, initial encounter
		S21.341A	Puncture wound with foreign body of right front wall of thorax with penetration into thoracic cavity, initial encounter
		S21.342A	Puncture wound with foreign body of left front wall of thorax with penetration into thoracic cavity, initial encounter
		S21.351A	Open bite of right front wall of thorax with penetration into thoracic cavity, initial encounter
		S21.352A	Open bite of left front wall of thorax with penetration into thoracic cavity, initial encounter
		S21.401A	Unspecified open wound of right back wall of thorax with penetration into thoracic cavity, initial encounter
		S21.402A	Unspecified open wound of left back wall of thorax with penetration into thoracic cavity, initial encounter
		S21.411A	Laceration without foreign body of right back wall of thorax with penetration into thoracic cavity, initial encounter
(Continued on next page)		S21.412A	Laceration without foreign body of left back wall of thorax with penetration into thoracic cavity, initial encounter

ICD-9-CM		ICD-10-CM	
862.9	Injury to multiple and unspecified intrathoracic organs with open wound into cavity *(Continued)*	S21.421A	Laceration with foreign body of right back wall of thorax with penetration into thoracic cavity, initial encounter
		S21.422A	Laceration with foreign body of left back wall of thorax with penetration into thoracic cavity, initial encounter
		S21.431A	Puncture wound without foreign body of right back wall of thorax with penetration into thoracic cavity, initial encounter
		S21.432A	Puncture wound without foreign body of left back wall of thorax with penetration into thoracic cavity, initial encounter
		S21.441A	Puncture wound with foreign body of right back wall of thorax with penetration into thoracic cavity, initial encounter
		S21.442A	Puncture wound with foreign body of left back wall of thorax with penetration into thoracic cavity, initial encounter
		S21.451A	Open bite of right back wall of thorax with penetration into thoracic cavity, initial encounter
		S21.452A	Open bite of left back wall of thorax with penetration into thoracic cavity, initial encounter

The transition to ICD-10-CM requires that the coder be able to pinpoint more specifics within the documentation. There will no longer be just one applicable code for multiple thoracic injuries; instead, the definition of the type of injury, the general location of the wound, and whether or not a foreign body was present will all play a part in code selection. Physicians may need to be educated about the need to report these specifics in the documentation.

Injuries of the Face and Neck

The injuries of the face and neck are also much more detailed in ICD-10-CM than in ICD-9-CM, not unlike the injuries to the chest wall. The new code set zeroes in on the specific location of the injury, as well as the tissues and/or organs affected.

Figure 10.11: Upper Respiratory System

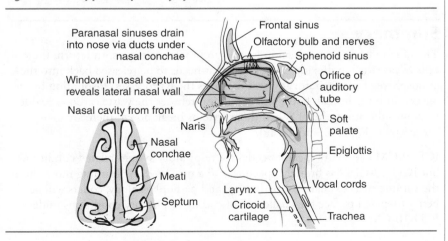

Fascia are fibrous sheets or bands of tissue that encase organs, muscles, and groups of muscles. The cervical trachea starts at the sixth cervical vertebra and extends to the sternum, where it divides into the bronchus. The vocal cords are a pair of strong bands of tissue located within the larynx. Their main purpose is to vibrate to produce sound for speaking or singing. They are also known as vocal folds, and injuries to these bands can obviously have a significant effect on a person's ability to communicate.

The thyroid gland is an endocrine gland located in the front of the lower neck composed of two lobes on either side of the trachea. The thyroid gland's main responsibility is secreting and storing the thyroid hormones that regulate metabolism.

The cervical esophagus connects the pharynx and stomach. This structure begins in the area of the fifth and sixth cervical vertebrae and runs to just above the sternum.

Coding for Other Injury of the Face and Neck

ICD-9-CM		ICD-10-CM	
959.09	Injury of face and neck, other and unspecified	S09.92xA	Unspecified injury of nose, initial encounter
		S09.93xA	Unspecified injury of face, initial encounter
		S16.8xxA	Other specified injury of muscle, fascia and tendon at neck level, initial encounter
		S16.9xxA	Unspecified injury of muscle, fascia and tendon at neck level, initial encounter
		S19.80xA	Other specified injuries of unspecified part of neck, initial encounter
		S19.81xA	Other specified injuries of larynx, initial encounter
		S19.82xA	Other specified injuries of cervical trachea, initial encounter
		S19.83xA	Other specified injuries of vocal cord, initial encounter
		S19.84xA	Other specified injuries of thyroid gland, initial encounter
		S19.85xA	Other specified injuries of pharynx and cervical esophagus, initial encounter
		S19.89xA	Other specified injuries of other specified part of neck, initial encounter
		S19.9xxA	Unspecified injury of neck, initial encounter

Summary

The human body uses oxygen in its cells to process nutrients. In return, these cells release carbon dioxide, a waste gas that needs to be released back into the atmosphere. The respiratory system manages these processes. Inspiration brings oxygen into the human body, and expiration releases the waste carbon dioxide back into the atmosphere. When these systems break down, there are many disease pathologies to understand.

ICD-9-CM had many specifics codes for respiratory system related conditions, but ICD-10-CM has brought specificity to a new level. By learning more about the various areas of anatomy, pathology, and pathophysiology, coders will be better prepared to face the challenges of coding respiratory conditions under ICD-10-CM.

Chapter 11. **Digestive System**

Anatomic Overview

The digestive system carries out the process of *digestion* and is composed of an alimentary canal, or the gastrointestinal tract, and accessory organs. The alimentary canal consists of the mouth, pharynx, esophagus, stomach, small intestine, large intestine, rectum, and anus. The accessory organs include the liver, gallbladder, and pancreas, as well as other structures such as the teeth, tongue, and salivary glands.

Digestion is a multistage process that can be divided into four main steps. The first—ingestion—involves placing food and liquids into the mouth. The second step—digestion—involves the breakdown of foods and can be divided into two subprocesses: chemical and mechanical. Mechanical digestion breaks larger pieces into smaller ones without altering their chemical composition, whereas chemical digestion breaks foods into simpler chemicals so that they can be absorbed into the bloodstream. The third step—absorption—involves the movement of nutrients from the digestive system to the circulatory and lymphatic systems through osmosis, active transport, or diffusion. The fourth and final step—excretion—involves removal of any undigested materials from the gastrointestinal tract through defecation.

	DEFINITIONS

digestion. Mechanical, chemical, and enzymatic process whereby ingested food is converted into material suitable for assimilation for synthesis of tissues or liberation of energy.

mastication. Process of chewing food to ready it for the digestive system.

peristalsis. Smooth muscle action of automatic contractions that propel substances through the body, such as urine into the bladder and food through the digestive tract.

Figure 11.1: Digestive System

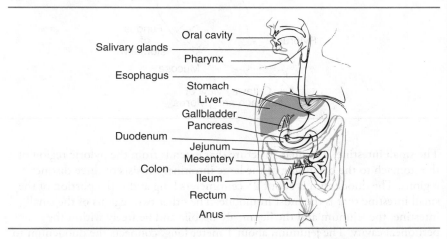

Digestion begins in the mouth where food is mechanically broken down in a process called *mastication*. The mouth or oral cavity is the chamber behind the lips and between the tongue and palate. The narrow space between the teeth, cheeks, and lips is called the vestibule. During mastication, the teeth grind the food into smaller particles while the tongue mixes the food with saliva. Once the food has been thoroughly chewed and mixed with saliva, the bolus is ready to be passed into the esophagus.

The esophagus is a straight, collapsible tube approximately 25 centimeters in length. It begins at the base of the pharynx, descends behind the trachea, and passes through the diaphragm until it reaches the stomach. Food is moved down the esophagus by a process called *peristalsis*. Peristalsis is a wavelike motion by which automatic smooth muscle contractions push the contents of tubular structures from one place in the tube to the place just ahead of it. No digestion occurs in the esophagus, as this tube merely functions as a passageway between the mouth and stomach.

The stomach is a small, J-shaped organ that hangs below the diaphragm in the upper portion of the abdominal cavity, mostly to the left of the median line. Its size and position are variable because an adult stomach is able to distend from a collapsed state to accommodate a volume of up to one liter or one and one-half liters, and it can be pushed up and down with inspiration and expiration.

There are three divisions of the stomach: the fundus, the body, and the pylorus. The fundus is the enlarged portion to the left above the cardiac sphincter. The body is the central part, and the pylorus is the lower narrowing portion. One of the primary critical functions of the stomach is to store partially digested food that is then churned, mixed, and moved into the duodenum. In addition, the stomach is a secretory organ that secretes gastric juices and an intrinsic factor to protect B12 before the vitamin's absorption. The stomach also absorbs some drugs, water, alcohol, and lactic fatty acids; produces gastrin hormone for digestive regulation; and helps destroy swallowed pathogenic bacteria.

Figure 11.2: Stomach and Pylorus

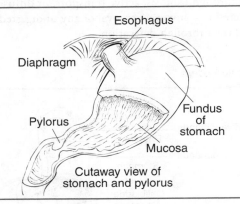

The small intestine, a tubular structure that extends from the pyloric region of the stomach to the beginning of the large intestine, consists of three distinct regions. The duodenum is about 25 centimeters long and is the portion of the small intestine that is the most immobile. The other two regions of the small intestine, the jejunum and the ileum, are mobile and lie freely within the peritoneal cavity. The jejunum, about 1 meter long, connects the duodenum to the final portion of the small intestine, the ileum. The ileum is about 2 meters long, and it connects the small intestine to the proximal end of the large intestine. Although the jejunum and the ileum are not distinctly separate parts, the diameter of the jejunum is greater than that of the ileum, and its wall is thicker, more vascular, and more active.

Figure 11.3: Duodenum

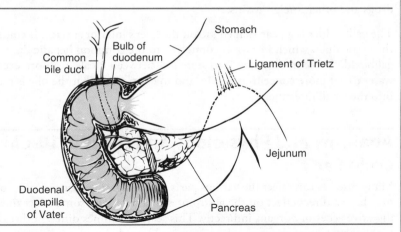

The small intestine plays an important role in digestion. It secretes digestive enzymes that aid in the complete digestion of carbohydrates, proteins, lipids, and nucleic acids. Not only does the small intestine secrete digestive enzymes, but about 90 percent of all the products of digestion are absorbed in the small intestine.

The next portion along the gastrointestinal tract is the large intestine. It joins the small intestines at the ileocecal sphincter and is about 15 meters long. The large intestine consists of the cecum, colon, rectum, and anal canal. The colon is further subdivided into four portions: the ascending, transverse, descending, and sigmoid.

The main role of the large intestine is to pass waste material from the body, although water and some nutrients such as sodium are absorbed in the large intestine. Mucus is secreted to protect the intestinal wall against the material passing through, and it also binds to the fecal matter. The undigested food, or chyme, entering the large intestine contains materials the small intestine did not digest or absorb. It also contains water, electrolytes, mucus, and bacteria. After the large intestine absorbs the water and electrolytes, the substances remaining in the tube become feces and are stored in the distal portion of the large intestine until they are excreted from the rectum.

Digestion occurs along the various portions of the gastrointestinal tract, but without the help of various accessory organs, certain substances could not be digested. The pancreas, for instance, is a glandular organ that has both an endocrine and exocrine function. It is more commonly known for its role in glucose maintenance and the production of insulin (see the endocrine chapter for more information on this role of the pancreas), yet it also plays an important role in digestion by secreting a fluid called pancreatic juice. This juice contains enzymes that digest carbohydrates, fats, proteins, and nucleic acids. The pancreas also helps neutralize the acidic chyme that leaves the stomach and enters the intestine.

The liver is a large, reddish-brown, glandular organ in the upper right portion of the abdominal cavity. The liver is enclosed by a fibrous covering and is divided into lobes by a thick layer of connective tissue. The liver produces bile, which aids digestion by breaking fats into smaller droplets, a process called emulsification, so that enzymes can break them down even further. Also, the liver processes carbohydrates and proteins absorbed by the small intestine and

 KEY POINT

- Peristalsis propels food content through the esophagus and the intestine.

- Mass peristalsis, which occurs only three to four times a day, moves the contents of the large intestine from one segment to the next.

- Reversed peristalsis occurs when the contractions occur in a direction that is opposite of normal, pushing the intestinal contents backwards.

 CLINICAL NOTE

The pancreas is both an endocrine and exocrine gland.

- The endocrine function involves the secretion of insulin, the hormone that plays a major role in glucose maintenance and has a direct relationship to diabetes mellitus.

- The exocrine function is the secretion of pancreatic juices, which help break down carbohydrates, fats, nucleic acids, and proteins.

acts as the detoxification center of the body by breaking down hormones and drugs and other foreign toxins.

The gallbladder is a pear-shaped sac on the liver's inferior surface. It connects to the cystic duct, which in turn is connected to the common hepatic duct. The gallbladder's role in digestion is to store *bile* between meals, reabsorb excess water to get more concentrated bile, and to contract so that the bile is released into the small intestine.

Anatomy and Physiology and the ICD-10-CM Code Set

Many diseases can affect the various parts of the digestive system. Some of them may have a direct effect on the gastrointestinal tract, and some affect the digestive accessory organs indirectly. This section outlines different diseases and highlights some of the areas where increased knowledge of anatomy and physiology is needed to understand the ICD-10-CM code set.

Diseases of the Accessory Digestive Organs

Tooth Loss

Teeth play a critical role in digestion because they begin the process of physically breaking down food into smaller particles. Tooth loss, also known as edentulism, signifies the loss of some or all natural teeth. Tooth loss is caused most commonly by periodontal disease and dental caries but can also be attributed to congenital conditions such as *Papillon–Lefèvre syndrome* (PLS), systemic conditions such as *Langerhans cell histiocytosis* (LCH), loss of supporting structures, and trauma.

Figure 11.4: Teeth

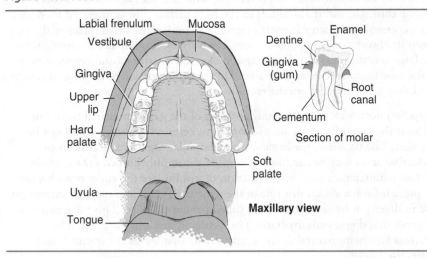

Maxillary view

Section of molar

Edentulism can be classified as partial, the loss of one or multiple teeth, or complete, the loss of all teeth. Edentulism is divided into four classes that differ in the level of difficulty or complexity in treatment for complete edentulism and how compromised the presenting diagnostic criteria are in partial edentulism. Class IV is the most debilitating, requiring reconstructive surgery when all teeth are missing, and has the most severely compromised edentulous area in partial edentulism.

Coding for tooth loss in ICD-9-CM requires the use of two codes: a code from category 525.1X represents the cause of the edentulism and 525.4X or 525.5X represents the class of edentulism. However, due to the increased granularity in ICD-10-CM, coding for tooth loss no longer requires multiple codes. There are now combination codes that represent both the cause and the class of the edentulism.

Coding for Edentulism

ICD-9-CM		ICD-10-CM	
525.11	Loss of teeth due to trauma	K08.111	Complete loss of teeth due to trauma, class I
		K08.112	Complete loss of teeth due to trauma, class II
		K08.113	Complete loss of teeth due to trauma, class III
		K08.114	Complete loss of teeth due to trauma, class IV
		K08.119	Complete loss of teeth due to trauma, unspecified class
		K08.411	Partial loss of teeth due to trauma, class I
		K08.412	Partial loss of teeth due to trauma, class II
		K08.413	Partial loss of teeth due to trauma, class III
		K08.414	Partial loss of teeth due to trauma, class IV
		K08.419	Partial loss of teeth due to trauma, unspecified class
525.12	Loss of teeth due to periodontal disease	K08.121	Complete loss of teeth due to periodontal disease, class I
		K08.122	Complete loss of teeth due to periodontal disease, class II
		K08.123	Complete loss of teeth due to periodontal disease, class III
		K08.124	Complete loss of teeth due to periodontal disease, class IV
		K08.129	Complete loss of teeth due to periodontal disease, unspecified class
		K08.421	Partial loss of teeth due to periodontal disease, class I
		K08.422	Partial loss of teeth due to periodontal disease, class II
		K08.423	Partial loss of teeth due to periodontal disease, class III
		K08.424	Partial loss of teeth due to periodontal disease, class IV
		K08.429	Partial loss of teeth due to periodontal disease, unspecified class
525.42	Complete edentulism class II	K08.102	Complete loss of teeth, unspecified cause, class II
		K08.112	Complete loss of teeth due to trauma, class II
		K08.122	Complete loss of teeth due to periodontal disease, class II
		K08.132	Complete loss of teeth due to caries, class II
		K08.192	Complete loss of teeth due to other specified cause, class II
525.52	Partial edentulism class II	K08.402	Partial loss of teeth, unspecified cause, class II
		K08.412	Partial loss of teeth due to trauma, class II
		K08.422	Partial loss of teeth due to periodontal disease, class II
		K08.432	Partial loss of teeth due to caries, class II
		K08.492	Partial loss of teeth due to other specified cause, class II

Sialoadenitis

The salivary glands secrete saliva, a predominantly alkaline fluid that moistens the mouth, softens food particles, and aids in chemical digestion. There are three pairs of major salivary glands. The first, and largest, pair is called the parotids, which secrete a clear, watery fluid rich in amylase, an enzyme that aids in breaking down carbohydrates. The second pair is the submandibular glands, which secrete a fluid containing a mixture of watery and mucus-type fluids that are slightly more viscous than the fluids secreted by the parotids. The third pair is the sublingual glands, which secrete a thick, mucus-type fluid containing the enzyme lysozyme, which aids in the destruction of bacteria that may enter the oral cavity.

Figure 11.5: Saliva Glands

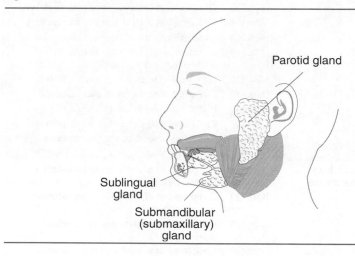

Parotid gland

Sublingual gland

Submandibular (submaxillary) gland

Sialoadenitis is a bacterial infection of one of the salivary glands, usually due to an obstruction or gland hyposecretion. It is characterized by swelling, pain, redness, and tenderness. The most common causal organism is *Staphylococcus aureus*, but sialoadenitis has also been known to be caused by streptococci, coliforms, and various other anaerobic bacteria.

Coding for sialoadenitis in ICD-9-CM is straightforward—there is only one code, 527.2, for this disease. However, in ICD-10-CM, coders need to know more than just that the disease is present.

Coding for Sialoadenitis in ICD-10-CM

> **K11.20**   **Sialoadenitis unspecified**
>
> **K11.21**   **Acute sialoadenitis**
>
> **K11.22**   **Acute recurrent sialoadenitis**
>
> **K11.23**   **Chronic sialoadenitis**

To code this disease accurately in ICD-10-CM, coders need to know if it is acute, acute recurrent, chronic, or unspecified. Because this is a new concept for this disease, providers may not be documenting required information. For this reason, it may be a good idea to start reviewing those concepts that are new in ICD-10-CM now and begin educating providers on documentation needs.

Hepatitis and Cirrhosis of the Liver

Cirrhosis of the liver is a chronic, progressive disease characterized by damage to the hepatic parenchymal cells and nodular regeneration, fibrosis formation, and disturbance of the normal architecture. Two different types of cirrhosis have been described based on the amount of regenerative activity in the liver. There is chronic sclerosing cirrhosis, in which the liver is small and hard, and nodular cirrhosis, in which the liver may be quite large initially.

Chronic alcohol use can lead to both hepatitis and cirrhosis. The conditions may have similar features, and both can occur without the use of alcohol. However, alcoholic cirrhosis accounts for about 60 percent of all cirrhosis cases, and the risk appears to rise with the amount of alcohol consumed daily.

Figure 11.6: Liver

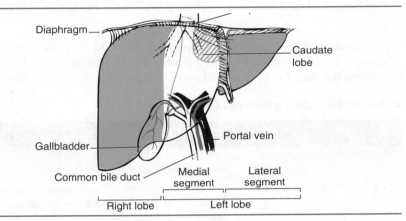

Hepatitis is the inflammation of the liver and may be caused by alcohol abuse or viruses. Alcoholic hepatitis is caused by prolonged excessive intake of alcohol and can be mild with only liver enzyme elevation or severe with symptoms that may include development of ascites or jaundice, prolonged prothrombin time, enlarged liver, and even liver failure. Many who consume excessive alcohol become malnourished due to the empty calories from alcohol, poor appetite, and poor absorption of nutrients. This condition is diagnosed by complete blood count (CBC), liver biopsy, and liver function test; and treatment includes alcohol cessation, rehabilitation and counseling programs, and vitamin B-complex and folic acid to help reverse the malnutrition.

Hepatitis due to viral infections, or viral hepatitis, is most commonly caused by one of the five unrelated hepatotropic viruses. Hepatitis A (HAV) is a picornavirus commonly found in children and young adults. It can be spread through person-to-person contact, consumption of raw shellfish, and drinking contaminated water. This form of hepatitis does not have a chronic stage and is the most common cause of acute viral hepatitis.

Hepatitis B (HBV) is a hepadnavirus that has both acute and chronic forms. HBV is the second most common cause of acute viral hepatitis, but its route of transmission is through contaminated blood, blood products, sexual contact, and via mother to child by breastfeeding. Routine screening for hepatitis B surface antigen (HbsAg) has nearly eliminated transmission via blood transfusion. However, needle sharing by drug users, sharing shaving accessories within closed institutions, and touching wounds of infected persons are still modes of transmission.

Hepatitis C (HCV) is a flavivirus that has six major subtypes. HCV infection is most often transferred through blood via needle sharing, tattoos, and body piercings. Transmission through sexual contact and from mother to baby is very rare, and HCV infection generally remains asymptomatic in patients for decades.

Hepatitis D (HDV), also called delta agent, has similar characteristics to a viroid as it can replicate only in the presence of HBV. HVD infection occurs as a coinfection with acute HBV or as a new infection in patients with chronic hepatitis B.

Hepatitis E (HEV) is an RNA virus that produces symptoms similar to HAV. Outbreaks of acute HEV infections have been linked to fecal contamination of the water supply and have occurred in China, India, Mexico, Pakistan, Peru, Russia, and central and northern Africa. Like hepatitis A, HEV does not have a chronic stage and does not produce chronic hepatitis or further develop into cirrhosis.

Codes for alcoholic cirrhosis and hepatitis in ICD-9-CM are in category 571 Chronic liver disease and cirrhosis. However, in ICD-10-CM coding for these conditions has been further specified as occurring with or without ascites.

Coding for Alcoholic Hepatitis and Cirrhosis

ICD-9-CM		ICD-10-CM	
571.1	Acute alcoholic hepatitis	K70.10	Alcoholic hepatitis without ascites
		K70.11	Alcoholic hepatitis with ascites
571.2	Alcoholic cirrhosis of the liver	K70.2	Alcoholic fibrosis and sclerosis of the liver
		K70.30	Alcoholic cirrhosis of liver without ascites
		K70.31	Alcoholic cirrhosis of liver with ascites

Ascites is an accumulation of fluid in the peritoneal cavity. The most common cause of ascites is advanced liver disease or cirrhosis. Approximately 81 percent of the ascites cases are thought to be due to cirrhosis and, of that number, 65 percent are attributed to alcohol use. Although the exact mechanism of ascites development is not completely understood, most theories suggest portal hypertension, which is an increased pressure in the liver blood flow, as the main contributor.

It is important to note that several conditions coded to 573.3 Unspecified hepatitis, in ICD-9-CM have their own codes in ICD-10-CM, as the list below indicates. Toxic liver disease refers to liver damage that is chemical- or drug-induced. Because this type of hepatitis is caused by a chemical, in both ICD-9-CM and ICD-10-CM instructional notes guide the coder to also identify the drug or toxic agent. Nonalcoholic steatohepatitis, or NASH, is a common, often "silent," liver disease. It resembles alcoholic liver disease but occurs in people who drink little or no alcohol. The major feature in NASH is fat in the liver, along with inflammation and damage. NASH can be severe and can lead to cirrhosis, in which the liver is permanently damaged and scarred and no longer able to work properly. Peliosis hepatitis is an uncommon condition characterized by randomly distributed multiple blood-filled cystic cavities throughout the liver. It is usually asymptomatic but has been known to develop into overt liver disease and can even cause rupture with hemorrhage. Mild cases are generally detected incidentally when liver function tests show abnormal results or when the cysts are seen on ultrasound.

Coding for Other Hepatitis Conditions in ICD-10-CM

K71.0		**Toxic liver disease with cholestasis**
	K71.10	**Toxic liver disease with hepatic necrosis, without coma**
	K71.11	**Toxic liver disease with hepatic necrosis, with coma**
K71.2		**Toxic liver disease with acute hepatitis**
K71.3		**Toxic liver disease with chronic persistent hepatitis**
K71.4		**Toxic liver disease with chronic lobular hepatitis**
	K71.50	**Toxic liver disease with chronic active hepatitis without ascites**
	K71.51	**Toxic liver disease with chronic active hepatitis with ascites**
K71.6		**Toxic liver disease with hepatitis NEC**
K71.7		**Toxic liver disease with fibrosis and cirrhosis of liver**
K71.8		**Toxic liver disease with other disorders of liver**
K71.9		**Toxic liver disease, unspecified**
K75.2		**Nonspecific reactive hepatitis**
K75.3		**Granulomatous hepatitis not elsewhere classified**
	K75.81	**Nonalcoholic steatohepatitis (NASH)**
	K75.89	**Other specified inflammatory liver diseases**
K75.9		**Inflammatory liver disease, unspecified**
K76.4		**Peliosis hepatitis**

The code descriptions include several manifestations with toxic liver disease. For instance, cholestasis refers to the impairment of bile flow, which has been known to be caused by many different drugs. Also mentioned is necrosis, the pathologic death of one or more cells, or of a portion of tissue or organ; in the liver this most commonly refers to the parenchymal cells. In toxic liver disease, necrosis is classified with or without coma. Lobular hepatitis is an inflammation localized to one of the lobes of the liver, and ascites is an accumulation of fluid in the peritoneal cavity and, as previously mentioned, is commonly caused by advanced liver disease or cirrhosis.

Acute or Chronic Pancreatitis

Pancreatitis is the inflammation of the pancreas and is classified as acute or chronic. The acute form is sudden, while chronic pancreatitis is recurring or persistent abdominal pain. Chronic pancreatitis is characterized by tissue changes that are irreversible and progressive and that result in a considerable amount of pancreatic function. Patients with chronic pancreatitis may have a flare-up of acute disease.

Figure 11.7: Pancreas

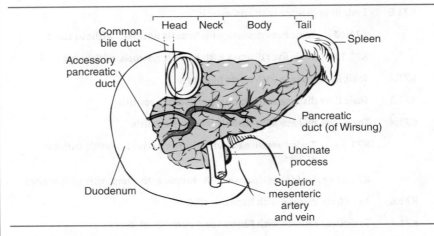

In ICD-9-CM, coding for pancreatitis is divided between two codes, 577.0 Acute pancreatitis, and 577.1 Chronic pancreatitis. ICD-10-CM still has two main categories of the disease, but the code range has been expanded to include the cause of the pancreatitis.

Patients who have had any type of procedure that requires cannulation or injection of the pancreatic ducts are at slightly higher risk for developing pancreatitis. The condition is also a major risk for patients who have undergone endoscopic retrograde cholangiopancreatography, which involves endoscopic and radiographic exam of the pancreatic and common bile ducts and is used to diagnose and treat conditions of the pancreatic and biliary ductal systems. During the procedure, the physician passes an endoscope through the oropharynx, esophagus, and small intestine where contrast material is injected through the ampulla of Vater in a direction opposite of normal flow. The common bile duct, biliary tract, and gallbladder are then visualized and imaged. Pancreatitis resulting from ERCP can be mild but can also require hospitalization and be life-threatening in rare cases.

Pancreatitis can also arise from *cytomegalovirus*, which can cause infections ranging widely in severity. Cytomegaloviral pancreatitis is coded from category B25 in ICD-10-CM.

The most common cause of acute pancreatitis is the presence of gallstones, small, pebble-like substances made of hardened bile that cause inflammation in the pancreas as they pass through the common bile duct. Excessive alcohol and drug use are two of the most common causes of chronic pancreatitis and can also be a contributing factor in acute pancreatitis.

 DEFINITIONS

cytomegalovirus. Large herpesvirus, also known as *human herpesvirus 5*, that remains mostly latent in leukocytes and replicates very slowly. CMV is spread from direct person-to-person contact and is usually harmless but can cause severe disease in people with compromised immune systems.

Coding for Pancreatitis

ICD-9-CM		ICD-10-CM	
577.0	Acute pancreatitis	B25.2	Cytomegaloviral pancreatitis
		K85.0	Idiopathic acute pancreatitis
		K85.1	Biliary acute pancreatitis
		K85.2	Alcohol induced acute pancreatitis
		K85.3	Drug induced acute pancreatitis
		K85.8	Other acute pancreatitis
		K85.9	Acute pancreatitis, unspecified
577.1	Chronic pancreatitis	K86.0	Alcohol-induced chronic pancreatitis
		K86.1	Other chronic pancreatitis

Disease of the Gastrointestinal Tract

Esophageal Diseases and Complications

Gastroesophageal reflux disease, more commonly referred to as GERD, is characterized by incompetence of the lower esophageal sphincter that allows reflux of gastric acid into the esophagus. GERD is a fairly common disease, occurring in 30 to 40 percent of adults. Treatment involves lifestyle modification, acid suppression, and, in some instances, surgery. Coding for this disease in both ICD-9-CM and ICD-10-CM is straightforward, and there is a one-to-one mapping correlation between the two code sets. The only difference between the descriptions is that ICD-10-CM clarifies that no esophagitis is present.

Coding for Gastroesophageal Reflux Disease

ICD-9-CM		ICD-10-CM	
530.81	Esophageal reflux	K21.9	Gastro-esophageal reflux disease without esophagitis

Figure 11.8: Esophagus

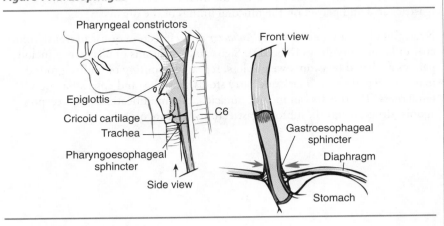

There may be an exact mapping relationship for GERD, but there are a few esophageal disorders with clinical differences in the code sets between ICD-9-CM and ICD-10-CM.

Barrett's esophagus refers to an abnormal change, known as *metaplasia*, in the cells of the inferior portion of the esophagus. The condition occurs due to

> **DEFINITIONS**
>
> **metaplasia.** Transformation of one type of mature differentiated cell type into another mature differentiated cell type. Examples include squamous metaplasia of the columnar epithelial cells of salivary gland ducts when stones are present and squamous metaplasia of the transitional epithelium of the bladder when stones are present.

chronic inflammation, usually caused by GERD. The chronic exposure of the cells in the lower esophagus to gastric acid damages those cells, resulting in the metaplasia. While there is no relationship between the severity of the reflux disease and the development of Barrett's esophagus, there is a relationship between chronic GERD and the development of Barrett's esophagus.

Coding for Barrett's Esophagus

ICD-9-CM	ICD-10-CM	
530.85 Barrett's esophagus	K22.70	Barrett's esophagus without dysplasia
	K22.710	Barrett's esophagus with low grade dysplasia
	K22.711	Barrett's esophagus with high grade dysplasia
	K22.719	Barrett's esophagus with dysplasia, unspecified

DEFINITIONS

dysplasia. Term used in pathology to refer to abnormal tissue development.

In addition to coding the Barrett's esophagus, coders need to familiarize themselves with the different grades of *dysplasia*. Dysplasia is defined as abnormal tissue development and is the earliest form of precancerous lesion recognizable in a biopsy. The cells of Barrett's esophagus can be classified into four general categories: nondysplastic, low-grade dysplasia, high-grade dysplasia, and frank carcinoma. High-grade dysplasia and frank carcinoma patients are generally advised to undergo surgical treatment. Nondysplastic and low-grade patients are generally advised to undergo annual observation with endoscopy. In high-grade dysplasia, the risk of developing cancer might be at 10 percent or greater per patient-year.

Ulcers

An ulcer is defined as a lesion through the skin or mucous membrane resulting from loss of tissue, usually with inflammation. Ulcers can occur in various places along the gastrointestinal tract, including within the oral cavity, esophagus, and gastrointestinal mucosa. A gastric ulcer is a condition formed by discreet tissue destruction within the lumen of the stomach. Duodenal ulcers form in the duodenum and typically occur about five times more frequently than gastric ulcers. Both conditions are a result of the increased activity of hydrochloric (gastric) acid and pepsin on the mucosal linings of the organs.

Nearly all ulcers are caused by *Helicobacter pylori* infection or use of nonsteroidal anti-inflammatory drugs (NSAID). Signs and symptoms of ulcers may include pain exacerbated by eating, weight loss, repeated vomiting of "coffee ground" material, hematemesis, black and tarry stools, burning, and epigastria tenderness. Treatments can include antacids, diet modifications, H_2 receptor agonist drugs, bismuth, subtotal gastrectomy, and vagotomy.

KEY POINT

NSAIDs are nonsteroidal anti-inflammatory drugs commonly used to treat the following:

- Inflammatory arthropathies
- Metastatic bone pain
- Mild-to-moderate pain due to inflammation and tissue injury
- Postoperative pain
- Pyrexia (fever)
- Rheumatoid arthritis

Figure 11.9: Stomach

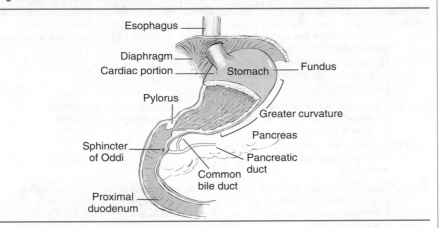

The four categories of codes for gastrointestinal ulcers in ICD-9-CM are divided based on the specified site of the ulcer. Gastric ulcers are coded using category 531, duodenal ulcers are coded using category 532, gastrojejunal ulcers are coded using 534, and ulcers where the site is unspecified or documented as peptic ulcers are coded using category 533. In ICD-10-CM, there are still four distinct categories for the specified sites, but the coder no longer needs to indicate via a fifth digit if an obstruction has occurred.

Coding for Gastrointestinal Ulcers

ICD-9-CM		ICD-10-CM	
531.00	Acute gastric ulcer with hemorrhage, without mention of obstruction	K25.0	Acute gastric ulcer with hemorrhage
531.01	Acute gastric ulcer with hemorrhage and obstruction		
531.10	Acute gastric ulcer with perforation, without mention of obstruction	K25.1	Acute gastric ulcer with perforation
531.11	Acute gastric ulcer with perforation and obstruction		
531.20	Acute gastric ulcer with hemorrhage and perforation, without mention of obstruction	K25.2	Acute gastric ulcer with both hemorrhage and perforation
531.21	Acute gastric ulcer with hemorrhage, perforation, and obstruction		
531.30	Acute gastric ulcer without mention of hemorrhage, perforation, or obstruction	K25.3	Acute gastric ulcer without hemorrhage or perforation
531.31	Acute gastric ulcer without mention of hemorrhage or perforation, with obstruction		
531.40	Chronic or unspecified gastric ulcer with hemorrhage, without mention of obstruction	K25.4	Chronic or unspecified ulcer with hemorrhage
531.41	Chronic or unspecified gastric ulcer with hemorrhage and obstruction		
531.50	Chronic or unspecified gastric ulcer with perforation, without mention of obstruction	K25.5	Chronic or unspecified gastric ulcer with perforation
531.51	Chronic or unspecified gastric ulcer with perforation and obstruction		

ICD-9-CM		ICD-10-CM	
531.60	Chronic or unspecified gastric ulcer with hemorrhage and perforation, without mention of obstruction	K25.6	Chronic or unspecified gastric ulcer with both hemorrhage and perforation
531.61	Chronic or unspecified gastric ulcer with hemorrhage, perforation, and obstruction		
531.70	Chronic gastric ulcer without mention of hemorrhage, perforation, without mention of obstruction	K25.7	Chronic gastric ulcer without hemorrhage or perforation
537.71	Chronic gastric ulcer without mention of hemorrhage or perforation, with obstruction		
531.90	Gastric ulcer, unspecified as acute or chronic, without mention of hemorrhage, perforation, or obstruction	K25.9	Gastric ulcer, unspecified as acute or chronic, without hemorrhage or perforation
531.91	Gastric ulcer, unspecified as acute or chronic, without mention of hemorrhage or perforation, with obstruction		

The table above identifies the crosswalk for only category 531 Gastric ulcers. There are similar crosswalks for duodenal, peptic, and gastrojejunal ulcers.

When an ulcer causes scarring or swelling and this swelling prevents the contents of the stomach from properly entering into the duodenum, this condition is known as gastric outlet obstruction. In ICD-9-CM, unlike ICD-10-CM, code selection for ulcer is based on whether there was an obstruction. The only two complications of ulcers included in the code descriptions for ICD-10-CM are hemorrhage and perforation. The most common ulcer complication is gastrointestinal bleeding or hemorrhage, which occurs when the ulcerated tissue of the organ grows so thin that the gastric acids begin to erode the GI blood vessels. *Perforation* occurs when the ulcer erodes the wall of the GI organ, potentially spilling the stomach or intestinal contents into the abdominal cavity. Further complications from the spillage can lead to more serious conditions, such as peritonitis, pancreatitis, and penetration.

Diverticular Disease

Diverticula are saclike out-pouchings of colonic mucosa and submucosa that protrude outward. Diverticulosis is the condition of having multiple diverticula in the colon. This disease can occur anywhere along the intestine but is most often found in the sigmoid colon. It has been suggested that diverticula are caused by increased intraluminal pressure, leading to mucosal extrusion through weaknesses in the muscle layer of the colon wall. About 70 percent of diverticula are asymptomatic, 15 to 25 percent are painful and become inflamed, and 10 to 15 percent bleed painlessly. The inflammation of diverticula is commonly referred to as diverticulitis.

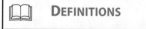

DEFINITIONS

perforation. Abnormal opening in a hollow organ or viscus.

Figure 11.10: Volvulus and Diverticulitis

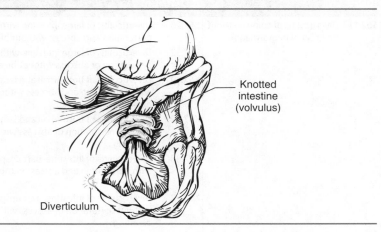

Knotted
intestine
(volvulus)

Diverticulum

Diverticulitis occurs when a perforation occurs within a diverticulum and releases intestinal bacteria. For about 75 percent of the patients with this condition, the resultant inflammation remains localized. For the other 25 percent, this condition can progress and cause abscess, free intraperitoneal perforation, bowel obstruction, or fistulas.

Coding for diverticular disease is a bit more complex in ICD-10-CM than in ICD-9-CM. ICD-9-CM coders need to consider only the site of the diverticular disease and whether hemorrhage was present. In ICD-10-CM, coders also need to identify whether or not any additional complications exist.

Coding for Diverticular Disease

ICD-9-CM		ICD-10-CM	
562.00	Diverticulosis of small intestine (without mention of hemorrhage)	K57.10	Diverticulosis of small intestine without perforation or abscess without bleeding
562.01	Diverticulitis of small intestine (without mention of hemorrhage)	K57.00	Diverticulitis of small intestine with perforation and abscess without bleeding
		K57.12	Diverticulitis of small intestine without perforation or abscess without bleeding
562.02	Diverticulosis of small intestine with hemorrhage	K57.11	Diverticulosis of small intestine without perforation or abscess with bleeding
		K57.51	Diverticulosis of both small and large intestine without perforation or abscess with bleeding
562.03	Diverticulitis of small intestine with hemorrhage	K57.01	Diverticulitis of small intestine with perforation and abscess with bleeding
		K57.13	Diverticulitis of small intestine without perforation or abscess with bleeding
		K57.41	Diverticulitis of both small and large intestine with perforation and abscess with bleeding
		K57.53	Diverticulitis of both small and large intestine without perforation or abscess with bleeding
562.10	Diverticulosis of colon (without mention of hemorrhage)	K57.30	Diverticulosis of large intestine without perforation or abscess without bleeding

ICD-9-CM		ICD-10-CM	
562.11	Diverticulitis of colon (without mention of hemorrhage)	K57.20	Diverticulitis of large intestine with perforation and abscess without bleeding
		K57.32	Diverticulitis of large intestine without perforation or abscess without bleeding
		K57.40	Diverticulitis of both small and large intestine with perforation and abscess without bleeding
		K57.52	Diverticulitis of both small and large intestine without perforation or abscess without bleeding
		K57.80	Diverticulitis of intestine, part unspecified, with perforation and abscess without bleeding
		K57.92	Diverticulitis of intestine, part unspecified, without perforation or abscess without bleeding
562.12	Diverticulosis of colon with hemorrhage	K57.31	Diverticulosis of large intestine without perforation or abscess with bleeding
		K57.51	Diverticulosis of both small and large intestine without perforation or abscess with bleeding
		K57.91	Diverticulosis of intestine, part unspecified, without perforation or abscess with bleeding
562.13	Diverticulitis of colon with hemorrhage	K57.21	Diverticulitis of large intestine with perforation and abscess with bleeding
		K57.33	Diverticulitis of large intestine without perforation or abscess with bleeding
		K57.41	Diverticulitis of both small and large intestine with perforation and abscess with bleeding
		K57.53	Diverticulitis of both small and large intestine without perforation or abscess with bleeding
		K57.81	Diverticulitis of intestine, part unspecified, with perforation and abscess with bleeding
		K57.93	Diverticulitis of intestine, part unspecified, without perforation or abscess with bleeding

CODING AXIOM

The physician's diagnostic statement often includes both terms diverticulosis and diverticulitis. In ICD-9-CM, a diagnosis of diverticulitis assumes the presences of diverticula and only one code is needed for both conditions. This is further defined by the inclusion terms for codes 562.01, 562.11, and by alphabetic index.

Code selection in ICD-10-CM begins the same as in ICD-9-CM. Coders need to first identify if the patient has diverticulosis or if the condition has progressed to diverticulitis. Unlike in ICD-9-CM, however, the coder needs not only to know whether there is a hemorrhage, but also to look for additional documentation on whether there is a perforation or abscess. These complications are what distinguish codes within each subcategory under category K57 Diverticular disease of the intestine.

Enteritis and Colitis

Regional enteritis is an inflammatory disease of the intestine characterized by a chronic *granulomatous* disease. It is chronic and can affect any part of the gastrointestinal tract but most commonly affects the ileum and colon. Also known as Crohn's disease, regional enteritis is identified by its characteristic cobblestone appearance where segments of diseased bowel are located between regions of healthy bowel tissue, hence the name regional enteritis.

There are five types of regional enteritis:

- Ileitis affects the ileum alone.
- Ileocolitis is the most common form and affects the lowest part of the small intestine (ileum) and the large intestine (colon).

DEFINITIONS

granulomatous. Having to do with granuloma, which are nodular inflammatory lesions, usually small or granular, firm, persistent, and containing compactly grouped modified phagocytes.

- Jejunoileitis causes spotty patches of inflammation in the top half of the small intestine (jejunum).

- Crohn's (granulomatous) colitis affects only the large intestine.

- In some rare cases, gastroduodenal Crohn's disease causes inflammation in the stomach and first part of the small intestine, called the duodenum.

Figure 11.11: Large Intestine

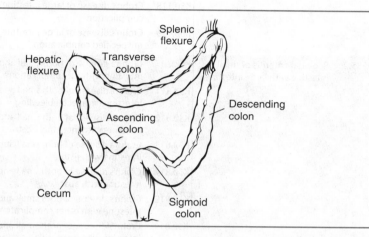

To code for this condition in ICD-10-CM, it is important to remember that the category title has changed. In ICD-9-CM, category 555 is entitled "Regional enteritis." The alphabetic index and the inclusion notes under the category title alert coders that this category also includes the coding for Crohn's disease and granulomatous enteritis. In ICD-10-CM, the opposite is true—the category title is Crohn's disease, and the alphabetic index and inclusion notes alert the coder that regional enteritis is coded under the category.

Another important difference between ICD-9-CM and ICD-10-CM is that coding for Crohn's disease and any of its complications no longer requires multiple codes. There is now one combination code that represents both conditions.

Coding for Regional Enteritis

ICD-9-CM		ICD-10-CM	
555.0	Regional enteritis of small intestine	K50.00	Crohn's disease of small intestine without complication
		K50.011	Crohn's disease of small intestine with rectal bleeding
		K50.012	Crohn's disease of small intestine with intestinal obstruction
		K50.013	Crohn's disease of small intestine with fistula
		K50.014	Crohn's disease of small intestine with abscess
		K50.018	Crohn's disease of small intestine with other complication
		K50.019	Crohn's disease of small intestine with unspecified complication

ICD-9-CM		ICD-10-CM	
555.1	Regional enteritis of large intestine	K50.10	Crohn's disease of large intestine without complication
		K50.111	Crohn's disease of large intestine with rectal bleeding
		K50.112	Crohn's disease of large intestine with intestinal obstruction
		K50.113	Crohn's disease of large intestine with fistula
		K50.114	Crohn's disease of large intestine with abscess
		K50.118	Crohn's disease of large intestine with other complication
		K50.119	Crohn's disease of large intestine with unspecified complication
555.2	Regional enteritis of small intestine with large intestine	K50.80	Crohn's disease of both small and large intestine without complications
		K50.811	Crohn's disease of both small and large intestine with rectal bleeding
		K50.812	Crohn's disease of both small and large intestine with intestinal obstruction
		K50.813	Crohn's disease of both small and large intestine with fistula
		K50.814	Crohn's disease of both small and large intestine with abscess
		K50.818	Crohn's disease of both small and large intestine with other complication
		K50.819	Crohn's disease of both small and large intestine with unspecified complications
555.9	Regional enteritis of unspecified site	K50.90	Crohn's disease, unspecified, without complications
		K50.911	Crohn's disease, unspecified, with rectal bleeding
		K50.912	Crohn's disease, unspecified, with intestinal obstruction
		K50.913	Crohn's disease, unspecified, with fistula
		K50.914	Crohn's disease, unspecified, with abscess
		K50.918	Crohn's disease, unspecified, with other complication
		K50.919	Crohn's disease, unspecified, with unspecified complications

Crohn's disease can lead to several complications, including obstruction, abscess, fistula, and hemorrhage. The formation of strictures and adhesions that narrow the lumen can block the passageway of intestinal contents and cause an intestinal obstruction. In Crohn's disease, fistulae, abnormal passages from one epithelial surface to another, can develop between two loops of bowel, between the bowel and bladder, between the bowel and vagina, and between the bowel and skin. Commonly found in the abdominal and perianal of Crohn's disease sufferers are abscesses, collections of pus that has accumulated in a cavity formed by the tissues containing the pus. Abscesses are frequently associated with swelling and other signs of inflammation

In ICD-9-CM, coders need to know only the specific site of the disease. Any documented Crohn's disease complication is reported with a separate code. However, coding for Crohn's disease and its complications in ICD-10-CM largely depends on selecting the appropriate fifth and sixth characters. The fifth character 0 (zero) indicates that there are no complications. The fifth character 1 indicates that there are complications, described by the sixth characters from the following list.

1   Rectal bleeding

2   Intestinal obstruction

3   Fistula

4   Abscess

8   Other complication

9   Unspecified complication

Regional enteritis is not the only intestinal disease that has been expanded in ICD-10-CM to include complications like abscess, obstruction, and fistulas. ICD-9-CM category 556 Ulcerative colitis has also undergone a similar expansion.

Ulcerative colitis causes inflammation and ulcers in the top layers of the lining of the large intestine. The inflammation usually occurs in the rectum and lower part of the colon but can affect other areas of the colon. Ulcerative colitis is a chronic, intermittent disease, with periods of exacerbated symptoms and periods that are relatively symptom-free. The symptoms of ulcerative colitis can sometimes diminish on their own, but they often require treatment to induce remission.

Coding for ulcerative colitis in ICD-10-CM is based on whether there is a complication and, if there is one, what it is. This is a new concept for this condition in ICD-10-CM. In ICD-9-CM, when a complication is documented, coders choose an additional code to represent it.

Coding for Ulcerative Colitis

ICD-9-CM		ICD-10-CM	
556.3	Ulcerative (chronic) proctosigmoiditis	K51.30	Ulcerative (chronic) rectosigmoiditis without complications
		K51.311	Ulcerative (chronic) rectosigmoiditis with rectal bleeding
		K51.312	Ulcerative (chronic) rectosigmoiditis with intestinal obstruction
		K51.313	Ulcerative (chronic) rectosigmoiditis with fistula
		K51.314	Ulcerative (chronic) rectosigmoiditis with abscess
		K51.318	Ulcerative (chronic) rectosigmoiditis with other complication
		K51.319	Ulcerative (chronic) rectosigmoiditis with unspecified complications
556.4	Pseudopolyposis of colon	K51.40	Inflammatory polyps of colon without complications
		K51.411	Inflammatory polyps of colon with rectal bleeding
		K51.412	Inflammatory polyps of colon with intestinal obstruction
		K51.413	Inflammatory polyps of colon with fistula
		K51.414	Inflammatory polyps of colon with abscess
		K51.418	Inflammatory polyps of colon with other complication
		K51.419	Inflammatory polyps of colon with unspecified complications

Note that a few of the code descriptions in this category have been renamed. For example, ulcerative proctosigmoiditis in ICD-9-CM is now ulcerative chronic rectosigmoiditis. The terms recto and procto are sometimes used interchangeably, but both are considered medical terminology for the rectum.

Pseudopolyposis is a condition of numerous pseudopolyps in the colon and rectum, due to longstanding inflammation. In ICD-10-CM, the code description for this condition has been changed to "inflammatory polyps of colon." In fact, the term pseudopolyposis has been completely retired in ICD-10-CM. This term has been removed from both the code description and the alphabetic index. The only way to code this condition in ICD-10-CM is to be familiar with the new clinical concept of inflammatory polyps of the colon.

Colostomy and Enterostomy Complications

A colostomy is a procedure in which a portion of the large intestine is divided and the open end is secured to the skin to drain bowel contents outside the body. An enterostomy is similar to the colostomy but is performed to create a passageway into the patient's small intestine through the abdomen with an opening for drainage or to insert a tube for feeding. Enterostomies are often classified according to the part of the small intestine that is used to create the stoma. Documentation may reflect ileostomies, jejunostomies, and often physicians use the word "ostomy" to describe all types of enterostomies.

Figure 11.12: Colostomy

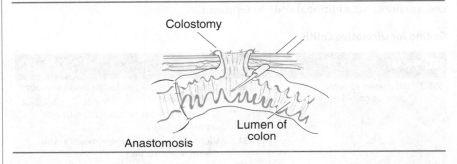

Formation of colostomies and enterostomies are surgical procedures and just as with any other surgical procedure, complications can occur. These can be both mechanical and other specified complications, such as infection or hemorrhage. Coding for the complications of colostomy and enterostomies in ICD-9-CM requires the coder to know only that a complication was present. However, in ICD-10-CM coders need to consider the anatomy of the intestine and be familiar with the names of the parts of the small and large intestines.

Coding for Colostomy and Enterostomy Complications

ICD-9-CM		ICD-10-CM	
569.60	Unspecified complication of colostomy or enterostomy	K94.00	Colostomy complication, unspecified
		K94.10	Enterostomy complication, unspecified
569.61	Infection of colostomy or enterostomy	K94.02	Colostomy infection
		K94.12	Enterostomy infection
569.62	Mechanical complication of colostomy and enterostomy	K94.03	Colostomy malfunction
		K94.13	Enterostomy malfunction

ICD-9-CM		ICD-10-CM	
569.69	Other complication of colostomy or enterostomy	K94.01	Colostomy hemorrhage
		K94.09	Other complication of colostomy
		K94.11	Enterostomy hemorrhage
		K94.19	Other complication of enterostomy

Some of the common complications of colostomies and enterostomies include skin irritation or infection caused by stool that leaks under the bag, peristomal hernias, parastomal fistulas, narrowing bowel, and prolapse of the stoma. In ICD-9-CM, colostomy and enterostomy complications are grouped together under category 569.6. In ICD-10-CM, these are split into two separate categories. Coders need to pay close attention to the specific part of the intestine with the complication. Was the procedure documented as a colostomy, jejunostomy, ileostomy, or did the documentation just say ostomy?

Infectious Diseases of the Digestive System

The digestive system is a common and easily accessible portal of entry for microorganisms. As a result, microbes or their toxins that have entered the digestive system through the gastrointestinal tract can often cause infection, inflammation, or disease. Sources of GI infections may include an overgrowth of normal flora, contaminated food or water, contact with contaminated soil, or oral contact with fecal matter.

Typhoid fever is an acute generalized illness caused by the microorganism *Salmonella typhi*. Important clinical features include fever, headache, abdominal pain, cough, toxemia, *leucopenia*, abnormal pulse, rose spots on the skin, bacteremia, hyperplasia of the intestinal lymph nodes, and *Peyer's patches* in the intestines. Typhoid fever is generally transmitted through food or water that has been contaminated with fecal matter but can also be contracted through close contact with an infected individual. Typhoid infections are treated with antimicrobial therapy, which shortens the clinical course of the infection and reduces the risk of death. However, one of the frequent complications of therapy is the development of antibiotic resistance.

Coding for typhoid fever infections in ICD-10-CM is a bit more complex than in ICD-9-CM due to the inclusion of various complications within the code descriptions. In ICD-9-CM, there is only one code option for typhoid fever, 002.0. The complications of the disease are coded elsewhere. However, in ICD-10-CM, there are seven possible code selections for this infection.

Coding for Typhoid Fever in ICD-10-CM

A01.00   **Typhoid fever, unspecified**

A01.01   **Typhoid meningitis**

A01.02   **Typhoid fever with heart involvement**

A01.03   **Typhoid pneumonia**

A01.04   **Typhoid arthritis**

A01.05   **Typhoid osteomyelitis**

A01.09   **Typhoid fever with other complications**

To select the appropriate code in ICD-10-CM, the coder must look for documentation that describes the associated typhoid complication. Documentation of meningitis, pneumonia, arthritis, osteomyelitis, and any cardiac condition that is due to *Salmonella typhi* or typhoid fever would be

DEFINITIONS

leukopenia. Condition in which the total numbers of leukocytes circulating in the blood are less than normal.

Peyer's patches. Aggregations of lymphoid tissue that are found in the ileum of humans and are used to visually differentiate the ileum from the jejunum and duodenum.

considered a complication of typhoid fever. For example, meningitis is an inflammation of the meninges, the covering over the brain and spinal cord. Documentation that this inflammation is due to *Salmonella typhi* or with typhoid fever would indicate typhoid meningitis. Coders need to understand the physiology behind the disease process and its complications to select the appropriate typhoid fever code in ICD-10-CM.

Amebiasis, ICD-9-CM code category 006, is defined as an infection of the large intestine caused by *Entamoeba histolytica*. In amebiasis, protozoa can live in the large intestine without causing symptoms or can invade the colon wall, causing severe colitis, acute dysentery, or chronic diarrhea. The infection may spread through the blood to the liver, lungs, brain, or other organs and often causes abscesses in the various organs.

There are many similarities between ICD-9-CM and ICD-10-CM when coding for amebiasis infections and the complications. All but one of the codes in ICD-9-CM has an exact mapping to a code in ICD-10-CM. The same amebiasis complications available in ICD-9-CM are also available in ICD-10-CM.

Coding for Amebiasis

ICD-9-CM		ICD-10-CM	
006.0	Acute amebic dysentery without mention of abscess	A06.0	Acute amebic dysentery
006.1	Chronic intestinal amebiasis without mention of abscess	A06.1	Chronic intestinal amebiasis
006.2	Amebic nondysenteric colitis	A06.2	Amebic nondysenteric colitis
006.3	Amebic liver abscess	A06.4	Amebic liver abscess
006.4	Amebic lung abscess	A06.5	Amebic lung abscess
006.5	Amebic brain abscess	A06.6	Amebic brain abscess
006.6	Amebic skin ulceration	A06.7	Cutaneous amebiasis
006.9	Unspecified amebiasis	A06.9	Amebiasis, unspecified

The one exception within this code category is for code 006.8 Other specified amebic infections. In ICD-10-CM this code has been expanded to identify some additional complications.

A06.3   **Ameboma of intestine**

A06.81   **Amebic cystitis**

A06.82   **Other amebic genitourinary infections**

A06.89   **Other amebic infections**

Amoebas usually remain in the host's gastrointestinal tract, but they can spread elsewhere. The expansion of the other specified category enables the coder to identify other specified sites where amebic infections may occur.

Intestinal trichomoniasis is characterized by colitis, diarrhea, or dysentery and is caused by the protozoan *Trichomonas*. A protozoan is a eukaryotic organism that is classified as parasitic to humans. Trichomoniasis is usually transmitted through sexual intercourse and is primarily an infection of the urogenital tract. The most common site of infection is the urethra and the vagina in women, but this protozoan may also colonize and infect the oropharynx, duodenum, and colon.

The ICD-9-CM code description for this infection is 007.3 Intestinal trichomoniasis. In ICD-10-CM, this condition does not have its own code but is coded using AØ7.8 Other specified protozoal intestinal diseases.

Coding for Intestinal Trichomoniasis

ICD-9-CM		ICD-10-CM	
007.3	Intestinal trichomoniasis	AØ7.8	Other specified protozoal intestinal diseases

To code this condition in ICD-10-CM, coders need to know that *Trichomonas* is classified as a protozoan. Intestinal trichomoniasis is listed as an includes term along with other protozoan intestinal diseases like microsporidiosis, sarcocystosis, and sarcosporidiosis.

Ascariasis is an intestinal infection that occurs when the eggs of the parasitic round worm, *Ascaris lumbricoides*, are ingested. Patients often remain asymptomatic, but the illness may cause visceral damage, peritonitis, enlargement of the liver and spleen, toxicity, and pneumonia. Infections are generally treated for one to three days with antiparasitic medications and, in cases of heavy infections, patients may require surgery to repair intestinal damage and remove the worms.

In ICD-9-CM, one code, 127.0, is used to report ascariasis and any complications must be coded separately. However in ICD-10-CM, the complications of the infection are also included in the code for infection.

Coding for Ascariasis in ICD-10-CM

B77.Ø   **Ascariasis with intestinal complications**

B77.81   **Ascariasis pneumonia**

B77.89   **Ascariasis with other complications**

B77.9   **Ascariasis, unspecified**

Another parasitic infection that has been expanded in ICD-10-CM is strongyloidiasis, caused by the roundworm *Strongyloides stercoralis*. Some common symptoms include gastric pain, vomiting, and diarrhea. Drug therapy for this condition includes ivermectin, but because the medication kills only the adult worm, repeat dosing is necessary to completely eradicate the infection.

Strongyloidiasis may infect a number of sites, including the skin and intestinal track, or may be disseminated throughout the body. In the ICD-10-CM coding system, correct code assignment is not only dependent on the infection, but also the infection site.

Coding for Strongyloidiasis in ICD-10-CM

B78.Ø   **Intestinal strongyloidiasis**

B78.1   **Cutaneous strongyloidiasis**

B78.7   **Disseminated strongyloidiasis**

B78.9   **Strongyloidiasis, unspecified**

Pulmonary symptoms can occur when the larvae migrate into the lungs. Cutaneous symptoms may include urticarial rashes in the buttock and waist areas. If the infection becomes chronic and the patient becomes immunosuppressed, a potentially fatal condition called disseminated strongyloidiasis can occur. Symptoms include abdominal pain, distention, shock, pulmonary and neurologic complications, and septicemia.

☛ **INTERESTING A & P FACT**

The condition microsporidiosis is classified as a protozoal disease in ICD-10-CM, but microsporidia is in the fungi family.

Summary

The digestive system interacts closely with other organ systems to carry out the process of digestion. It is important to learn about the anatomy and physiology of the digestive tract, and the varied differences between ICD-9-CM and ICD-10-CM coding. Discovering areas where there are major anatomy, physiology, and disease pathology differences between the two code sets will help prepare coders for the ICD-10-CM transition.

Chapter 12. **Urinary System**

Anatomic Overview

The urinary system is a collection of various organs, tubes, muscles, and nerves whose function is to create, store, and transport urine out of the body. It comprises two kidneys, two ureters, the bladder, two sphincter muscles, and the urethra.

Figure 12.1: Urinary System

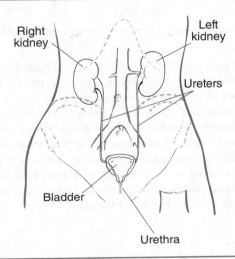

The body absorbs needed nutrients to maintain body function, including energy and self-repair from food. Once the body has the appropriate amount of nutrition, resulting waste products must be eliminated from the body. The urinary system, in conjunction with the lungs, skin, and intestines, excretes waste and keeps chemicals and water in the body in balance.

Specifically, the urinary system removes urea from the blood. Urea is generated when foods containing proteins (meat, poultry, and some vegetables) break down in the body.

The kidneys, bean-shaped organs approximately the size of a fist, perform the majority of the work within the urinary system, acting as a filter to remove waste and other foreign substances from the blood. The two main areas of the kidneys are the renal cortex and the renal medulla. The renal cortex is a superficial, light red, smooth-textured area that extends from the renal capsule to the base of the renal pyramids and into the spaces between them. The renal medulla is a darker reddish brown area made up of multiple cone-shaped renal pyramids; the base or wider end of each pyramid faces the renal cortex and its apex or narrower end points toward the renal hilum.

Figure 12.2: Kidney

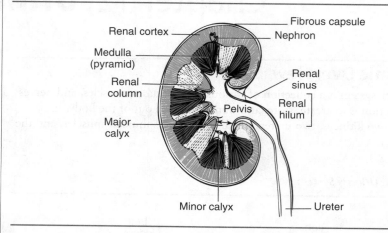

Blood comes into the kidneys by way of arteries that branch within the kidneys into small clusters of looping blood vessels. These clusters are called glomeruli, the tiny units in the kidney where blood is cleaned. Approximately 1 million glomeruli (filters) are in each kidney. Each glomerulus is attached to the opening of a small, fluid-collecting tube known as the tubule. Every glomerulus and tubule unit combined is called a nephron, or the functional unit of the kidneys. Each kidney contains approximately 1 million nephrons. The glomerulus functions as a filter keeping normal proteins and cells in the bloodstream while allowing extra fluid and wastes to pass through. Urea, combined with water, other waste materials, and excess salt, forms urine.

Figure 12.3: Nephron

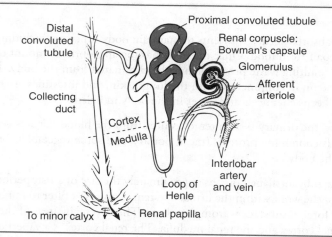

The kidneys also perform other necessary functions, including:

- Regulate:
  - blood ionic composition
  - blood pH
  - blood pressure
  - blood glucose level

- Produce three important hormones:
  - **erythropoietin (EPO):** Stimulates bone marrow to produce red blood cells.
  - **renin:** Regulates blood pressure.
  - **calcitriol:** An active form of vitamin D, this hormone helps to maintain calcium for bones and normal chemical balance in the body.

Once the urine is formed, it passes through the nephrons and down the renal tubules of the kidney and is subsequently funneled from the renal pelvis, the area at the center of the kidney, into the ureters, which then transport the urine to the bladder. The ureters are tube-shaped structures approximately 8 to 10 inches long that connect the kidney to the urinary bladder. Muscles within the ureters continually contract and relax in order to force urine downward into the urinary bladder. The glomerular membrane separates the blood vessel from the tubule, allowing waste products and extra water to pass into the tubule while at the same time keeping blood cells and protein in the bloodstream.

The urinary bladder is a triangular or pear-shaped, expandable hollow organ located in the pelvic area, held in place by ligaments that bind to the pelvic bones. It is the organ in the urinary system that stores urine and allows urination to be infrequent and voluntary. The urinary bladder muscles relax in order to allow urine to enter from the ureters and contract to excrete urine from the body by way of the urethra. Layers of muscle tissue stretch to house urine, with a capacity of 400 to 600 mL being considered normal. Note that in the average healthy adult, approximately two cups, or 400 to 500 mL, of urine can be stored in the bladder for approximately two to five hours. Once the urinary bladder is full, nerves within the bladder signal the brain the need to urinate. To release urine, the muscles in the urinary bladder contract.

> **CLINICAL NOTE**
>
> Urine is excreted from the kidneys every 10 to 15 seconds and collected in the bladder.

Figure 12.4: Bladder

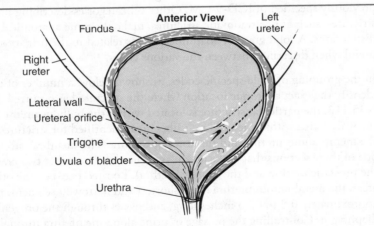

The urethra is the tube through which urine is drained from the bladder. In men, the urethra is approximately 20 cm long. In women, the urethra is approximately 4 cm long. There are two sphincters associated with the urethra: the internal sphincter, which surrounds the urethra at the top where it meets the bladder, and the external sphincter, which surrounds the urethra at the pelvic floor. These two sphincters control urinary voiding, allowing the flow of urine through the urethra.

> **INTERESTING A & P FACT**
>
> Approximately 440 gallons of blood passes through the kidneys of a healthy adult on a daily basis, resulting in about 1.5 liters of urine.

Anatomy and Physiology and the ICD-10-CM Code Set

The urinary system can be affected by many disease states, including aging, illness, and injury. Aging, in particular, can affect the structure of the kidneys and thereby cause a loss of ability to remove wastes from the blood. Furthermore, the muscles within the ureters, bladder, and urethra often tend to lose some of the elasticity or strength, which can lead to an increase in urinary infections due to the bladder's inability to empty completely. This lack of elasticity and strength in the muscles can also cause incontinence, an unwanted leakage of urine. Injuries such as blunt force trauma or penetrating wounds or illness can also lead to the kidneys being unable to filter blood completely or even blocking the passage of urine. Additionally, in the case of injuries, other complications can occur such as bleeding or the leakage of urine to surrounding tissues, which can cause infection.

The ICD-10-CM coding system offers more detail in code selection pertaining to the urinary system. In this section, a number of common conditions or disease processes that afflict the urinary system will be discussed. Attention is focused on conditions that have notable coding distinctions or differences from ICD-9-CM to ICD-10-CM.

Urethral Strictures

ICD-9-CM code 598.00 reports a urethral stricture as the result of an unspecified infection. A urethral stricture is a narrowing of the urethra, the tube that allows urine to exit the body. As indicated in the aforementioned code, this condition can be attributed to infection; however, it can also be caused by inflammation, injury, disease, or even scar tissue from prior surgeries. ICD-10-CM identifies where the stricture occurs within the urethra, such as the meatus, the external opening where urine passes out of the body, and also details the stricture as postinfective or occurring after the infection, which was not previously specified in ICD-9-CM. Other subcategories describing urethral strictures, such as posttraumatic strictures, make the same anatomical distinctions. A solid grasp of anatomical terms related to the urinary system is useful when discerning between the various codes.

In the grouping of male-specific codes, as shown below, a number of terms identify the exact anatomic location where the stricture has occurred. In code N35.112, the particular stricture is located within the bulbous urethra, which is the widest area within the urethra. Other areas identified for strictures include the membranous urethra and the anterior urethra. The membranous urethra is one of three sections that make up the male urethra (the other two areas include the prostatic urethra and the spongy urethra). Located between the other two areas, the membranous urethra is the shortest and narrowest segment, measuring approximately 0.5 to 0.75 inches long, and passes through the urogenital diaphragm. Controlling the passage of urine along the urethra through the urogenital diaphragm is the external urethral sphincter. This circular muscle is under voluntary control, meaning that urine can be stopped in midstream at this passageway. An anterior urethral stricture describes a narrowing of the portion of the urethra that is the furthest from (distal) the urogenital diaphragm.

Coding for Urethral Strictures Due to Unspecified Infection

ICD-9-CM	ICD-10-CM	
598.00 Urethral stricture due to unspecified infection	N35.111	Postinfective urethral stricture, not elsewhere classified, male, meatal
	N35.112	Postinfective bulbous urethral stricture, not elsewhere classified
	N35.113	Postinfective membranous urethral stricture, not elsewhere classified
	N35.114	Postinfective anterior urethral stricture, not elsewhere classified
	N35.119	Postinfective urethral stricture, not elsewhere classified, male, unspecified
	N35.12	Postinfective urethral stricture, not elsewhere classified, female

Other categories of urethral strictures in ICD-10-CM include traumatic and postoperative; the distinctions noted and described above include the same anatomical terms and descriptions and are divided into the male and female categories as well.

Glomerular Diseases

A large number of conditions within the urinary system affect the *glomeruli* and hinder the filtering efficacy of the kidneys. The two most common conditions that affect the glomeruli are nephritic and nephrotic syndromes.

Nephritic syndrome is a type of glomerulonephritis or an inflammation of the glomeruli. It is often associated with an immune response that resulted from an infection or other disease process but, in rare cases, can be hereditary in origin. Basically antibodies attach directly to the kidney cells or to antigens outside of the kidney and are then carried to the kidney through the bloodstream. The antigens get trapped in the glomeruli, causing inflammation. When enough of the glomeruli are damaged, blood filtering is decreased and waste products build up in the blood. Scarring may develop, which also impairs filtering.

In nephrotic syndrome, damage to the glomeruli allows large amounts of protein to be lost from the blood into the urine, which results in a blood protein deficiency. The condition arises when, instead of circulating, fluid begins to accumulate in the tissues of the body, causing swelling and puffiness. When nephritic syndrome is due to an inflammatory process, there are large numbers of red blood cells in the urine, whereas in noninflammatory nephrotic syndrome, there are no red blood cells present in the urine. In severe cases of nephrotic syndrome, the glomeruli become scarred and kidney damage can occur.

Glomerular diseases include a number of conditions with a myriad of genetic and environmental causes. However, they can be separated into two major categories:

- **Glomerulonephritis:** Inflammation of the membrane tissue in the kidney that acts as a filter, separating wastes and extra fluid from the blood.

- **Glomerulosclerosis:** Scarring or hardening of the tiny blood vessels within the kidneys.

Both conditions can lead to kidney failure.

 DEFINITIONS

glomeruli. Clusters of microscopic blood vessels located within the kidneys containing small pores through which blood is filtered; tuft of capillaries situated within a Bowman's capsule at the end of a renal tubule in the kidney that filters waste products from the blood and subsequently forms urine. A single glomeruli is called a glomerulus.

These conditions are assigned to categories 580 to 583 in ICD-9-CM. Differentiation is often made between acute and chronic versions of these conditions. However, it should be noted that ICD-10-CM categories for these conditions refer to a number of terms not noted as relevant in ICD-9-CM.

For example, ICD-10-CM codes NØØ to NØ8 describe glomerular diseases, N1Ø to N16 are assigned to renal tubulo-interstitial diseases, and N17 to N19 are assigned to acute kidney failure and chronic kidney disease. In ICD-10-CM, specificity is now provided for the various *types* of glomerulonephritis and therefore a thorough understanding of the disease process is necessary to distinguish between the various code choices and to differentiate between acute, chronic, or recurrent and persistent conditions. In fact, codes within the section for glomerular diseases are first classified according to whether the condition is described as acute, rapid progressive, recurrent and persistent, chronic, or unspecified and then subsequently catalogued according to the specific type of glomerulonephritis (GN).

Acute glomerulonephritis (AGN), ICD-10-CM category NØØ, is a grouping of renal diseases caused by a number of immunologic reactions that cause inflammation and proliferation of glomerular tissue. Proliferation is defined as a rapid reproduction of tissue. This condition often presents with the sudden onset of blood or protein in the urine, known as hematuria or proteinuria, respectively, along with red blood cells. Hypertension, edema (swelling due to fluid retention), and impaired renal function may likely accompany these symptoms.

In AGN, the basic disease process involves deposits or in situ deposits of *immune complexes* in the glomeruli. As a result of this, the kidneys become enlarged and may increase to twice the size of normal kidneys.

AGN is often categorized based on whether it is proliferative or nonproliferative. Nonproliferative AGN is not associated with a large number of cells and consists of minimal change GN, membranous GN, and focal segmental glomerulosclerosis.

In contrast, proliferative AGN is significantly more cellular in nature, and conditions related to proliferative AGN often lead to renal failure. Conditions associated with proliferative AGN include IgA disease, commonly referred to as Berger's nephropathy, Henoch-Schönlein purpura (HSP), postinfectious GN, mesangiocapillary GN, and rapidly progressive or crescentic GN. Note that in ICD-10-CM, greater detail is provided as to the types of cells identified histologically as the result of biopsies (e.g., crescentic, etc).

Types of Glomerulonephritis

Focal Segmental Glomerulonephritis

Focal segmental glomerulosclerosis (FSGS) presents as a nephrotic syndrome. Nephrotic syndrome is, essentially, a collection of symptoms, including proteinuria, swelling, and low blood protein levels, and is caused by damage to the kidneys as the result of infection (e.g., strep throat, hepatitis, or mononucleosis), use of certain drugs, cancer, genetic disorders, immune disorders, or diseases that affect multiple body systems such as diabetes, systemic lupus erythematous (SLE), multiple myeloma, and amyloidosis. Often, nephrotic syndrome accompanies kidney disorders such as GN, focal and segmental glomerulosclerosis, and mesangiocapillary glomerulonephritis.

FSGS refers to scar tissue that has formed in the glomeruli. The term "focal" describes the part of the glomeruli that has become scarred while the rest

DEFINITIONS

immune complexes. Clusters of antigens and antibodies that are locked together. Under normal circumstances, the spleen removes these immune complexes from the blood; however, on occasion, they can continue to circulate and may become trapped in various body tissues, which causes inflammation and tissue damage.

remains normal. "Segmental" indicates that only a part of an individual glomerulus has been damaged.

It is estimated that FSGS contributes to approximately 10 to 15 percent of all nephrotic syndrome cases.

Membranous Glomerulonephritis

Membranous glomerulonephritis also presents as a nephrotic syndrome and is said to be the leading cause of nephrotic syndrome in adults. Typically, this specific type of GN is associated with cancer, yet most of the time it arises spontaneously without any known cause. No significant cellularity or growth in cells is noted in this specific type of GN despite the basement membrane thickening. As this condition progresses, the kidneys degenerate (waste away).

IgA (Berger's Nephropathy)

IgA (Berger's nephropathy) is the most common form of proliferative GN and the most common form of GN worldwide. It often presents with blood in the urine and can progress to nephrotic syndrome.

Henoch-Schönlein Purpura (HSP) is a variation of IgA, and its pathology, or origin, is a vasculitis of the small vessels.

Postinfectious GN

As indicated by its name, postinfectious GN is the type of AGN associated with streptococcal infections.

Mesangiocapillary GN

Mesangiocapillary GN is associated with systemic lupus erythematous (SLE), viral hepatitis, and hypocomplementemia, a condition in which one or another component of complement is lacking or reduced in amount. It is associated with immune complex diseases and cases of membranoproliferative glomerulonephritis in which nephritic factor is present. Complement is a group of proteins that move throughout the bloodstream freely, work with the immune system, and contribute to the development of inflammation within the body.

Rapidly Progressive GN (Crescentic GN)

As the name implies, rapidly progressive GN is characterized by a rapid decrease in the glomerular filtration rate (GFR) of 50 percent or more over a relatively short period of time; typically, anywhere from a few days to three months. The crescentic adjective in the name is attributed to pathological findings, after biopsy, of extensive glomerular crescent formation. Goodpasture's syndrome, Wegener's granulomatosis, and polyarteritis are all conditions categorized to this type of GN.

In the following table, note the use of the following terms to differentiate the various types of glomerulonephritis: focal, segmental, and crescentic. These terms are used to describe scattered variations of renal disease identified by histologic study.

Endocapillary Glomerulonephritis

Endocapillary glomerulonephritis is usually referred to as "diffuse" endocapillary GN but in some instances can be segmental or focal. It is described as a cellular proliferation affecting mesangial areas and capillary lumens. In other words, the number of cells increases due to cell growth and division, specifically mesangials, endothelials, and circulating inflammatory cells that have migrated to the capillary tuft. As a result of the cellular proliferation and subsequent endothelial cells edema, there is often an occlusion, or blockage, of capillary lumens. Sometimes, this can be accompanied by extracapillary proliferation (crescents).

Mesangial Proliferative Glomerulonephritis

Mesangial proliferative glomerulonephritis is a rare form of GN that typically presents as nephrotic syndrome and upon biopsy is identified histologically by the appearance of diffuse glomerular increases in endocapillary and mesangial cells and in mesangial matrix. Also called diffuse mesangial proliferation, characteristics of this disease process include blood in the urine caused by a particular type of inflammation inside the kidneys. Abnormalities within the immune system can lead to abnormal immune deposits in the mesangial cells (part of the capillaries inside the kidneys) of the kidneys. As a result, the mesangial cells become bigger and their numbers increase.

Dense Versus Diffuse

In addition to the particular descriptive types of GN described above, references to the terms "dense" and "diffuse" are also noted throughout this section in ICD-10-CM. The word "dense" is generally used when a thick or closely packed group of cells is noted on histologic examination; likewise, the term "diffuse" represents a more dispersed or scattered group of cells.

Codes are also subdivided into conditions described as acute, chronic, recurrent or persistent, and rapidly progressive. When a condition is defined as "acute," it refers to the rapid onset and/or worsening of that condition, whereas a "chronic" condition develops and worsens over time.

The following table is an example of the increased code choices in ICD-10-CM for glomerulonephritis and demonstrates the use of many of the aforementioned terms. The increased specificity is a common theme throughout the section on glomerular diseases, which includes nephritic and nephrotic syndrome, as well as nephropathy.

Coding for Acute Glomerular Disease with Lesion of Proliferative GN

ICD-9-CM		ICD-10-CM	
580.0	Acute glomerulonephritis with lesion of proliferative glomerulonephritis	N00.0	Acute nephritic syndrome with minor glomerular abnormality
		N00.1	Acute nephritic syndrome with focal and segmental glomerular lesions
		N00.2	Acute nephritic syndrome with diffuse membranous glomerulonephritis
		N00.3	Acute nephritic syndrome with diffuse mesangial proliferative glomerulonephritis
		N00.4	Acute nephritic syndrome with diffuse endocapillary proliferative glomerulonephritis
		N00.5	Acute nephritic syndrome with diffuse mesangiocapillary glomerulonephritis
		N00.6	Acute nephritic syndrome with dense deposit disease
		N00.7	Acute nephritic syndrome with diffuse crescentic glomerulonephritis

Nephrotic Syndrome

Nephrotic syndrome results in excessive amounts of protein being excreted in the urine and typically leads to the accumulation of fluid in the body, as well as low levels of protein albumin and high levels of fats in the blood due to glomeruli damage.

Nephrotic syndrome can be congenital, primary (affecting only the kidneys), or secondary (caused by a disease process that affects other parts of the body such as diabetes mellitus or system lupus erythematosus). It may also be caused by viral infections or glomerulonephritis. Nephrotic syndrome is classified to category 581 Nephrotic syndrome in the ICD-9-CM system but is classified to several categories in the ICD-10-CM system, depending on etiology, including:

N02	**Noncongenital or primary**
N04	**Congenital**
E08	**Due to or associated with diabetes mellitus**
E09	**Drug induced**

Renal Tubulointerstitial Diseases

When diseases affecting the kidney involve structures outside the glomerulus, they are broadly referred to as tubulointerstitial, or involving the tubules and/or interstitium of the kidneys. A tubule is a small, fluid-filled collecting tube at the end of each glomerulus. The glomerulus and tubule unit combined is called a nephron, or the functional unit of the kidneys. Each kidney contains approximately 1 million nephrons.

Tubulointerstitial kidney diseases can present as acute or chronic and often involve a number of varied etiologies. Generally, acute tubulointerstitial nephritis (ATIN) involves allergic reactions to different types of medications, including antibiotics and nonsteroidal anti-inflammatory drugs (NSAID), immune system diseases such as lupus or Goodpasture's syndrome, organ transplant rejection, and infections (e.g., bacterial, viral, fungal, or parasitic).

Tubulointerstitial nephritis, also called interstitial nephritis, is caused by damage to the tubules of the kidneys and the tissues around them, called interstitial tissue. Essentially, kidney tubules help return filtered substances such as sodium and water to the blood. Drugs such as penicillin also move through the tubules and leave the body through the urine. Tubulointerstitial nephritis may be acute or chronic in nature and can cause kidney failure.

Acute tubulointerstitial nephritis (ATIN) is the sudden onset of the condition and is often triggered by certain types of drugs such as analgesics, lithium, diuretics, and cyclosporine; certain infections including bacterial (streptococcus, staphylococcus, and salmonella); and viruses such as Epstein Barr, cytomegalovirus (CMV), and human immunodeficiency virus (HIV); or it may be idiopathic.

Chronic tubulointerstitial nephritis (CTIN) arises when recurrent chronic tubular attacks cause gradual interstitial infiltration and fibrosis, tubular atrophy and dysfunction, and a gradual deterioration of renal function, usually over years. Glomerular involvement (glomerulosclerosis) is much more commonly noted when categorized as chronic rather than acute. CTIN can be attributed to a number of causes, including hereditary renal diseases, exogenous or metabolic toxins, autoimmune disorders, and neoplastic disorders.

There is no category specific to this condition in the ICD-9-CM coding system; however, the ICD-10-CM system is much more specific with three categories classifying the condition. Categories N10, N11, and N12 classify tubulointerstitial and tubular conditions according to acute or chronic. Note that when the documentation does not describe the condition as acute (rapid onset) or chronic (a more long-term condition), category N12 Tubulo-interstitial nephritis, not specified as acute or chronic, is used.

N10	**Acute tubulo-interstitial nephritis**
N11	**Chronic tubulo-interstitial nephritis**
N12	**Tubulo-interstitial nephritis, not specified as acute or chronic**

Uropathy

Types of Uropathy

Obstructive uropathy involves blocked urine flow and the inability to drain urine through a ureter, causing it to back up and injure one or both kidneys. Swelling can occur in the kidneys, referred to as hydronephrosis.

Reflux uropathy describes a condition in which urine backs up into the ureters with the remaining amount emptying through the urethra. This can occur for a few reasons, including:

- Sphincter muscle at the junction of the bladder and the ureter is abnormally tight
- Inability of the bladder muscles to close off the opening to the ureters due to weakness
- Bladder infection or irritation
- Ureteral congenital abnormality

This condition can impact one or both ureters and can be classified as mild or severe. It is associated more commonly with children than adults and boys more so than girls.

Vesicoureteral-reflux (VUR) describes the abnormal flow of urine from the bladder back into the ureters. There are two types of VUR: primary and secondary.

Primary VUR usually occurs when a child is born with an impaired valve and the ureter connects to the bladder as the result of the ureters not growing long enough during development in utero. Because the valve does not close properly, urine backs up (refluxes) from the bladder to the ureters, and eventually to the kidneys. Primary VUR may improve or dissipate entirely as the child gets older because the ureter gets longer during the growth period and the function of the valve improves.

Secondary VUR is associated with a blockage anywhere within the urinary system. Blockages can be caused by a bladder infection that subsequently triggers swelling of the ureters and a reflux of urine to the kidneys.

Hydroureter is a term used with category N13.4 Hydroureter, and is also referenced in category N13.7 Vesicoureteral-reflux.

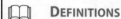

DEFINITIONS

hydroureter. Distention (enlargement, swelling) of the ureter with urine due to blockage or obstruction.

reflux. Return or backward flow.

Coding for Vesicoureteral Reflux

ICD-9-CM	ICD-10-CM	
593.71 Vesicoureteral reflux with reflux nephropathy, unilateral	N13.721	Vesicoureteral-reflux with reflux nephropathy without hydroureter, unilateral
	N13.731	Vesicoureteral-reflux with reflux nephropathy with hydroureter, unilateral

Note that ICD-10-CM specifies whether a hydroureter is present, whereas ICD-9-CM does not.

Below is another example of the terms previously discussed and their use in ICD-10-CM to provide greater coding specificity.

Coding for Vesicoureteral Reflux with Reflux Nephropathy NOS

ICD-9-CM	ICD-10-CM	
593.73 Vesicoureteral reflux with reflux nephropathy, NOS	N13.729	Vesicoureteral-reflux with reflux nephropathy without hydroureter, unspecified
	N13.739	Vesicoureteral-reflux with reflux nephropathy with hydroureter, unspecified
	N13.9	Obstructive and reflux uropathy, unspecified

A clear understanding and comprehension of these specific terms assist in appropriate code selection.

Pyelonephritis and Pyonephrosis

Pyelonephritis is a type of kidney infection caused by bacteria that primarily affects the interstitial area of the kidney, as well as the renal pelvis or, less often, the renal tubules. In ICD-9-CM, there is one code for unspecified pyelonephritis (590.80), which encompasses both pyelitis NOS and pyelonephritis NOS. ICD-10-CM uses three codes to describe the same condition.

Coding for Unspecified Pyelonephritis

ICD-9-CM	ICD-10-CM	
590.80 Pyelonephritis, unspecified	N11.9	Chronic tubulo-interstitial nephritis, unspecified
	N12	Tubulo-interstitial nephritis, not specified as acute or chronic
	N13.6	Pyonephrosis

Pyonephrosis

Pyonephrosis is distention of the kidney with infected pus-producing urine in an obstructed collecting system. Similar in nature to an abscess, pyonephrosis is typically associated with fever, chills, and flank pain; though patients can present as asymptomatic. This condition may be caused by a broad spectrum of pathologic conditions involving a urinary tract infection or the spread of a bacterial pathogen in the bloodstream.

Coding for Malignant Neoplasms of the Kidney and Other and Unspecified Urinary Organs

Unlike ICD-9-CM codes, ICD-10-CM codes indicate laterality for the right or left sides. Coders should therefore determine from the documentation which kidney or other urinary organ has been treated. When documentation does not specify the right or left side, an unspecified code is available in urinary malignant neoplasm category C64 for the kidney, C65 for the renal pelvis, and C66 for the ureters.

Coding for Neurogenic Bladder, NOS

Category 596.54 in ICD-9-CM is assigned for a nonspecific dysfunctional bladder due to a lesion in the central or peripheral nervous system that causes incontinence, residual urine retention, urinary infection, stones, and renal failure. ICD-10-CM describes three types of dysfunctional bladder.

An uninhibited neuropathic bladder is an abnormal condition that disrupts the normal inhibitory control of the detrusor muscle function by the central nervous system due to underdevelopment or impairment (usually by a lesion), resulting in urgency, frequent involuntary urination, uncontrolled urine leakage or *anuresis*. Simply put, a patient with this condition often does not realize the bladder has filled until urine begins to empty from it.

Reflex neuropathic (neurogenic) bladder is an interruption in both the sensory and motor bladder pathways in the spinal cord, just above the sacral segments. Bladder sensations are absent as the result of lesions above the lower thoracic cord. As a result, the detrusor muscle contracts spontaneously and the sphincter muscles may completely relax, resulting in incontinence. Reflex neuropathic bladder is often associated with spinal cord injuries. In such cases, patients can develop a condition called detrusor sphincter dyssynergia with detrusor hyperreflexia (DSD-DH), or the inability to completely empty the bladder due to overactivity in the bladder and sphincter muscles.

Neuromuscular dysfunction of the bladder is a general term that describes the loss of normal bladder function because of damage to an area of the nervous system. The ICD-10-CM code for this condition is assigned a fourth character of 9 and is the most generic code of the three. If documentation is not specific enough to assign one of the aforementioned codes, this code is the most likely choice.

DEFINITIONS

anuresis. Inability to urinate or the retention of urine in the bladder.

Coding for Neuromuscular Dysfunction of Bladder, NEC

ICD-9-CM	ICD-10-CM	
596.54 Neurogenic bladder, NOS	N31.0	Uninhibited neuropathic bladder, not elsewhere classified
	N31.1	Reflex neuropathic bladder, not elsewhere classified
	N31.9	Neuromuscular dysfunction of bladder, unspecified

Urinary Incontinence

Urinary incontinence is a loss of bladder control resulting from weakened or overactive bladder muscles. The severity of incontinence can range from mild leaking of urine to uncontrollable wetting. While commonly associated with aging, urinary incontinence can be diagnosed in any age group. Weak bladder muscles can contribute to "accidents" when sneezing, laughing, or lifting heavy objects because the muscles are unable to keep the opening to the bladder closed. Bladder muscles that are too active give the strong urge to use the bathroom when, in fact, very little urine is actually in the bladder.

Urinary incontinence is not a disease; rather, it is a symptom. It is often caused by everyday habits, or an underlying medical condition. Some causes of temporary urinary incontinence include alcohol or caffeine consumption, overhydration, dehydration, bladder irritation, and certain medications. In addition, there are some easily treated medical conditions that may also cause urinary incontinence, such as a urinary tract infection. More chronic, persistent types of urinary incontinence are often attributed to pregnancy and childbirth, aging, hysterectomy, interstitial cystitis, prostate conditions (prostatitis, enlarged prostate, prostate cancer), bladder cancer or stones, neurological disorders, or obstructions.

Treatment for urinary incontinence are wide ranging, including behavioral techniques (bladder training, scheduled toilet trips, or fluid and diet management), physical therapy (pelvic floor exercises or electrical stimulation), medications (anticholinergics, topical estrogen, or Imipramine), special devices (urethral inserts, pessary), therapies (radiofrequency therapy, botulinum toxin type A, bulking material injections, or sacral nerve stimulation), or surgery (sling procedures, bladder neck suspension, artificial urinary sphincter).

Types of Urinary Incontinence

There are many types of urinary incontinence, such as:

- Stress incontinence
- Urge incontinence
- Overflow incontinence
- Mixed incontinence
- Functional incontinence
- Gross total incontinence

Stress Incontinence

Stress incontinence describes a loss of urine when the bladder is stressed by coughing, sneezing, laughing, exercising, or lifting something heavy. It is caused by weak sphincter muscles of the bladder due to physical changes from pregnancy and childbirth or menopause in women; in men, removal of the prostate gland can cause this type of incontinence.

Urge Incontinence

Urge incontinence is an unexpected, powerful urge to urinate followed by a small involuntary loss of urine. This type of incontinence is described as bladder muscle contractions that afford only a few seconds to a minute of warning before those afflicted need to use the bathroom. Patients with urge incontinence often indicate a frequent need to urinate, including throughout the night. This type of incontinence is often attributed to urinary tract infections (UTI), bladder irritants, bowel problems, Parkinson's or Alzheimer's disease, stroke, injury, or nervous system damage associated with multiple sclerosis (MS). When no known etiology can be identified, urge incontinence is also called overactive bladder.

Overflow Incontinence

Incontinence described as a frequent or constant dribble of urine is called overflow incontinence and is the inability to fully empty one's bladder. Patients with this type of incontinence often feel as though they can never completely empty their bladder, producing only a weak stream of urine. Often, overflow incontinence is associated with a damaged bladder, blocked urethra, or nerve damage from diabetes mellitus or, in men, prostate gland problems.

Mixed Incontinence

When symptoms from more than one type of urinary incontinence are present, such as stress and urge incontinence, a patient is described as having mixed incontinence. Mixed incontinence is most commonly found in women. The cause of the two forms may or may not be related.

Functional Incontinence

Functional incontinence is the inability to make it to the toilet in time due to a physical or mental impairment, such as in the case of a person with severe arthritis not being able to unbutton his or her pants quickly enough. This type of incontinence is commonly noted in older adults, especially those residing in nursing homes. It is the most common type of incontinence among older adults with arthritis, Parkinson's disease, or Alzheimer's disease. Patients with this type of incontinence are often unable to control their bladder before reaching the bathroom due to limitations in moving, thinking, or communicating.

Gross Total Incontinence

Gross total incontinence is continuous leaking of urine, both day and night, or periodic uncontrollable leaking of large volumes of urine. Essentially, this indicates the bladder is incapable of storing urine. This type of incontinence is typically seen in patients born with an anatomical defect with injuries to the spinal cord or urinary system, or with an abnormal opening (fistula) between the bladder and an adjacent structure, such as the vagina.

Male Urinary Incontinence

Urinary incontinence in men is typically limited to the following three types: stress, urge, and overflow incontinence, generally associated with nerve or prostate problems. In order for the urinary system to function, muscles and nerves must work together to contain urine in the bladder and release it at the appropriate time. Nerve problems are defined as any disease, condition, or injury that impairs the nerves, leading to problems with urination. For example, male patients with diabetes mellitus can develop nerve damage that affects bladder control. Strokes, Parkinson's disease, and multiple sclerosis can all affect the brain and nervous system, thereby impacting bladder function. Overactive bladder, or urge incontinence, can often be caused by nervous damage or it can occur with unknown etiology. Spinal cord injuries also can interrupt nerve signals required for bladder control.

As discussed in the male reproductive chapter, the prostate gland is approximately the size and shape of a walnut and surrounds the urethra just beneath the bladder. Its function is to add fluid to semen prior to ejaculation. One prostate condition that can contribute to urinary incontinence is benign prostatic hyperplasia (BPH), which is an enlarged prostate. When the prostate becomes enlarged, pressure is applied to the urethra, thereby affecting urine flow. The term for urinary symptoms associated with BPH is lower urinary tract symptoms (LUTS). BPH with LUTS typically occurs in men aged 60 to 80 years old. Note that while it is common to have hesitation, interrupted or weak urine stream, urgency, or leaking, as well as urge and frequency with urination, particularly at night, this does not necessarily mean an enlarged prostate is the cause.

Male patients who have undergone radical prostatectomy or external beam radiation for prostate cancer can also experience impotence and incontinence.

Female Urinary Incontinence

Incontinence occurs in females twice as often than in men, due largely in part to the anatomical structure of the female urinary tract, pregnancy and childbirth, as well as menopause. Additionally, older female patients tend to experience urinary tract-related problems more frequently than do younger female patients. Common types of incontinence associate with females include stress, urge (overactive bladder), functional, overflow, and mixed.

As previously stated, urinary incontinence is not a disease process but a symptom and as such, is coded to the signs, symptoms, and ill-defined conditions section in ICD-9-CM. Codes in this section are classified to category 788.3 with a fifth-digit subclassification assigned for the specific type of incontinence, including:

788.30	**Urinary incontinence, unspecified**
788.31	**Urge incontinence**
788.32	**Stress incontinence, male**
788.33	**Mixed incontinence (male) (female)**
788.34	**Incontinence without sensory awareness**
788.35	**Post-void dribble**
788.36	**Nocturnal enuresis**
788.37	**Continuous leakage**
788.38	**Overflow incontinence**
788.39	**Other urinary incontinence**

In ICD-10-CM, equivalent mapping is available for the ICD-9-CM codes. For example, 788.30 Urinary incontinence, unspecified, is mapped to R32 Unspecified urinary incontinence.

Urinary incontinence codes in ICD-10-CM are classified to category N39 Other disorders of urinary system, with stress incontinence assigned to N39.3 and the remaining types assigned to category N39.4 with a fifth character identifying the specific type. Other specified urinary incontinence is assigned to category N39.49 with a sixth character identifying the specific type as N39.490 Overflow incontinence, or N39.498 Other specified urinary incontinence. See the table below for equivalent mapping.

Coding for Urinary Incontinence

ICD-9-CM		ICD-10-CM	
788.31	Urge incontinence	N39.41	Urge incontinence
788.32	Stress incontinence, male	N39.3	Stress incontinence (female) (male)
788.33	Mixed incontinence (male) (female)	N39.46	Mixed incontinence
788.34	Incontinence without sensory awareness	N39.42	Incontinence without sensory awareness
788.35	Post-void dribble	N39.43	Post-void dribbling
788.36	Nocturnal enuresis	N39.44	Nocturnal emesis
788.37	Continuous leakage	N39.45	Continuous leakage
788.38	Overflow incontinence	N39.490	Overflow incontinence
788.39	Other urinary incontinence	N39.498	Other specified urinary incontinence

Note that female stress urinary incontinence is coded in ICD-9-CM to category 625 Pain and other symptoms associated with female genital organs, with the fifth digit specifying stress incontinence, female. However, in ICD-10-CM, female stress urinary incontinence is not separately distinguished but rather is included in the same category as male stress urinary incontinence N39.3 Stress incontinence (female) (male).

Injury to the Kidneys and Pelvic Organs

An injury to the kidney can involve a laceration, contusion, hematoma, or an unspecified injury. ICD-9-CM category 866 Injury to kidney is further subdivided into two subcategories: injury to kidney without mention of open wound into cavity and injury to kidney with open wound into cavity. A fifth-digit subclassification is provided for use with this category to provide greater specificity as follows:

- Unspecified injury

- Hematoma without rupture of capsule

- Laceration

- Complete disruption of *kidney parenchyma*

ICD-10-CM provides laterality codes that permit coders to indicate *which* specific kidney has been injured and also allows coders to note the type of encounter. In the examples below, "A" indicates the initial visit. However, other seventh-character codes are available, including "D" for subsequent encounter and "S" for sequela.

Coding for Injury to the Kidney without Mention of Open Wound into the Cavity, Unspecified

ICD-9-CM	ICD-10-CM
866.00 Unspecified kidney injury without mention of open wound into cavity	S37.001A Unspecified injury of right kidney, initial encounter
	S37.002A Unspecified injury of left kidney, initial encounter
	S37.009A Unspecified injury of unspecified kidney, initial encounter

ICD-9-CM code 866.01 Kidney hematoma without rupture of capsule or mention of open wound into cavity, does not enable the coder to specify laterality; ICD-10-CM, however, does provide laterality choices, along with a seventh character noting the encounter. Additional terms are also used to describe the contusion (hematoma) as major or minor. No option is provided to the coder for a contusion not described as major or minor; therefore, documentation needs to indicate the severity of the hematoma.

DEFINITIONS

kidney parenchyma. Primary, essential, and functional units of the kidney, specifically the nephrons.

Coding for Kidney Hematoma without Rupture of Capsule or Mention of Open Wound in Cavity

ICD-9-CM		ICD-10-CM	
866.01	Kidney hematoma without rupture of capsule or mention of open wound into cavity	S37.011A	Minor contusion of right kidney, initial encounter
		S37.012A	Minor contusion of left kidney, initial encounter
		S37.019A	Minor contusion of unspecified kidney, initial encounter
		S37.021A	Major contusion of right kidney, initial encounter
		S37.022A	Major contusion of left kidney, initial encounter
		S37.029A	Major contusion of unspecified kidney, initial encounter

ICD-9-CM code 866.02 follows a similar mapping to ICD-10-CM codes as the tables above, with the ICD-10-CM code specifying both the laterality and type of encounter, as well as whether the laceration was considered minor or moderate, or was unspecified. Major lacerations involve a complete disruption of the kidney parenchyma (866.03).

There is an interesting difference in coding between ICD-9-CM and ICD-10-CM when it comes to injuries to the kidney that involve an *open wound* into the cavity. Note in the table below that *two* codes are necessary in ICD-10-CM to describe a condition assigned only one code in ICD-9-CM.

ICD-9-CM codes 866.11, 866.12, and 866.13 map to two ICD-10-CM codes: one that specifies laterality, encounter type, and whether the hematoma was minor or major, and a secondary code that more adequately describes the severity of the hematoma, laceration, or disruption of the kidney parenchyma, and the open wound into the cavity. Seventh characters in ICD-10-CM identify the type of encounter, with "A" indicating the initial encounter, "D" indicating subsequent encounters, and "S" used for sequela.

Coding for Kidney Hematoma without Rupture of Capsule, with Open Wound into Cavity

ICD-9-CM		ICD-10-CM	
866.11	Kidney hematoma, without rupture of capsule, with open wound into cavity	S37.019A	Minor contusion of unspecified kidney, initial encounter
		S37.029A	Major contusion of unspecified kidney, initial encounter
		AND	
		S31.001A	Unspecified open wound of lower back and pelvis with penetration into retroperitoneum, initial encounter

Another example is shown below.

Coding for Kidney Laceration with Open Wound into Cavity

ICD-9-CM		ICD-10-CM	
866.12	Kidney laceration with open wound into cavity	S37.039A	Laceration of unspecified kidney, unspecified degree, initial encounter
		S37.049A	Minor laceration of unspecified kidney, initial encounter
		S37.059A	Moderate laceration of unspecified kidney, initial encounter
		AND	
		S31.001A	Unspecified open wound of lower back and pelvis with penetration into retroperitoneum, initial encounter

ICD-9-CM code 866.13 maps to ICD-10-CM codes S37.069A Major laceration, unspecified kidney, initial encounter, and S31.001A Unspecified open wound of lower back and pelvis with penetration into the retroperitoneum, initial encounter.

ICD-9-CM category 867 Injury to pelvic organs, includes categories for other organs within the urinary system. For example, 867.0 and 867.1 describe an injury to the bladder and urethra, with or without mention of an open wound into the cavity, respectively. Likewise, categories are provided for an injury to the ureter with (867.3) and without (867.2) open wound into the cavity. No fifth-digit subclassification is provided for use with category 867. In ICD-10-CM, codes for injuries to the bladder or urethra without mention of an open wound include the specific type of injury (contusion, laceration, other, or unspecified) and a seventh character identifying the encounter type.

Coding for Injury to the Bladder or Urethra without Mention of an Open Wound into Cavity

ICD-9-CM		ICD-10-CM	
867.0	Bladder and urethra injury without mention of open wound into cavity	S37.20xA	Unspecified injury of bladder, initial encounter
		S37.22xA	Contusion of bladder, initial encounter
		S37.23xA	Laceration of bladder, initial encounter
		S37.29xA	Other injury of bladder, initial encounter
		S37.30xA	Unspecified injury of urethra, initial encounter
		S37.32xA	Contusion of urethra, initial encounter
		S37.33xA	Laceration of urethra, initial encounter
		S37.39xA	Other injury of urethra, initial encounter

As for injuries to the kidney, for injuries to the bladder and urethra involving an open wound into the retroperitoneal cavity (ICD-9-CM code 867.1), two ICD-10-CM codes are required: the code for the anatomic site of the injury (bladder or urethra) and code S31.001A Unspecified open wound of lower back and pelvis with penetration into the retroperitoneum. This mapping also applies to injuries of the ureters with open wound into the cavity.

Summary

The urinary system's main function is to create, store, and transport urine out of the body. This is a complex process, managed by the main organs of the urinary system, as well as a series of tubules. It is important and necessary to pay close attention to the differences between the two coding systems from an anatomy and pathology perspective. ICD-10-CM includes increased specificity, so taking the time to explore the additional areas of anatomy, physiology, and disease pathology is an important step in the transition to ICD-10-CM.

Chapter 13. **Reproductive Systems**

Note: This chapter includes both the male and female reproductive systems, as well as a separate section on pregnancy, childbirth, and the puerperium. For ease of use, each section is discussed separately, beginning with the male reproductive system.

Anatomic Overview: Male Reproductive System

Three primary organs make up the external male reproductive system: the penis, scrotum, and testicles (testes). Internal organs, also referred to as accessory organs, include:

- Bulbourethral glands
- Ejaculatory ducts
- Epididymis
- Prostate gland
- Seminal vesicles
- Urethra
- Vas deferens

External Organs

The first primary external organ is the penis and it has three parts: the root, which attaches to the wall of the abdomen; the body (shaft); and the glans, the cone-shaped part at the end of the penis, often referred to as the head of the penis (glans penis). At birth, this area is covered with a loose layer of skin called the foreskin. The urethral opening is at the tip of the penis and, as discussed in the urinary section, is the tube that transports urine from the body. In the male reproductive system, semen is also transported through the urethra. In addition, the penis also contains a number of sensitive nerve endings.

Figure 13.1: Male Genitalia

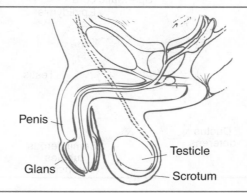

📁 **CLINICAL NOTE**

Circumcision is a procedure involving the surgical removal of the foreskin, the tissue covering the head of the penis. The procedure involves the freeing of the foreskin, or prepuce, from the head of the penis (glans), and clipping the excess foreskin off. When performed on a newborn, the procedure takes approximately five to 10 minutes; adults may take one hour. Healing occurs usually within five to seven days.

The scrotum is an external reproductive organ since temperatures inside the human body are too high for sperm to survive.

Figure 13.2: Glans Penis

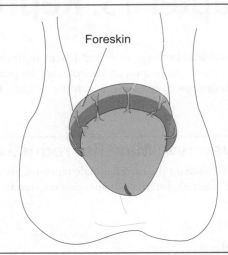

Foreskin

Behind and just below the penis lies a loose, pouch-like sac of skin known as the scrotum, which houses the testicles, commonly known as the testes. A number of nerves and blood vessels are located within the scrotum. The main function of the scrotum is to control the temperature of the testes to that of a slightly lower-than-normal body temperature in order to ensure healthy sperm development. The scrotum wall contains special muscles that contract and relax, thereby allowing the testicles to move closer to the body as necessary for warmth or further away in order to cool the temperature back down.

The last of the external male sex organs are the testicles (testes), which function to make the primary male sex hormone, testosterone, and to generate sperm. Most men have two testes. The testicles are oval in shape and approximately the size of large olives, protected at either end by the spermatic cord. Within the testes lie the *seminiferous tubules,* which produce sperm cells.

DEFINITIONS

seminiferous tubules. Small tubes found in the testes where the spermatozoa develop.

Figure 13.3: Testis and Sperm Generation

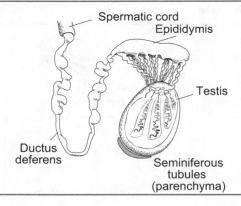

Spermatic cord
Epididymis
Testis
Ductus deferens
Seminiferous tubules (parenchyma)

Internal Organs

The epididymis, a long, firm tube that lies on the backside of each testicle, coils in order to stay contained within its small space. It is approximately 20 feet in length and functions as a storage area for sperm, allowing room and time for sperm emerging from the testes to mature. The epididymis comprises three sections: the head or expanded upper end, the body, and the pointed tail. It is the task of the epididymis to nourish the sperm by absorbing fluid and adding substances that help the sperm reach maturity in order to be capable of fertilization. During sexual arousal, contractions of the epididymis force sperm into the vas deferens.

As the excretory duct of the testicles, the vas deferens is a continuation of the epididymis canal. Often referred to as the ductus deferens or the seminal duct, the vas deferens is a long, muscular tube that transports mature sperm to the urethra in preparation for ejaculation. Starting at the lower part of the epididymis tail, it moves into the pelvic cavity, located behind the bladder. The structure of the vas deferens, or ductus deferens, consists of three "coats": an external or areolar coat, a muscular coat, and an internal or mucous coat. In the larger part of the tube, the muscular coat is made up of two layers of unstriped muscular fiber: an outer layer, longitudinal in direction, and an inner, circular layer. At the beginning area of the ductus, a third layer is present, encompassing longitudinal fibers between the circular stratum and the mucous membrane. The internal or mucous coat is light in color and runs lengthwise.

There are two ejaculatory ducts, approximately 2 cm in length, formed by the fusing of the vas deferens and the seminal vesicles. The ducts begin at the base of the prostate, running both forward and downward between the middle and lateral lobes, as well as along the sides of the prostatic utricle and ending just within the utricle margins, diminishing in size as they do so. The coats of the ejaculatory ducts are extremely thin and consist of a fibrous outer layer, muscular fibers made up of a thin circular outer layer, and a longitudinal inner layer as well as mucous membrane.

As discussed in the urinary chapter, the tube that carries urine from the bladder is called the urethra. In males, the urethra has the additional responsibility of ejaculating semen upon orgasm. During intercourse, the penis is erect and the flow of urine is blocked from the urethra, thereby permitting only the release of semen upon orgasm.

A pair of small, tubular glands in the male genitourinary system, seminal vesicles appear as sac-like pouches attached to the vas deferens near the bladder's base. The seminal vesicles produce a fructose-rich seminal fluid that is a component of semen. This fluid is a source of energy, assisting the sperm to move, and makes up a significant amount of the volume of a man's ejaculate. The seminal vesicles can very often be an early location for metastasis from prostate cancer.

The prostate gland is comparable in size to a walnut and is located below the urinary bladder, in front of the rectum, surrounding the neck of the bladder and urethra. It has a muscular and glandular makeup and ducts that open into the prostatic portion of the urethra. It consists of three lobes: right, left, and middle. The primary function of the prostate gland is to secrete an additional fluid that makes up part of the ejaculate. Additionally, during orgasm, muscular glands of the prostate help force prostate fluid, including sperm produced in the testicles, into the urethra.

Figure 13.4: Prostate and Seminal Vesicles

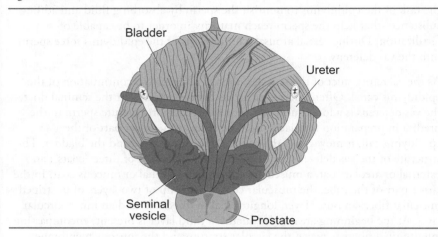

Bulbourethral glands, also known as Cowper's glands, are small, pea-sized, yellowish colored, lobular-like bodies located behind and to the sides of the urethra, below the prostate gland. These glands produce a transparent, slick fluid that serves as a lubricant to the urethra, as well as a neutralizing agent to any acid left behind by urine droplets in the urethra. Each gland contains an excretory duct, approximately 2.5 cm in length, that empties directly into the urethra.

The male reproductive system relies on hormones—chemicals produced by the body to help regulate the various functions of a myriad of different cell types or organs. Hormones primarily involved in regulating the male reproductive system include follicle-stimulating hormone (FSH), luteinizing hormone (LH), and testosterone. Each of the three hormones is necessary for sperm production, though testosterone is also responsible for developing many male characteristics, such as facial hair growth, voice changes, body muscle mass size and strength, fat distribution, and sex drive.

Anatomy and Physiology and the ICD-10-CM Code Set: Male Reproductive System

The human reproductive system, like all complex organ systems, is affected by a number of disease processes that can be grouped into four main categories: congenital abnormalities, cancers, infections including sexually transmitted diseases (STD), and functional problems brought about by injury or physical damage, environmental factors, psychological issues, autoimmune disorders, or other causes. There are some reproductive diseases that often present as a sign or symptom of another disease or disorder or have multiple causes of unknown etiology, creating difficulty when trying to classify or categorize them.

The ICD-10-CM coding system allows for greater specificity when assigning codes related to the reproductive system, in part through the use of more descriptive terms within the code descriptors that ensure improved accuracy and significantly more detail in code selection. Throughout the ICD-10-CM coding system, there are minimal or minor distinctions, such as in the case of ICD-9-CM code 601.0 Acute prostatitis, listed under the category for inflammatory diseases of the prostate. In ICD-10-CM, there are now two codes to choose from: Acute prostatitis with or without hematuria (blood in the urine). In order to select the appropriate code, it is necessary to understand the meaning of the term "hematuria," as well as whether the documentation indicated that the patient had blood in his urine in addition to the acute prostatitis. This section focuses on disease processes identified as having an obvious and significant coding distinction or difference between the current ICD-9-CM coding system and ICD-10-CM.

Other Specified Disorders of the Prostate

Within the ICD-9-CM coding system, there is one code (602.8) designated for other specified disorders of the prostate; however, ICD-10-CM provides three code options under the same titled category: prostatodynia syndrome, prostatosis syndrome, and other specified disorders of the prostate. As a result, the coder must know and understand the difference between the two different syndromes before resorting to the least specific of the three codes.

Figure 13.5: Male Urinary and Reproductive Systems

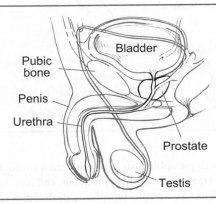

Prostatodynia syndrome describes a deep burning or aching type of pain that appears to originate from the prostate. Many times, prostate pain is diagnosed as prostatitis, an inflammatory condition often caused by infection. Patients with prostatodynia feel the prostate pain radiate into the rectum, which can sometimes lead to an incorrect clinical diagnosis of proctalgia, a term that refers to pain in the rectum. Difficulty urinating or pain during voiding may accompany prostatodynia. The term prostatosis is somewhat ambiguous, general in nature and means "a condition of the prostate." Pain emanating from the prostate without an accompanying infection is considered more of a symptom. The terms prostatosis and prostatodynia are often used interchangeably. While these two conditions are often characterized by many of the same symptoms associated with chronic bacterial prostatitis, no bacteria are identified in the patient's urine and prostatic fluid cultures are negative.

Coding for Other Specified Disorders of the Prostate

ICD-9-CM		ICD-10-CM	
602.8	Other specified disorder of the prostate	N42.81	Prostatodynia syndrome
		N42.82	Prostatosis syndrome
		N42.89	Other specified disorders of the prostate

Redundant Prepuce and Phimosis

Phimosis is a constriction, or tightening, of the prepuce (foreskin). In this condition, the foreskin contracts and is not able to be retracted or pulled back behind the glans or tip of the penis. Often, phimosis is caused from chronic infections of the foreskin. However, it may also be congenital, or present at birth. Circumcision is a common treatment for phimosis.

Figure 13.6: Slitting of Prepuce

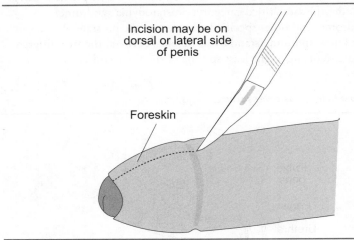

In contrast to phimosis, paraphimosis is considered a urological emergency requiring immediate treatment. In this condition, the foreskin retracts and tightens below the glans. As a result, lymphatic drainage is compromised, causing the glans to swell. If the condition is left untreated, blood flow within the penis is hindered by the ever-tightening band of foreskin, thereby causing increased swelling of the glans penis. The lack of oxygen associated with the decreased blood flow can lead to necrosis, or tissue death.

The term "adherent prepuce" describes a condition whereby a growth or adhesion blocks the foreskin from pulling back off the glans penis. This condition is considered an indication for circumcision. A "deficient" foreskin is one in which the prepuce is considered incomplete or inadequate. Finally, adhesions of the prepuce and penis may occur following circumcision if the residual skin is not pulled back after healing. During a circumcision, normal intact tissue is divided and, without proper care, it is possible for the tissue at the area of the removal to reattach to glans tissue, creating an adhesion or scar tissue. These adhesions can often be easily freed by simply cutting through the scar tissue. In some cases, however, the tissues have fused together in such a way that further intervention may be required.

Coding for Redundant Prepuce and Phimosis

ICD-9-CM		ICD-10-CM	
605	Redundant prepuce and phimosis	N47.Ø	Adherent prepuce newborn
		N47.1	Phimosis
		N47.2	Paraphimosis
		N47.3	Deficient foreskin
		N47.4	Benign cyst of prepuce
		N47.5	Adhesions of prepuce and glans penis
		N47.7	Other inflammatory disease of prepuce
		N47.8	Other disorders of prepuce

Male Infertility: Azoospermia and Oligospermia

Azoospermia is a condition in which there is total absence of sperm in the ejaculate fluid. Blockage within the testes or a missing duct can lead to a lack of sperm during ejaculation despite sperm being produced. In other cases, sperm may not be produced as the result of a hormonal issue or a *varicocele.*

Oligospermia, or low sperm count, occurs when semen contains fewer sperm than normal. Abnormal sperm count is defined as fewer than 20 million sperm per milliliter of semen. There are a number of medical conditions that can contribute to oligospermia, including but not limited to:

- Hormonal imbalance
- Infection
- Sperm duct defect
- Tumors
- Undescended testicle
- Varicocele

In addition, environmental and lifestyle factors can also lead to a low sperm count, including exposure to pesticides or radiation/x-rays, prolonged cycling, overheating of the testicles from excessive hot tub or sauna use, smoking, alcohol or drug abuse, age, weight, and emotional stress.

The need to understand the various causes and factors associated with male infertility becomes increasingly more important with the adoption of ICD-10-CM.

In the ICD-9-CM coding system, under category 606 Male infertility, four subcategories are provided: 606.0 Azoospermia, 606.1 Oligospermia, 606.8 Infertility due to extratesticular causes, and 606.9 Male infertility, unspecified.

However, in ICD-10-CM, under category N46 Male infertility, there are two main subcategories: azoospermia and oligospermia. Both subcategories are further divided into two classifications: organic and due to extratesticular causes. Additional characters are provided to indicate the "extratesticular causes" as shown in the following table.

Note that code N46.8 Other male infertility is mapped to ICD-9-CM code 606.8 Infertility due to extratesticular causes, despite also being incorporated into the new classifications for N46.Ø Azoospermia, and N46.1 Oligospermia; however, N46.9 Male infertility, unspecified, directly corresponds to existing ICD-9-CM code 606.9.

DEFINITIONS

varicocele. Abnormal enlargement of the veins in the scrotum, most commonly seen on the left side, that prevents proper blood flow, leading to swelling and widening of the veins, essentially creating varicose veins. Varicoceles are slow to develop, typically seen in males between the ages of 15 to 25, and are often a cause of male infertility.

Coding for Male Infertility: Azoospermia and Oligospermia

ICD-9-CM		ICD-10-CM	
606.0	Azoospermia	N46.01	Organic azoospermia
		N46.021	Azoospermia due to drug therapy
		N46.022	Azoospermia due to infection
		N46.023	Azoospermia due to obstruction of efferent ducts
		N46.024	Azoospermia due to radiation
		N46.025	Azoospermia due to systemic disease
606.1	Oligospermia	N46.11	Organic oligospermia
		N46.121	Oligospermia due to drug therapy
		N46.122	Oligospermia due to infection
		N46.123	Oligospermia due to obstruction of efferent ducts
		N46.124	Oligospermia due to radiation
		N46.125	Oligospermia due to systemic disease
		N46.129	Oligospermia due to other extratesticular causes
606.8	Infertility due to extratesticular causes	N46.029	Azoospermia due to other extratesticular causes
		N46.8	Other male infertility
606.9	Unspecified male infertility	N46.9	Male infertility, unspecified

Other Specified Disorders of Penis: Impotence of Organic Origin/Male Erectile Dysfunction

Impotence, or as it is now more commonly termed, erectile dysfunction, is the failure to attain or maintain an erection when sexually aroused. It may be the result of psychological factors (e.g., guilt, anxiety, conflict, depression) or due to organic or physical causes. Since organic causes impede any erection, the occurrence of any normal erections would rule out impotence of organic origin.

In the current coding system, erectile dysfunction (ED) due to physiological causes is classified under the category 607.84 Impotence of organic origin. No further specificity is provided. In ICD-10-CM, category N52 Male erectile dysfunction, is further divided into six subcategories:

N52.0   **Vasculogenic erectile dysfunction**

N52.1   **Erectile dysfunction due to diseases classified elsewhere**

N52.2   **Drug-induced erectile dysfunction**

N52.3   **Post-surgical erectile dysfunction**

N52.8   **Other male erectile dysfunction**

N52.9   **Male erectile dysfunction, unspecified**

Furthermore, subcategories N52.0 Vasculogenic erectile dysfunction, and N52.3 Post-surgical erectile dysfunction, also contain additional classifications to allow for greater detail and specificity as to the exact type of vascular condition or surgery causing the impotence.

Vasculogenic Erectile Dysfunction

Three specific conditions are identified under category N52.0: ED due to arterial insufficiency, corporo-venous occlusive ED, and combined arterial insufficiency and corporo-venous occlusive ED. Correct code assignment necessitates a clear understanding of these conditions, as well as the differences between them. A discussion of each condition follows.

Simply put, arterial insufficiency means there is not enough blood flowing through the arteries to meet the needs of the tissue. When arterial flow to the penis is impeded, a decrease in venous pressure results that subsequently leads to an inadequate erection. A number of factors can contribute to a decline in arterial flow including, but not limited to, peripheral artery disease (PAD). Peripheral artery disease is often directly linked to common risk factors such as smoking, high blood pressure, diabetes mellitus, and high cholesterol. However, other environmental or outside causes do exist, as well, including injury or radiation to the pelvic region. A patient presenting with ED of organic origin would be evaluated to determine the risk and possibility of peripheral or coronary artery disease (CAD).

The corpora cavernosa are two compartments made of spongy tissue within the penis that run lengthwise against the organ. Blood flows into the space and fills the open areas in the spongy tissue, causing an erection. Corporal veno-occlusive dysfunction (CVOD) is one of the most common forms of erectile dysfunction and is noted to be associated with aging. Other disease processes can also be associated with the corpora cavernosa and contribute to venous *occlusive* ED. The term "venous occlusive" means blocked veins that impede circulation to the penis.

In addition to understanding the differences in these various conditions, it is also necessary for the medical record documentation to clearly identify the specific procedure performed when ED is considered a postoperative condition related to the prior surgery in order to ensure correct code assignment.

DEFINITIONS

occlusive. Having to do with constriction, closure, or blockage of a passage.

Figure 13.7: Penis

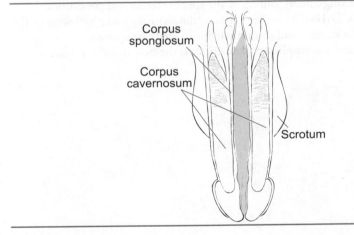

Coding for Male Erectile Dysfunction

ICD-9-CM		ICD-10-CM	
607.84	Impotence of organic origin	N52.01	Erectile dysfunction due to arterial insufficiency
		N52.02	Corporo-venous occlusive erectile dysfunction
		N52.03	Combined arterial insufficiency and corporo-venous occlusive erectile dysfunction
		N52.1	Erectile dysfunction due to diseases classified elsewhere
		N52.2	Drug-induced erectile dysfunction
		N52.31	Erectile dysfunction following radical prostatectomy
		N52.32	Erectile dysfunction following radical cystectomy
		N52.33	Erectile dysfunction following urethral surgery
		N52.34	Erectile dysfunction following simple prostatectomy
		N52.39	Other post-surgical erectile dysfunction
		N52.8	Other male erectile dysfunction
		N52.9	Male erectile dysfunction, unspecified

Summary: Male Reproductive System

The conditions discussed in this section were just a few of the common disease processes associated with the male reproductive system. As previously mentioned, being vigilant and prudent when reviewing and selecting codes within the ICD-10-CM coding system is vitally important to ensure accuracy. This requires a strong understanding of the specific terms and conditions detailed within ICD-10-CM as they relate to the anatomy and physiology of the male reproductive system, and certainly helps to facilitate a more straightforward and uncomplicated transition to the new coding system.

Anatomic Overview: Female Reproductive System

The female reproductive system comprises external and internal structures. External structures include the labia majora, labia minora, Bartholin's glands, and the clitoris. These organs allow sperm to enter the body, as well as to safeguard the internal genital organs from infection. The internal reproductive organs consist of the following:

- Fallopian tubes
- Ovaries
- Uterus
- Vagina

Several functions take place within the female reproductive system, including the production of egg cells, called ova or oocytes, the transport of the ova to the fallopian tubes for conception, and then the transport of the ova to the uterus for fetal development, all part of the menstrual cycle. In the event that egg fertilization does not occur, the system commences menstruation—the monthly shedding of the uterine lining. Other functions of the female reproductive system involve production of female sex hormones necessary for maintaining the reproductive cycle.

External Organs

The labia majora are two large, fleshy, longitudinal, cutaneous folds that extend downward and backward from the mons pubis to the perineum, and are the counterpart to the scrotum in a male. They contain sweat and oil-secreting glands. Pubic hair covers the labia majora after puberty begins. The smaller labia minora lie on the inside of the labia majora surrounding the opening to the vagina and urethra and are approximately 2 inches wide. The Bartholin's glands lie next to the vaginal opening and produce mucus. The clitoris, a collection of nerves approximately the size of a pea located where the two labia minora meet, is highly sensitive to stimulation and is responsible for feelings of sexual pleasure. Similar to foreskin on the glans penis, the clitoris is covered by a skin fold called the prepuce. The clitoris is the counterpart to the penis in the male reproductive system.

Figure 13.8: Female External Genitalia

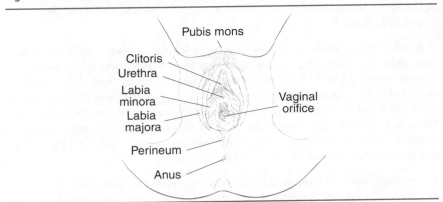

☞ **INTERESTING A & P FACT**

During the course of fetal development, approximately 6 to 7 million eggs are generated with no further eggs to be produced; at birth only about 1 million eggs remain. By the time a woman reaches puberty, it is estimated that only 300,000 to 400,000 eggs remain. Of these, an average of 300 to 400 will be ovulated over the course of a woman's reproductive lifetime.

Internal Organs

The vagina or birth canal is a passageway that adjoins the lower part of the uterus, called the cervix, to the outside of the body. The hollow, pear-shaped organ, which houses the fetus during development, is called the uterus. It has two parts: the cervix or lower portion as described above and the corpus or main body. Naturally, the corpus is designed to expand to accommodate a developing baby. The cervix contains a channel that permits sperm to enter and menstrual blood to exit when fertilization does not occur. On either side of the uterus lie small, oval-shaped glands called ovaries that produce eggs and hormones. The fallopian tubes attach to the upper part of the uterus and are the means by which the egg cells travel from the ovaries to the uterus. Conception, fertilization of an egg by a sperm, typically occurs in the fallopian tubes, whereupon the egg continues down the tube to the uterus, where it implants in the uterine wall.

Figure 13.9: Female Reproductive System

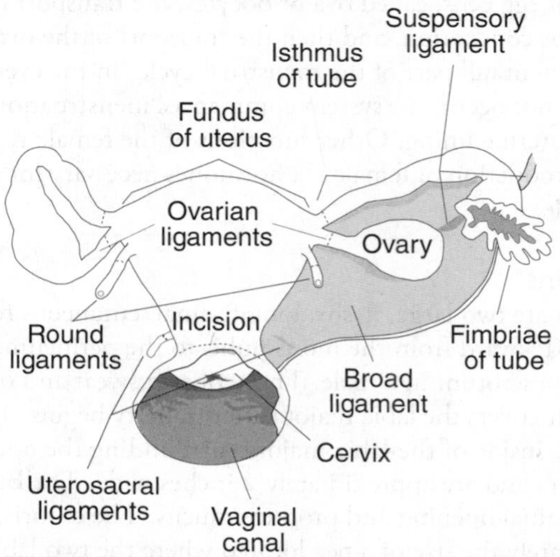

Breasts

Breasts are considered a part of the female reproductive system in large part due to the role they play in providing nourishment to a newborn baby, as well as for the sexual stimulation generated during intercourse. Breast development begins in puberty with the release of estrogen and later progesterone, triggering changes in the breast form, usually over a three- to four-year period and typically completed by age 16.

A female breast is made up of four structures: lobules or glands, milk ducts, fat, and connective tissue. A grouping of lobules form a larger unit called a lobe. Approximately 15 to 20 lobes are in each breast, emanating from the nipple and areolar area, that appear to be arranged in a wheel-spoke pattern. Distribution of the lobes is not even, and there is a predominate amount of glandular tissue in the upper and outer portions of the breast. This accounts for the tenderness experienced by many women prior to the menstrual cycle. Note that this is the site of more than half of all diagnosed breast cancers.

Lobes empty into milk ducts that course through the breast towards the nipple/areolar region, converging into about 6 to 10 larger ducts called collecting ducts. These collecting ducts enter at the base of the nipple and connect to the outside of the body. During lactation, which is the production and secretion of milk by the mammary glands, the breast milk is emptied via this course on its way to the infant.

Of course, each woman is different; therefore, it makes sense that breast lobes would vary from woman to woman. However, as a general rule, glandular tissue has a firm, almost nodular feel to it, and fat surrounds the glandular portion of the breast. In contrast, fat is almost always soft. Ducts are not usually palpable unless engorged with milk, inflamed, or containing a tumor or mass. All components of the breast structure are affected by female hormones, though glandular tissue is the most sensitive.

There are a number of congenital abnormalities of the breast, with the most common being accessory nipples and/or breast tissue, which occurs in about 2 to 6 percent of the population. Severe underdevelopment or absence of one or both breasts is another congenital abnormality but is extremely rare.

Menstrual Cycle

The menstrual cycle is the process by which a woman's body prepares for the possibility of pregnancy. The term "menstru" means monthly; hence the word menstruation describes the monthly shedding of the uterine lining. On average, a menstrual cycle is 28-days long and takes place in three phases as described below.

Follicular Phase

The first day of the cycle (period) commences the follicular phase. During this phase, two of the four major hormones involved in the menstrual cycle are released: follicle stimulating hormone (FSH) and luteinizing hormone (LH). These hormones travel through the bloodstream to the ovaries to stimulate the development of several ovarian follicles. FSH and LH also activate the production of estrogen, a third hormone involved in the menstrual cycle. As levels of estrogen rise, it deactivates the FSH, thereby allowing the body to limit the number of follicles that reach maturity. Each follicle contains one egg. As FSH levels decrease, only one follicle in one ovary continues to develop. This dominant follicle stifles all other follicles within the group, causing them to cease growing and subsequently die. This dominant follicle continues producing estrogen.

Ovulation

The second phase in the menstrual cycle is called the ovulatory phase, or more commonly ovulation, which occurs approximately 14 days after the follicular phase began. This is considered the midpoint of the menstrual cycle. Typically, the next period starts within two weeks from this point. An increase in estrogen levels from the dominant follicle then generates a surge in luteinizing hormone. The increase in LH stimulates the release of an egg from the ovary (ovulation), which is then collected by the finger-like projections protruding from the ends of the fallopian tubes (fimbriae). The actions of the fimbriae sweep the egg into the fallopian tube. Estrogen levels peak during the surge, and the progesterone level starts to increase. An increase in the amount and thickness of mucus produced by the cervix also occurs so that if a woman were to engage in sexual intercourse during this phase, the thicker mucus would help to collect the male sperm, nourish it, and move it toward the egg for fertilization.

Luteal Phase

The third and final phase in the menstrual cycle begins after the release of the egg, when the empty follicle begins transforming into a new structure called the corpus luteum. The corpus luteum emits the hormones estrogen and progesterone. As the fourth hormone in the menstrual cycle, progesterone prepares the uterus for the possibility of receiving a fertilized egg to implant. Progesterone and estrogen stimulate the endometrium (lining of the uterus) to thicken, filling it with fluids and nutrients necessary to nourish the fetus. Progesterone also prompts the mucus in the cervix to thicken, making it less likely that sperm or bacteria can enter the uterus. Finally, it triggers the body temperature to slightly rise and remain elevated until the menstrual period begins. If an egg is not fertilized, it passes down through the uterus and, because the endometrium is no longer needed to support a pregnancy, it begins to break down and shed, beginning menstruation.

The consistency of the breasts is dramatically affected by the menstrual cycle as well, most notably just prior to menstruation when the levels of estrogen and progesterone are peaking. After menstruation, when hormone levels are at their lowest, breasts become softer and less tender, making it the recommended time to perform breast self-examination or to have a mammogram.

Anatomy and Physiology and the ICD-10-CM Code Set: Female Reproductive System

As mentioned previously in the male reproductive section, the human reproductive system is affected by various disease processes, such as congenital abnormalities, cancers, infections including sexually transmitted diseases (STD), and functional problems brought about by injury or physical damage, environmental factors, psychological-related issues, autoimmune disorders, or other causes. Further complicating matters are reproductive diseases or disorders, such as endometriosis, with multiple or unknown causes that make classification difficult.

This section discusses conditions that afflict the female reproductive system with an emphasis on diagnoses that contain noteworthy coding distinctions and differences between ICD-9-CM and ICD-10-CM.

Note that in conditions pertaining to the breasts, an option is now available in ICD-10-CM that provides for laterality coding; that is, a code is available that specifically describes the side of the body being evaluated or treated. For example, ICD-9-CM category 610 Benign mammary dysplasias, has six subcategories. For each of those six subcategories, there are three codes in ICD-10-CM specifying right breast, left breast, and unspecified breast.

Coding for Benign Mammary Dysplasia

ICD-9-CM		ICD-10-CM	
610.0	Solitary cyst of breast	N60.01	Solitary cyst of right breast
		N60.02	Solitary cyst of left breast
		N60.09	Solitary cyst of unspecified breast

The laterality coding option shown above is the same format that would be applied to the other codes under this category for diffuse cystic mastopathy, fibroadenosis of breast, fibrosclerosis of breast, mammary duct ectasia, other specified benign mammary dysplasias, and benign mammary dysplasia, unspecified.

Inflammatory Disease of Ovary, Fallopian Tube, Pelvic Cellular Tissue, and Peritoneum

Infection and *inflammation* involving the fallopian tubes is called salpingitis; when the ovaries are involved, the term is oophoritis. In the current coding system, the two conditions are combined into single code categories to indicate acute, chronic, or unspecified. However, in ICD-10-CM, an individual code is available for salpingitis, oophoritis, or salpingitis and oophoritis combined; again, separate categories designate acute, chronic, or unspecified.

📖 **DEFINITIONS**

inflammation. Cytologic and chemical reactions that occur in affected blood vessels and adjacent tissues in response to injury or abnormal stimulation from a physical, chemical, or biologic agent.

Figure 13.10: Ovary and Fallopian Tube

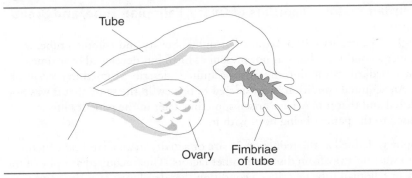

Coding for Inflammatory Diseases of Female Pelvic Organs

ICD-9-CM		ICD-10-CM	
614.0	Acute salpingitis and oophoritis	N70.01	Acute salpingitis
		N70.02	Acute oophoritis
		N70.03	Acute salpingitis and oophoritis
614.1	Chronic salpingitis and oophoritis	N70.11	Chronic salpingitis
		N70.12	Chronic oophoritis
		N70.13	Chronic salpingitis and oophoritis
614.2	Salpingitis and oophoritis not specified as acute, subacute, or chronic	N70.91	Salpingitis, unspecified
		N70.92	Oophoritis, unspecified
		N70.93	Salpingitis and oophoritis, unspecified

Other codes under category 614 Inflammatory disease of ovary, fallopian tube, pelvic cellular tissue, and peritoneum, generally show a one-to-one coding designation with ICD-10-CM with the exception of code 614.9 Unspecified inflammatory disease of female pelvic organs and tissues. In this example, ICD-10-CM contains three options: A56.11 Chlamydial female pelvic inflammatory disease, N73.5 Female pelvic peritonitis, unspecified, and N73.9 Female pelvic inflammatory disease, unspecified.

Inflammatory Disease of Cervix, Vagina, and Vulva

Similar to the codes for salpingitis and oophoritis, the codes for vaginitis and vulvovaginitis are also assigned ICD-10-CM codes that separate the two conditions into distinct categories, as well as individual codes to indicate whether the condition is acute or subacute and chronic.

Vaginitis is a condition that encompasses symptoms such as swelling, itching, and burning in the vagina, often accompanied by an abnormal discharge that can be caused by several different kinds of germs. The term vaginitis is often used to describe any infection or inflammation of the vagina. When the infection or inflammation also involves the vulva, the term used is vulvovaginitis.

Coding for Inflammatory Diseases of Female Pelvic Organs

ICD-9-CM		ICD-10-CM	
616.10	Unspecified vaginitis and vulvovaginitis	N76.0	Acute vaginitis
		N76.1	Subacute and chronic vaginitis
		N76.2	Acute vulvitis
		N76.3	Subacute and chronic vulvitis

Noninflammatory Disorders of Ovary, Fallopian Tube, and Broad Ligament

ICD-9-CM category 620.3 Acquired atrophy of ovary and fallopian tube, describes a condition that was not present at birth but developed over time. From a medical standpoint, the word "acquired" describes something recent or new. An acquired condition is considered to be new in the sense that it was not inherited and that it may have arisen sometime later in the patient's life as opposed to the patient being born with it.

Atrophy is defined as the reduction in size or activity in an anatomic structure, due to wasting away from disease or other factors. Thus, acquired atrophy of the ovary or fallopian tube describes a condition that developed over time and that has caused a decrease or decline in the size or function of that structure.

As with previously discussed codes, the ICD-10-CM coding system divides the conditions into distinct code categories for ovary, fallopian tube, and a combination of both anatomical sites.

Coding for Acquired Atrophy of Ovary and Fallopian Tube

ICD-9-CM		ICD-10-CM	
620.3	Acquired atrophy of ovary and fallopian tube	N83.31	Acquired atrophy of ovary
		N83.32	Acquired atrophy of fallopian tube
		N83.33	Acquired atrophy of ovary and fallopian tube

Torsion of Ovary, Ovarian Pedicle, or Fallopian Tube

As the fifth most common gynecologic emergency, torsion, or twisting of the ovary, affects females of all age ranges. However, most cases tend to present in patients in their early reproductive years. Children younger than age 15 have an increased risk for this condition. Most often, an ovarian torsion occurs on one side, with 60 percent of cases occurring on the right side. Delay in diagnosing and treating ovarian torsion can lead to the torsion worsening and cutting off arterial blood flow into and venous blood flow out of the ovary. When this happens, the result is necrosis (death) of the ovarian tissue. The ovarian (vascular) pedicle is the area of the ovary containing the ovarian artery and vein. Cysts and neoplasms often cause the ovary to swing on its vascular pedicle much more easily than normal, and the larger the cyst or mass, the greater the potential for torsion unless the mass develops to such a size that movement is hindered.

Torsion of the fallopian tube is a much rarer event but has been reported in both normal and pathological fallopian tubes. A number of possible causes can be attributed to this condition, such as tubal ligation, hematosalpinx (bleeding into the tubes), congenital hydrosalpinx (blockage at the end of the tube with fluid that causes swelling), and neoplasms, as well as trauma, pregnancy, adhesions, and ovarian tumors.

Torsion of the fallopian tube is usually accompanied by torsion of the ovary with an ovarian mass being present in approximately 50 to 60 percent of fallopian tube torsion cases. As in the case with an ovarian torsion, the right side is more commonly affected than the left.

ICD-9-CM currently encompasses torsion involving the ovary, ovarian pedicle, and fallopian tube under one code, 620.5, but as evidenced with other code sets, ICD-10-CM provides for greater specificity by splitting ovarian and ovarian pedicle torsion into one code and torsion of the fallopian tube into its own code category. A third code category has been developed to describe cases in which the torsion occurs in all three areas

Coding for Torsion of Ovary, Ovarian Pedicle, and Fallopian Tube

ICD-9-CM		ICD-10-CM	
620.5	Torsion of ovary, ovarian pedicle, or fallopian tube	N83.51	Torsion of ovary and ovarian pedicle
		N83.52	Torsion of fallopian tube
		N83.53	Torsion of ovary, ovarian pedicle and fallopian tube

Dysplasia of Vagina

Dysplasia describes abnormal changes in the cells found on the surface of the vagina. It is categorized by three stages: mild, moderate, and severe. The most common form of dysplasia is mild, and more than 65 percent of cases diagnosed as mild tend to return to a normal state of tissue without any intervention. Mild dysplasia is defined as only involving approximately 25 percent of the thickness of the cell layer overlying the vagina. Unfortunately, moderate and severe forms of dysplasia rarely resolve without intervention and have an increased chance of developing into cancer. Moderate dysplasia is defined as having 50 percent involvement of the cell layer, and severe dysplasia generally means that most, if not all, of the full-thickness of the cell layer covering the vagina have abnormal cells present.

ICD-9-CM describes only the mild and moderate forms of this condition, whereas ICD-10-CM identifies whether the dysplasia is classified as mild, moderate, or unspecified. Severe dysplasia is coded in ICD-9-CM to code 233.31 Carcinoma in situ of breast and genitourinary system, other and unspecified female genital organs, vagina, and is mapped to ICD-10-CM code D07.2 Carcinoma in situ of other and unspecified genital organs, carcinoma in situ of vagina.

Coding for Other Noninflammatory Disorders of the Vagina

ICD-9-CM		ICD-10-CM	
623.0	Dysplasia of vagina	N89.0	Mild vaginal dysplasia
		N89.1	Moderate vaginal dysplasia
		N89.3	Dysplasia of vagina, unspecified

Summary: Female Reproductive System

Careful review of the terms and descriptions used in the ICD-10-CM coding system helps ensure accurate code assignment. Not all conditions associated with the female reproductive system have been addressed; however, many of the common disease processes within the female reproductive system with notable distinctions between the two coding systems were discussed to demonstrate the areas coders should focus on during the transition to ICD-10-CM.

Anatomic Overview: Pregnancy, Childbirth, and the Puerperium

This section represents only those conditions that relate to, or are aggravated by, pregnancy, childbirth, and the puerperium. Many coding concepts in ICD-9-CM remain consistent in ICD-10-CM. For example, guidelines state that codes from this chapter (15) in ICD-10-CM continue to take precedence over codes from other chapters. However, additional codes can be used in conjunction with codes from this chapter to add further specificity to the reporting of conditions.

Providers must state whether any condition the patient is being treated for affects the pregnancy; when this information is not stated, it is presumed that the condition does impact pregnancy and is reported with a code from chapter 15 in ICD-10-CM.

Anatomy and Physiology and the ICD-10-CM Code Set: Pregnancy, Childbirth, and the Puerperium

Delivery Status

In ICD-9-CM, delivery status is reported with a fifth-digit classification system that is not used in ICD-10-CM. Instead, most codes in chapter 15 require the assignment of a final character to indicate the pregnancy trimester **at the time of the encounter.**

The three trimesters include:

- First: Less than 14 weeks, 0 days
- Second: 14 weeks, 0 days to less than 28 weeks, 0 days
- Third: 28 weeks, 0 days until delivery

Example:

> **O26.0   Excessive weight gain in pregnancy**

Fifth-character choices:

> **O26.00   Excessive weight gain in pregnancy, unspecified trimester**
> **O26.01   Excessive weight gain in pregnancy, first trimester**
> **O26.02   Excessive weight gain in pregnancy, second trimester**
> **O26.03   Excessive weight gain in pregnancy, third trimester**

⚬ CODING AXIOM

Chapter 15 codes should be reported only on the maternal record, never on the newborn record.

A number of coding categories are affected by this particular change, including but not limited to 641.01 Placenta previa without hemorrhage, 641.11 Hemorrhage from placenta previa, and 641.21 Premature separation of the placenta. Note that ICD-9-CM codes with a fifth-digit subclassification of 1 or 3 indicate the codes within ICD-10-CM with the greater specificity by trimester. This is explained by the fact that in ICD-9-CM, the number one (1) describes a subclassification for "delivered, with or without mention of antepartum condition" and the number three (3) describes an "antepartum condition or complication" episode of care. The other two fifth-digit subclassifications are already encompassed in the trimester definitions shown above.

Additional Categories Designating Trimesters and Conditions During Childbirth or Affecting the Puerperium

ICD-10-CM guidelines also differ from those for ICD-9-CM in that they have categories that designate trimesters, as well as specific codes for conditions that occur during childbirth or that affect the puerperium.

Example:

O99.3 **Mental disorders and disease of the nervous system complicating pregnancy, childbirth, and the puerperium**

Additional character choices:

O99.31 **Alcohol use complicating pregnancy, childbirth, and the puerperium**
Use additional code(s) from F1Ø to identify the manifestations of the alcohol use

O99.31Ø **Alcohol use complicating pregnancy, unspecified trimester**

O99.311 **Alcohol use complicating pregnancy, first trimester**

O99.312 **Alcohol use complicating pregnancy, second trimester**

O99.313 **Alcohol use complicating pregnancy, third trimester**

O99.314 **Alcohol use complicating childbirth**

O99.315 **Alcohol use complicating the puerperium**

Note: A new guideline in 2010 was issued stating that whenever delivery occurs during the current admission and there is an "in childbirth" option for the obstetric complication being coded, the "in childbirth" code should be assigned.

Coding for Trimester

Trimester is not always a component of a code, either because the trimester is not applicable or because the condition always occurs in a specific trimester. For example, for O32 Maternal care for malpresentation of fetus, malpresentation is a condition associated with delivery and, therefore, would not apply to the first and second trimesters.

Seventh-Character Extensions for Multiple Gestations

A seventh-character extension for multiple gestations in categories that designate maternal care for a fetal anomaly, damage, or other problem is required in order to indicate the affected fetus. Using the aforementioned example, category O32 Maternal care for malpresentation of fetus, states that a seventh-digit character is to be assigned to each code under this category with "Ø," indicating a single gestation or a multiple gestation where the fetus is unspecified. Characters 1 through 9 are used for multiple gestations to identify the fetus to which the code applies. In addition, a code from category O3Ø Multiple gestation, must also be assigned if a code is reported from category O32 with a seventh character of 1 through 9.

Character	Fetus
1	1
2	2
3	3
4	4
5	5
9	Other fetus

Gestational Diabetes

In ICD-10-CM, gestational diabetes (GD) is divided into three subcategories: pregnancy, childbirth, and the puerperium, with final subdivision of these codes specifying whether the GD is diet controlled, insulin controlled, or unspecified control. Trimester is not applicable to these codes but does apply where preexisting Type I or Type 2 diabetes in pregnancy is noted and would be subdivided by trimester.

ICD-9-CM code 648.8 Abnormal glucose tolerance, is the category under which gestational diabetes is located. A fifth-digit subclassification denotes the episode of care. Under ICD-10-CM, codes are classified to category O24.4 Gestational diabetes mellitus, with the three aforementioned subcategories, O24.41 Gestational diabetes in pregnancy, O24.42 Gestational diabetes in childbirth, and O24.43 Gestational diabetes in the puerperium. Under each subcategory, three subclassifications are denoted by characters 0, 4, or 9, indicating whether the gestational diabetes is diet controlled, insulin controlled, or unspecified, respectively.

Coding for Abnormal Glucose Tolerance: Gestational Diabetes

ICD-9-CM		ICD-10-CM	
648.8[0-4]	Abnormal maternal glucose tolerance, complicating pregnancy, childbirth, or the puerperium	O24.410	Gestational diabetes mellitus in pregnancy, diet controlled
		O24.414	Gestational diabetes mellitus in pregnancy, insulin controlled
	5th Character meanings for codes as indicated 0 *Unspecified as to episode of care* 1 *Delivered, with or without mention of antepartum condition* 2 *Delivered, with current postpartum complication* 3 *Antepartum condition or complication* 4 *Previous postpartum condition or complication*	O24.419	Gestational diabetes mellitus in pregnancy, unspecified control
		O24.420	Gestational diabetes mellitus in childbirth, diet controlled
		O24.424	Gestational diabetes mellitus in childbirth, insulin controlled
		O24.429	Gestational diabetes mellitus in childbirth, unspecified control
		O24.430	Gestational diabetes mellitus in the puerperium, diet controlled
		O24.434	Gestational diabetes mellitus in the puerperium, insulin controlled
		O24.439	Gestational diabetes mellitus in the puerperium, unspecified control
		O99.810	Abnormal glucose complicating pregnancy
		O99.814	Abnormal glucose complicating childbirth
		O99.815	Abnormal glucose complicating the puerperium

Spontaneous Abortion

A spontaneous abortion is the premature expulsion or removal of the products of conception from the uterus, often referred to as a miscarriage. In ICD-9-CM, this condition is coded to category 634 with a fourth digit identifying the subcategory and a fifth digit identifying the stage, such as complete, incomplete, or unspecified. For the most part, these subcategories have a one-to-one mapping in ICD-10-CM; however, code 634.7 Spontaneous abortion with other specified complications, unspecified (∅), incomplete (1), and complete (2) are combined differently in ICD-10-CM. The unspecified spontaneous abortion and complete abortion codes are described by a single set of codes: O∅3.8 Other and unspecified complications following complete or unspecified spontaneous abortion.

Coding for Other and Unspecified Complications Following Complete or Unspecified Spontaneous Abortion

ICD-9-CM	ICD-10-CM	
634.7[0, 2] Spontaneous abortion with other specified complications **5th Character meanings for codes as indicated** **0 Unspecified 2 Complete**	O03.85	Other venous complications following complete or unspecified spontaneous abortion
	O03.86	Cardiac arrest following complete or unspecified spontaneous abortion
	O03.87	*Sepsis* following complete or unspecified spontaneous abortion
	O03.88	Urinary tract infection following complete or unspecified spontaneous abortion
	O03.89	Complete or unspecified spontaneous abortion with other complications

ICD-9-CM code 634.71 Incomplete spontaneous abortion with other specified complications has its own category in ICD-10-CM, O∅3.3 Other and unspecified complications following incomplete spontaneous abortion, with a fifth character identifying the specific type of complication.

Coding for Other and Unspecified Complications Following Incomplete Spontaneous Abortion

ICD-9-CM	ICD-10-CM	
634.71	Incomplete spontaneous abortion with other specified complications	O03.35	Other venous complications following incomplete spontaneous abortion
		O03.36	Cardiac arrest following incomplete spontaneous abortion
		O03.38	Urinary tract infection following incomplete spontaneous abortion
		O03.39	Incomplete spontaneous abortion with other complications

Legally Induced Abortion

A legally induced abortion is the intentional expulsion of the products of conception from the uterus performed by a medical professional within the boundaries of the law. This often occurs by the patient's choice (elective), through a court order or other mandated action (legal), or for reasons such as the mother's health or life is at risk (therapeutic). These codes are categorized similarly to the spontaneous abortion codes. In ICD-9-CM, this condition is coded to category 635 with a fourth digit identifying the subcategory and a fifth

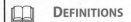

DEFINITIONS

septicemia/sepsis. Systemic disease associated with the presence and persistence of pathogenic microorganisms and their toxins in the blood. Septicemia is not interchangeable with sepsis, nor with bacteremia. Septicemia is a more acute illness than bacteremia and is also a clinically distinct condition presenting with a different clinical picture and outcome than sepsis. Septicemia is coded to ICD-9-CM category 038 with fourth- and fifth-digit assignment to identify the causal organism. Septicemia becomes sepsis when it is present with two or more manifestations of systemic inflammatory response syndrome.

digit identifying the stage, such as complete, incomplete, or unspecified. For the most part, these subcategories have a one-to-one mapping in ICD-10-CM; however, ICD-9-CM code 635.7 Legally induced abortion with other specified complications, unspecified (0), incomplete (1), and complete (2) is now described by a single set of codes in ICD-10-CM under category O04.8 (Induced) termination of pregnancy with other and unspecified complications.

Coding for Legally Induced Abortion With Other Specified Complications

ICD-9-CM	ICD-10-CM	
635.7[0, 2] Legally induced abortion with other specified complications	O04.85	Other venous complications following (induced) termination of pregnancy
5th Character meanings for codes as indicated *0 Unspecified* *1 Incomplete* *2 Complete*	O04.86	Cardiac arrest following (induced) termination of pregnancy
	O04.87	Sepsis following (induced) termination of pregnancy
	O04.88	Urinary tract infection following (induced) termination of pregnancy
	O04.89	(Induced) termination of pregnancy with other complications

Antepartum Hemorrhage Associated with Coagulation Defects

Antepartum hemorrhage associated with coagulation defects describes a condition in which the uterine hemorrhages prior to delivery. Coagulation defect is a general term for various conditions that disrupt the body's ability to control blood clotting.

Afibrinogenemia is an uncommon, inherited blood disorder that affects the blood's ability to clot by causing a serious deficiency in fibrinogen, a protein produced by the liver. This protein is required to stop bleeding by forming clots. In this condition, an abnormal gene is typically passed from both parents.

Disseminated intravascular coagulation (DIC) is a serious disorder in which the proteins that control blood clotting become abnormally active. It is normal for certain proteins in the blood to become active and travel in the bloodstream, such as when an injury occurs in order to stop bleeding. But for patients with DIC, the proteins become abnormally active and can result in the development of clots and more often severe bleeding. When small blood clots are formed within the blood vessels, blood supply can be cut off to the liver, brain, or kidneys. Once this happens, the organs cease to function. Additionally, clotting proteins in the blood can be exhausted, placing the patient at risk for severe bleeding from even a minor cut. The blood clots also have the potential to destroy healthy red blood cells. Some of the risk factors for this condition include cancer, especially certain types of leukemia (cancer of the blood); bacterial or fungal blood infections; complications of pregnancy, such as retained placenta after delivery; surgery/anesthesia; sepsis; and severe liver disease.

ICD-9-CM code 641.3 Antepartum hemorrhage associated with coagulation defects, is subdivided into categories by the episode of care. In ICD-10-CM, categories O46.00 Antepartum hemorrhage with coagulation defect, unspecified, O046.01 Antepartum hemorrhage with afibrinogenemia, O46.02 Antepartum hemorrhage with disseminated intravascular coagulation, and O46.09 Antepartum hemorrhage with other coagulation defects, enable coders to assign a code specific to the condition rather than to a general term such as coagulation defects. Understanding the specific terms referenced by

ICD-10-CM is the key to assigning and reporting the correct code within this category.

Coding for Antepartum Hemorrhage, Not Elsewhere Classified

ICD-9-CM		ICD-10-CM	
641.30	Antepartum hemorrhage associated with coagulation defects, unspecified as to episode of care	O46.009	Antepartum hemorrhage with coagulation defect, unspecified, unspecified trimester
		O46.019	Antepartum hemorrhage with afibrinogenemia, unspecified trimester
		O46.029	Antepartum hemorrhage with disseminated intravascular coagulation, unspecified trimester
		O46.099	Antepartum hemorrhage with other coagulation defect, unspecified trimester
641.3[1, 3]	Antepartum hemorrhage associated with coagulation defects	O46.001	Antepartum hemorrhage with coagulation defect, unspecified, first trimester
5th Character meanings for codes as indicated *1 With delivery* *3 Antepartum*		O46.002	Antepartum hemorrhage with coagulation defect, unspecified, second trimester
		O46.003	Antepartum hemorrhage with coagulation defect, unspecified, third trimester
		O46.011	Antepartum hemorrhage with afibrinogenemia, first trimester
		O46.012	Antepartum hemorrhage with afibrinogenemia, second trimester
		O46.013	Antepartum hemorrhage with afibrinogenemia, third trimester
		O46.021	Antepartum hemorrhage with disseminated intravascular coagulation, first trimester
		O46.022	Antepartum hemorrhage with disseminated intravascular coagulation, second trimester
		O46.023	Antepartum hemorrhage with disseminated intravascular coagulation, third trimester
		O46.091	Antepartum hemorrhage with other coagulation defect, first trimester
		O46.092	Antepartum hemorrhage with other coagulation defect, second trimester
		O46.093	Antepartum hemorrhage with other coagulation defect, third trimester

Postpartum Hemorrhage: Third Stage

A postpartum hemorrhage is defined as a blood loss of greater than 500 ml after the birth of a baby, and a severe postpartum hemorrhage constitutes blood loss of more than 1,000 ml after delivery.

The third stage of labor is the period of time between the birth of the baby and the expulsion of the placenta. It is during this time frame when the uterine muscles contract downward and the placenta begins to separate from the uterine walls. Blood loss depends on how long it takes the placenta to come apart from the uterine wall. When the uterus fails to begin normal contractions, known as uterine atony, blood vessels in the placenta stay open and can result in severe bleeding.

This condition is categorized to ICD-9-CM code 666.0 Third-stage hemorrhage, with a fifth-digit subclassification to indicate the current episode of care; fifth-digit choices in this category are limited to the delivery characters 2 delivered, with mention of postpartum complication, or 4 postpartum condition or complication.

In ICD-10-CM, two codes are required to accurately and correctly report this condition: O72.Ø Third-stage hemorrhage, and O43.21 Placenta accrete, O43.22 Placenta increta, or O43.23 Placenta percreta. In addition, a sixth character for each of the three categories is necessary to identify the trimester in which the hemorrhage occurred.

Coding for Third Stage Hemorrhage with Morbidly Adherent Placenta

ICD-9-CM	ICD-10-CM
666.0*[2,4]* Third-stage postpartum hemorrhage	O72.Ø Third-stage Hemorrhage

5th Character meanings for codes as indicated
  2 **With delivery**
  4 **Postpartum**
	AND
	O43.21[1–3]Placenta accreta
	OR
	O43.22[1–3]Placenta increta
	OR
	O43.23[1–3]Placenta percreta
	
	6th Character meanings for codes as indicated
	  1 **First trimester**
	  2 **Second trimester**
	  3 **Third trimester**

Placenta accreta, increta, and percreta all describe a condition whereby the placenta attaches too deeply into the uterine wall; the difference between the three depends on the severity of the attachment. The least invasive and most common is placenta accreta and accounts for approximately 75 percent of all cases. Placenta increta is a moderate form of the condition with a deeper attachment, penetrating into the uterine muscle. Placenta percreta is the most severe where the attached placenta penetrates through the entire uterine wall and actually attaches to another nearby organ, such as the bladder. It is rare, accounting for approximately 5 percent of all cases.

Summary: Pregnancy, Childbirth, and the Puerperium

The chapter on pregnancy, childbirth, and the puerperium encompasses a significant number of disease processes and disorders. As demonstrated in some of the earlier examples, many ICD-9-CM code categories have been expanded in ICD-10-CM to include a character indicating the trimester at the time of the encounter. It is important and necessary to pay close attention to the distinctions and differences between the two coding systems. The additional detail and specificity afforded by the ICD-10-CM coding system is certainly a benefit, though it is clear that proper code selection rests on thoroughly understanding the new terms referenced and how certain ICD-9-CM categories break out in ICD-10-CM.

Appendix A. **Knowledge Review**

Introduction to the Human Body

1. The following are all levels of structural organization *except*:
    a. Chemical
    b. Organ
    c. Organismal
    d. Anatomical

2. The principal parts of a cell are the _____, _____ and the _____.

3. All of the following are basic types of tissue found in the body, *except*:
    a. DNA
    b. Connective
    c. Muscle
    d. Nervous

4. Metabolism takes place in two parts: _____ and _____.

5. Growth refers only to adding additional cells to the body.
    a. True
    b. False

6. A patient that is face down on the examining room table would most likely be in the _____ position.

7. When the body is standing upright with palms forward, this is the _____ position.

8. Write the correct term or terms that denote relationships, compare positions, or denote movement.
    a. Toward the back of the body _____
    b. Toward the front of the body _____
    c. Farther from the middle _____
    d. Toward the middle _____
    e. Toward the top of the body _____
    f. Toward the lower part of the body _____
    g. Farthest from the point of origin _____
    h. Nearest to the point of origin _____
    i. Farthest from the center _____
    j. Nearest to the center _____
    k. Closest to the surface _____

l. Conveying toward the center _____

m. Conveying away from the center _____

n. The movement causing decreased angle of a joint _____

o. The movement causing straightening of a joint _____

p. Movement away from the median plane _____

q. Movement toward the median plane _____

r. Movement of lower arm that rotates the palm and forearm anteriorly
    _____

s. Movement of the lower arm that rotates the palm and forearm
    posteriorly _____

t. Movement of the foot at the ankle away from the medial plane
    _____

u. Movement of the foot at the ankle toward the medial plane _____

9. The left arm and left leg would be ipsilateral to one another.

    a. True

    b. False

10. When we consciously control our own muscle tissues, this type of muscle is
    often referred to as _____ muscle.

Integumentary System

1. A furuncle is also known as a _____ and is typically found in a
   _____.

2. The following are all layers of the skin and subcutaneous tissue, except:
   a. Epidermis
   b. Dermis
   c. Muscle and fascia
   d. Hypodermis

3. What is the key role of the sudoriferous glands in the body?
   a. Releasing oil onto the skins surface
   b. Releasing perspiration to cool the body
   c. Assisting in hair growth
   d. Serving as a sensory receptor

4. Which type of response to solar radiation causes hives or wheals in response to UV radiation?
   a. Drug photoallergic response
   b. Photocontact dermatitis
   c. Drug phototoxic response
   d. Solar urticaria

5. Lichenification is a _____ and _____ of the epidermis of the skin.

6. The most common form of psoriasis is:
   a. Psoriasis vulgaris
   b. Palmoplantar psoriasis
   c. Pustular psoriasis
   d. Guttate psoriasis

7. Acne vulgaris affects only adolescents, not adult patients.
   a. True
   b. False

8. Treatment for all types of alopecia is cosmetic in nature.
   a. True
   b. False

9. Which stage of pressure ulcer involves a full-thickness skin loss extending through the subcutaneous tissue but not to the muscle and bone?
   a. First stage
   b. Second stage
   c. Third stage
   d. Fourth stage

10. What is another name for a "pins and needles" feeling in the skin?

    a. Anesthesia

    b. Paraesthesia

    c. Hyperesthesia

    d. Skin disturbance

Skeletal Systems and Articulations

1. The mandible is the only bone in the face that moves.

    a. True

    b. False

2. The bony spine is also called the _____ column, named after the 24 individual bones that it comprises.

3. There are how many vertebrae in each section of spine?

    a. _____ cervical

    b. _____ thoracic

    c. _____ lumbar

4. The _____ and _____ form the shoulder girdle.

5. What is the lowest portion of the coxal bones called? _____

6. The acetabulum is where the head of the _____ sits to form the _____ joint.

7. Both the thumb and big toe have more phalanges than the other toes.

    a. True

    b. False

8. The two sections of skeleton are _____ and _____.

9. A ligament attaches bone to muscle.

    a. True

    b. False

10. The shoulder is a pivot joint.

    a. True

    b. False

11. There are two types of etiology of fractures: traumatic and _____.

12. A _____ of a fracture is when it has healed or is healing in an incorrect position.

13. A _____ of a fracture is when it has failed to heal.

14. A type IIIa open fracture requires skin grafting.

    a. True

    b. False

15. A peripheral meniscus tear affects the outer _____ of the meniscus.

16. When a joint becomes inflamed as a reaction to another disease, it is referred to as _____ arthropathy.

17. When osteoarthritis is due to the aging process, it is considered secondary.

    a. True

    b. False

18. Spondylosis is _____ of the spine.

19. Spinal stenosis is the _____ of the vertebral foramen, or space the spinal nerves occupy.

20. The three types of spinal curvature abnormalities are:

    a. _____

    b. _____

    c. _____

Muscular System

1. The three types of muscle are _____, _____, and _____.

2. Cardiac muscle is found only in the _____.

3. Smooth muscle is located _____.

4. The basic components of muscle are:

    - _____
    - _____
    - _____
    - _____

5. A tendon connects a muscle to _____.

6. An aponeurosis connects muscle to _____.

7. _____ are located where muscles and tendons make contact with the bone.

8. The four distinctions that determine a muscle's movement are:

    - _____
    - _____
    - _____
    - _____

9. Abduction is moving _____ midline, and adduction is moving _____ midline.

10. Skeletal muscles are usually named for one or more of the following characteristics:

    - _____
    - _____
    - _____
    - _____
    - _____

11. The muscles in the head are responsible only for facial expression.

    a. True
    b. False

12. The _____ is the dome-shaped muscle dividing the abdominal and thoracic cavities and aids in respiration.

13. The trapezius is found in both the _____ and _____ regions.

14. The intrinsic muscles of the hand move _____.

15. A sprain is an injury to _____ whereas a strain is an injury of _____.

16. A rotator cuff tear usually involves the _____ muscle.

17. Tendinitis and tenosynovitis are synonymous.
    a. True
    b. False

18. Calcification can occur without ossification.
    a. True
    b. False

19. A cramp is a more severe form of a _____.

20. An abnormal gait may be a symptom of _____ or muscular disease.

Nervous System

1. The central nervous system includes the _____ and the _____. The peripheral nervous system includes the _____ organs and the nerves linking the _____, _____, and _____ to the central nervous system.

2. The following are all elements of the central nervous system *except*:
   a. Brain
   b. Spinal cord
   c. Connective tissues associated to the brain and spinal cord
   d. Sensory organs

3. In the central nervous system, the brain and spinal cord _____, _____, and _____ information, whereas in the peripheral nervous system, the _____ and _____ nerves facilitate communication between the CNS and the rest of the body.

4. The peripheral nervous system may be subdivided into the _____ and the _____ nervous system.

5. The nervous system works closely with other anatomic systems within the body to maintain _____ function.

6. The myelin (e.g., myelin sheath) is a fatty-appearing insulating membrane that covers and protects _____ while serving as a conducting mechanism for transmission of electrical signals between _____. An example of a demyelinating disease is _____.

7. Diplacusis is commonly known as being "tone deaf."
   a. True
   b. False

8. Disorders specified as "extrapyramidal" refer to the conditions affecting the areas of the brain that coordinate _____.

9. _____, classified to the circulatory system in ICD-9-CM, has been reclassified to the nervous system in ICD-10-CM.

10. High intraocular pressure may be an indication of what disease?
    a. Hypotension
    b. Glaucoma
    c. Oscillopsia
    d. Madarosis

11. Codes for ophthalmic manifestations of diabetes mellitus in ICD-9-CM depend on _____, whereas in ICD-10-CM, they depend on _____.

12. ICD-10-CM codes have been restructured and refined to accurately describe disease processes by reflecting advancing medical technologies and study of the patient populations. For example, in the eye and adnexa section, the term _____, which has connotations of dementia, has been replaced with the term _____. In the ear and mastoid process chapter, central auditory processing disorder, which was classified as a _____ delay in ICD-9-CM, is reclassified as a disorder of the _____ organs in ICD-10-CM.

13. The entire ear works as a sensory system by which _____ are collected, amplified, and conducted to the brain for processing of the nervous impulses and to elicit a response. The three parts of the ear (the _____, _____, and _____ ear) work together to achieve this goal.

14. The following are all types of cataracts *except*:
    a. Descemet's
    b. Nuclear
    c. Posterior subcapsular
    d. Cuneiform

15. The left side of the brain controls the motor function on the left side of the body and vice versa.
    a. True
    b. False

Endocrine System

1. Where are the parathyroid glands located?

   a. Brain

   b. In the neck behind the thyroid

   c. On top of each kidney

   d. Abdomen

2. The thymus gland plays a role in which of the following?

   a. Digestion

   b. Immune defenses

   c. Insulin production

   d. Sexual and reproductive function

3. A goiter is an enlargement of what gland?

   a. Pituitary

   b. Parathyroid

   c. Thymus

   d. Thyroid

4. Low blood sugar is called:

   a. Hyperglycemia

   b. Hypoglycemia

   c. Hyperparathyroidism

   d. Thyroiditis

5. What causes Cushing's disease?

   a. High blood pressure

   b. Obesity

   c. Benign tumor/hyperplasia

   d. Malignant tumor

6. Hypoparathyroidism is due to an abnormally low amount of what hormone?

   a. Follicle stimulating hormone (FSH)

   b. Parathyroid hormone (PTH)

   c. Growth hormone (GH)

   d. Thyrotropin (TSH)

7. What part of the eye does a cataract affect?

   a. Retina

   b. Lens

   c. Choroid

   d. Sclera

8. What distinguishes Type 1 diabetes from Type II?

   a. Insulin injections are always required

   b. Age of patient

   c. Glucose blood level

   d. Hypoglycemia

9. What two types of glandular tissue is the endocrine system composed of?

   a. Epithelial

   b. Connective

   c. Muscle

   d. Exocrine and endocrine

10. What is the main cause of thiamine deficiency?

   a. Malabsorption

   b. Alcoholism

   c. Diabetes

   d. Hypothyroidism

Cardiovascular System

1. In addition to supplying oxygen and nutrients to the body and carrying away carbon dioxide and other waste products, the cardiovascular system is integral to:

    a. Stabilizing body temperature

    b. Maintaining pH balance

    c. Transporting hormones

    d. All of the above

2. The tricuspid valve is found:

    a. Between the atria of the heart

    b. Between the right atrium and the right ventricle

    c. Between the ventricles of the heart

    d. Between the left atrium and the left ventricle

3. The process whereby carbon dioxide is passed from the blood to the alveoli in the lungs to be exhaled and oxygen from the air is passed from the lungs into the blood is known as:

    a. Alveolar capillary exchange

    b. Homeostasis

    c. Reoxygenation

    d. Collateral circulation

4. Blood in the right ventricle is:

    a. Picked up by the pulmonary circulation to be reoxygenated via the pulmonary trunk

    b. Pumped into the systemic circulation

    c. Pumped to the aorta

    d. Collected in the vena cava

5. The microscopic arterioles function to control blood flow into the capillary networks. Changes at this level also affect blood pressure in the following way(s):

    a. Arteriole vasodilatation decreases blood pressure

    b. Arteriole vasoconstriction increases blood pressure

    c. A and B

    d. None of the above

6. Blood is supplied to the brain by the:

    a. Subclavian artery

    b. Brachiocephalic branch

    c. Ascending aorta

    d. Carotid and vertebral arteries

7. Rheumatic heart disease primarily affects which area(s) of the heart:

    a. Endocardium

    b. Coronary ostia

    c. Pulmonary vein

    d. Valves

8. Arteriosclerosis, also referred to as "hardening of the arteries," occurs when the arteries become narrowed due to atherosclerosis, and then become hardened by fibrous tissue and calcification. This condition can affect:

    a. Heart only

    b. Brain only

    c. Extremities only

    d. Every system in the body

9. Other names for unstable angina include all of the following with the exception of:

    a. Acute coronary insufficiency

    b. Prinzmetal's variant angina

    c. Preinfarction angina

    d. Intermediate syndrome

10. Once plaque begins to build up in an artery of the leg, the following changes take place:

    a. The flow of blood and oxygen is reduced

    b. The walls of the artery become stiff

    c. Arterial walls become unable to dilate

    d. All of the above

11. Which of the following statements is false concerning aortic dissection?

    a. A dissecting aneurysm occurs when there is deterioration of the middle layer of the artery

    b. Hypertension increases and extends the damage to the damaged aorta

    c. Arteriosclerosis is not related to aortic dissection

    d. Surgery may or may not be required

12. The single greatest risk factor for superficial venous thrombosis and DVT is:

    a. A past medical history of these conditions

    b. Varicose veins

    c. Stroke

    d. Pregnancy

13. The difference between the two pressures, the systolic and the diastolic, is referred to as:

    a. Perfusion gradient

    b. Pulse pressure

    c. Ventricular differential

    d. Stroke volume

14. Examining the dilated retina is integral to assessing damage sustained due to hypertension because it:

    a. Allows visualization of the inner arterial and venous systems (e.g., arteriole narrowing and vessel sclerosis)

    b. Indicates systemic disease prior to the onset of symptoms

    c. Can indicate malignant and accelerating hypertension

    d. All of the above

15. The precerebral arteries are designated as the:

    a. Left anterior descending, circumflex, and marginal branch

    b. Carotid, subclavian, and cerebral

    c. Basilar, carotid, and vertebral arteries

    d. Vertebral, mesenteric, anterior communicating

Blood and Blood-Forming Organs

1. What are the three main functions of blood?

    a. _____

    b. _____

    c. _____

2. What are the formed elements found in blood?

    a. _____

    b. _____

    c. _____

3. The _____ is the liquid that suspends the formed elements.

4. Erythrocytes are also known as _____.

5. The red blood cells' main function is to carry _____ to cells and transport some _____ away.

6. _____ is the protein responsible for the red color of blood.

7. What are the four blood types?

    a. _____

    b. _____

    c. _____

    d. _____

8. Rh-negative means there are negative antigens present on the surface of the red blood cell.

    a. True

    b. False

9. The main function of leukocytes is _____.

10. Name the three types of granulocytes.

    a. _____

    b. _____

    c. _____

11. Most lymphocytes are stored in the body's _____ tissue.

12. Thrombocytes are also called _____.

13. Plasma helps maintain the Ph of the blood.

    a. True

    b. False

14. Name the three steps in hemostasis.

    a. _____

    b. _____

    c. _____

15. Three examples of foods containing vitamin B12 are _____, _____, and _____.

16. Sickle cell anemia only occurs in patients who also have thalassemia.

    a. True

    b. False

17. Other than acute and chronic, what are the two main types of leukemia?

    a. _____

    b. _____

18. The three phases of leukemia are _____, _____, and _____.

Lymphatic System

1. What lymphatic structure is bean-shaped and encapsulated?
    a. Lymphatic nodules
    b. Spleen
    c. Adenoids
    d. Lymph nodes

2. What is the name of the fluid that flows through the lymphatic system?
    a. Interstitial fluid
    b. Lymph
    c. B-cells
    d. Microphages

3. What is the main purpose of the lymphatic system?
    a. Move fluid though the blood vessels
    b. Provide immunity to foreign substances
    c. Aid in development of leukocytes
    d. Provide nourishment to the spleen

4. Where is interstitial fluid found?
    a. In the tissues at the cell level
    b. In the lymphatic trunk
    c. In the thymus vessels
    d. In lymph nodules

5. What tissues do not contain lymphatic vessels?
    a. Cardiac
    b. Avascular
    c. Thymus
    d. Gastrointestinal

6. What role does the thymus play in immune response?
    a. T-cells mature within the thymus
    b. B-cells mature within the thymus
    c. Provides nutrients for the lymph nodes
    d. Both a and b

7. Lymph nodes are found along the lymphatic vessels and may be solitary or in groups.
    a. True
    b. False

8. What are the main categories of lymphatic cancer?

    a. Hodgkin's lymphoma and all other lymphomas

    b. Non-Hodgkin's lymphoma and Hodgkin's lymphoma

    c. Hodgkin's lymphoma and sarcoidosis

    d. All lymphomas are terminal

9. What is the primary function of microphages?

    a. Ingest and destroy foreign matter

    b. Destroy immune cells

    c. Ingest and destroy dead tissue and cells

    d. Both a and c

10. What organ contains red and white pulp?

    a. Adenoids

    b. Thymus

    c. Spleen

    d. Peyer's patches

11. What is hyposplenism?

    a. A reduction in the size of the spleen

    b. A reduction in spleen function

    c. An increase in spleen function

    d. An increase in the size of the spleen

12. Localized enlarged lymph nodes typically involve _____area(s) of the body, whereas generalized enlarged lymph nodes typically involve _____area(s) of the body.

13. What additional information do coders need to report infectious mononucleosis in ICD-10-CM?

    a. Type of virus, such as gammaherpesviral mononucleosis or cytomegaloviral mononucleosis

    b. Whether the patient incurred complications

    c. Both a and b

    d. None of the above

14. Match the types of follicular lymphoma grades with the types of cells involved:

    a. Grade I   _____Centrocytes are still present

    b. Grade II   _____< 5 centroblasts per high power field

    c. Grade III   _____> 15 centroblasts per high power field

    d. Grade IIIa   _____Follicles consist almost entirely of centroblasts

    e. Grade IIIb   _____6–15 centroblasts per high power field

15. Immune reconstitution syndrome is limited to HIV-positive patients.

    a. True

    b. False

Respiratory System

1. What is the function of cilia?

    a. They prompt the sneezing reaction

    b. They have no known function

    c. They trap particles entering with air and prevent them from entering further into the respiratory system

    d. They are the first step in the body's immune response system

2. Which structure is included in the upper respiratory tract?

    a. Diaphragm

    b. Alveoli

    c. Pharynx

    d. Lung

3. What is the primary function that occurs within the lungs?

    a. Oxygen and carbon dioxide exchange

    b. Fluid waste is expulsion

    c. Involuntary muscle contraction

    d. Absorption of dust particles

4. The trachea is commonly referred to as:

    a. Larynx

    b. Pharynx

    c. Esophagus

    d. Windpipe

5. How many bronchial tubes branch off into the lungs?

    a. One

    b. Two

    c. Three

    d. Four

6. Where is the carina located?

    a. In the lungs

    b. In the sinuses

    c. In the diaphragm

    d. In the trachea

7. How many lobes are in the left lung?

    a. Two

    b. Three

    c. One

    d. Five

8. What is aspergillosis?

    a. A virus

    b. An injury

    c. A genetic disorder

    d. A fungal infection

9. What physiological changes occur in emphysema?

    a. Deterioration of the bronchioles

    b. A pH imbalance

    c. Fluid accumulation within the lungs

    d. None of the above

10. What structures are responsible for speech?

    a. Vocal cords

    b. Pharynx

    c. Sinuses

    d. All of the above

11. Which body part houses the adenoids?

    a. Sinuses

    b. Nasopharynx

    c. Oropharynx

    d. Mouth

12. What is the common name of the disease caused by the *Bordetella pertussis* bacteria?

    a. Strep throat

    b. Asthma

    c. Ascariasis

    d. Whooping cough

13. What is the cure for pneumoconiosis?

    a. Removal of irritant causing the symptoms

    b. Antibiotics

    c. There is no cure

    d. Rest and plenty of fluids

14. What is one of the major complications of a pulmonary contusion?

    a. There are none, a contusion is a superficial injury

    b. Fluid accumulation within the alveoli

    c. High mortality rate

    d. A life-long, chronic lung condition

15. How can a physician differentiate a pleural friction rub from a pericardial rub?

    a. By a chest x-ray

    b. Grating sounds within the chest

    c. Absence of irregular sounds when the patient holds his or her breath

    d. Absence or presence of chest pain

Digestive System

1. The digestive system consists *only* of the mouth, pharynx, esophagus, small intestine, large intestine, and anus.

    a. True

    b. False

2. What are some examples of the digestive system accessory organs?

    a. Pancreas, liver, gallbladder

    b. Spleen, tonsils, lymph nodes

    c. Esophagus, stomach, large intestine

    d. All of the above

3. What are the wavelike movements of a tubular structure, where alternate contraction and relaxation occurs and the contents of the tube are propelled forward, an example of?

    a. Rhythm method

    b. Peristalsis

    c. Wave current

    d. Body wave locomotion

4. The secretion of pancreatic juices aid the digestive process by breaking down which substances?

    a. Carbohydrates

    b. Proteins and fats

    c. Nucleic acids

    d. All of the above

5. The cause of edentulism is no longer significant when selecting the appropriate code in ICD-10-CM.

    a. True

    b. False

6. What additional details must be documented to accurately code sialoadenitis?

    a. The presence of any obstructions

    b. Any additional complications

    c. Whether the disease is acute, chronic, or recurrent

    d. None of the above

7. What condition is now included in codes for alcoholic hepatitis and cirrhosis of the liver?

    a. Abscess

    b. AIDS

    c. Ascites

    d. Aggression

8. Peliosis hepatitis is one of several conditions that were included in the code for unspecified hepatitis in ICD-9-CM, but it now has its own code in ICD-10-CM.

    a. True

    b. False

9. What are some of the causal conditions of acute/chronic pancreatitis that are now important to know when coding pancreatitis?

    a. Drug/alcohol induced pancreatitis

    b. Iron deficiency pancreatitis

    c. Dysplastic pancreatitis

    d. None of the above

10. What is the major physiological difference between coding for Barrett's esophagus in ICD-9-CM as opposed to ICD-10-CM?

    a. Coders need to determine if dysplasia is present and identify the grade

    b. Coders need to identify the root cause of the condition

    c. Coders need to identify if esophagitis is present

    d. All of the above

11. What clinical concept from ICD-9-CM is no longer required in ICD-10-CM for selecting the correct code for the various types of gastric ulcers?

    a. With or without hemorrhage

    b. With or without obstruction

    c. With or without perforation

    d. All of the above

12. What new clinical concepts must be considered when coding in ICD-10-CM for diverticular disease?

    a. With or without abscess/perforation

    b. With or without hemorrhage

    c. With or without obstruction

    d. All of the above

13. What complications of Crohn's disease are identified by the sixth character of the codes?

    a. Rectal bleeding

    b. Intestinal obstruction

    c. Fistula or abscess

    d. All of the above

14. The ICD-9-CM code category regional enteritis has been renamed Crohn's disease in ICD-10-CM.

    a. True

    b. False

15. Why is it important that coders pay close attention to the specific location of the stomal malfunction/complication in ICD-10-CM?

    a. Complications occur only in certain parts of the intestine

    b. The specific part of the intestine determines which codes to use

    c. Colostomy and enterostomy complications are no longer included in the same code category

    d. Both B and C

16. What is an inflammation of the meninges due to *Salmonella typhi* or associated with typhoid fever?

    a. Typhoid pneumonia

    b. Typhoid arthritis

    c. Typhoid osteomyelitis

    d. Typhoid meningitis

17. Intestinal trichomoniasis is classified as a protozoal intestinal disease in ICD-10-CM.

    a. True

    b. False

Urinary System

1. Name the six organs of the urinary system.
   a. Two kidneys, two ureters, one bladder, and one urethra
   b. Two kidneys, two ureters, and two sphincter muscles
   c. Two kidneys, two sphincter muscles, and two urethras
   d. Two kidneys, two ureters, and two urethras

2. What is the primary function of the urinary system?
   a. Create, store, and transport urine
   b. Promote absorption of nutrients
   c. Regulate blood volume and pH
   d. Excrete hormones

3. Approximately how many nephrons does each kidney have?
   a. 100,000
   b. 500,000
   c. 1,000,000
   d. More than 1,000,000

4. What is the functional unit of the kidney?
   a. Medulla
   b. Calices
   c. Nephron
   d. Glomerulus

5. The kidneys:
   a. Help regulate blood volume
   b. Help control blood pressure
   c. Help control pH
   d. All of the above

6. What organ in the urinary system is the reservoir for urine?
   a. Kidneys
   b. Bladder
   c. Renal pelvis
   d. Ureters

7. What drains urine from the kidneys to the ureters?
   a. Sphincter muscles
   b. Nephrons
   c. Urethra
   d. Renal pelvis

8. The ureters are tube-shaped structures about _____ to _____ long and connect the kidneys to the bladder.

    a. 24–30 inches

    b. 10–20 inches

    c. 15–24 inches

    d. 8–10 inches

9. What is the capacity of an adult bladder?

    a. 400–500 mL

    b. 100–300 mL

    c. 700–900 mL

    d. Greater than 1,000 mL

10. All of the following belong in the urinary system, except:

    a. Bladder

    b. Prostate

    c. Ureters

    d. Urethra

Male Reproductive System

1. Which organs make up the external male reproductive system?
   a. Penis, prostate, and scrotum
   b. Penis, scrotum, and testicles
   c. Penis, testicles, and vas deferens
   d. Penis, seminal vesicles, and scrotum

2. Which is not considered an internal accessory organ of the male reproductive system?
   a. Bulbourethral gland
   b. Ejaculatory duct
   c. Epididymis
   d. Testicle

3. What are the three hormones primarily involved in the regulation of the male reproductive system?
   a. FSH, LH, and testosterone
   b. FSH, TSH, and LH
   c. TSH, LH, and testosterone
   d. ADH, LH, and testosterone

4. How many ejaculatory ducts are in the male reproductive system?
   a. Four
   b. Three
   c. Two
   d. One

5. What is phimosis?
   a. Abnormal enlargement of the scrotal veins
   b. Constriction or tightening of the prepuce or foreskin
   c. Urological emergency requiring immediate treatment
   d. Condition that describes a total absence of sperm in the ejaculate fluid

6. What organ in the male reproductive system controls the temperature of the testes to ensure normal sperm development?
   a. Epididymis
   b. Vas deferens
   c. Scrotum
   d. Bulbourethral glands

7. What organ has the task of ejaculating semen upon orgasm?

    a. Ejaculatory ducts

    b. Prostate

    c. Seminal vesicles

    d. Urethra

8. Which organ is described as small, pea-sized, and yellow in color?

    a. Bulbourethral gland

    b. Seminal vesicle

    c. Vas deferens

    d. Epididymis

9. What condition describes a burning or aching type of pain coming from the area of the prostate?

    a. Prostatosis syndrome

    b. Proctalgia

    c. Oligospermia

    d. Prostatodynia syndrome

10. Which organ makes testosterone and generates sperm?

    a. Testes

    b. Prostate

    c. Scrotum

    d. Vas deferens

Female Reproductive System

1. Which organs make up the external female reproductive system?
    a. Labia majora, labia minora, vagina, and clitoris
    b. Labia majora, labia minor, clitoris, and Bartholin's glands
    c. Bartholin's glands, clitoris, vagina, and uterus
    d. Vagina, clitoris, ovaries, and labia majora

2. Which is not an internal organ of the female reproductive system?
    a. Vagina
    b. Ovaries
    c. Fallopian tubes
    d. Bartholin's glands

3. What are the four hormones involved in the regulation of the female reproductive system?
    a. FSH, LH, estrogen, and progesterone
    b. FSH, TSH, LH, and estrogen
    c. TSH, LH, estrogen, and progesterone
    d. TSH, LDH, testosterone, and progesterone

4. How many lobes are in each female breast?
    a. 5–10
    b. 10–15
    c. 15–20
    d. Greater than 20

5. What is dysplasia?
    a. Twisting of ovarian artery and vein
    b. Abnormal changes in cells
    c. A gynecological emergency requiring immediate treatment
    d. Bleeding into the fallopian tubes

6. What organ in the female reproductive system is also referred to as the birth canal?
    a. Uterus
    b. Ovary
    c. Vagina
    d. Cervix

7. Which disorder is considered the fifth most common gynecological emergency condition?

   a. Torsion of the fallopian tube

   b. Moderate dysplasia

   c. Vulvovaginitis

   d. Torsion of the ovary

8. Which organ is described as pear-shaped and hollow?

   a. Uterus

   b. Fallopian tube

   c. Vagina

   d. Bartholin's glands

9. What common condition affecting the female reproductive system causes swelling, itching, and burning in the vagina, as well as an abnormal discharge from bacteria related to a variety of different kinds of germs?

   a. Dysplasia

   b. Acquired atrophy

   c. Acute salpingitis

   d. Vaginitis

10. Name the phases of the menstrual cycle.

   a. Follicular, ovulation, and luteal

   b. Follicular, luteal, and pregnancy

   c. Ovulation, luteal, and menstruation

   d. Follicular, ovulation, and menstruation

Pregnancy, Childbirth, and the Puerperium

1. What does the seventh character for multiple gestations indicate?
    a. The specific fetal anomaly affecting the fetus
    b. The identity of the affected fetus
    c. The episode of care
    d. None of the above

2. What is afibrinogenemia?
    a. A type of spontaneous abortion
    b. A protein required to stop bleeding
    c. An abnormal attachment by the placenta to the uterine wall
    d. A rare, inherited blood disorder

3. What degree of blood loss is considered a severe postpartum hemorrhage?
    a. 1,000 ml
    b. 500 ml
    c. 1,500 ml
    d. Between 500 and 1,000 ml

4. What is the third stage of labor?
    a. The period of time just before delivery
    b. The period of time immediately following delivery
    c. The period of time between the birth and expulsion of the placenta
    d. The period of time after expulsion of the placenta

5. What condition is defined as the premature removal of the products of conception from the uterus?
    a. Placenta increta
    b. Spontaneous abortion
    c. Placenta percreta
    d. Legally induced abortion

6. What is disseminated intravascular coagulation (DIC)?
    a. A type of gestational diabetes
    b. A postpartum hemorrhage
    c. A serious disorder in which proteins that control blood clotting become abnormally active
    d. An uncommon, inherited blood disorder that affects the blood's ability to clot by causing a serious deficiency in fibrinogen, a protein produced by the liver

7. What condition is defined as the intentional expulsion of the products of conception by a medical professional?

   a. Spontaneous abortion

   b. Placenta percreta

   c. Afibrinogenemia

   d. Legally induced abortion

8. What are the three subclassifications under gestational diabetes?

   a. Diet controlled, insulin controlled, and unspecified

   b. Pregnancy, childbirth, and the puerperium

   c. First, second, and third trimester

   d. Antepartum, delivered, and postpartum

Appendix B. **Knowledge Review Answers**

Introduction to the Human Body

1. The following are all levels of structural organization *except*:

    a. Chemical

    b. Organ

    c. Organismal

    d. Anatomical

    Rationale: Chemical, organ, and organismal are all levels of structural organization of the human body, but anatomical is not.

2. The principal parts of a cell are the plasma membrane, cytoplasm, and the nucleus.

    Rationale: The principal parts of a cell are the plasma membrane, the cytoplasm, and the nucleus, where DNA is housed. These cells are the building blocks for all of our organs, muscles, blood, and more.

3. All of the following are basic types of tissue found in the body, *except*:

    a. DNA

    b. Connective

    c. Muscle

    d. Nervous

    Rationale: DNA is not a tissue found in the body. It is genetic material found in the nucleus of a cell. Connective, muscle, and nervous are all types of tissue.

4. Metabolism takes place in two parts: catabolism and anabolism.

    Rationale: Catabolism and anabolism are the two elements of metabolism. Catabolism is the process of breaking down a very complex chemical substance into a more simple one, such as breaking down protein in food into its component parts such as amino acids. Anabolism is the opposite—it takes those smaller component parts and creates complex chemical substances.

5. Growth refers only to adding additional cells to the body.

    a. True

    b. False

    Rationale: Growth can occur by adding additional cells, by having existing cells grow larger, or by having the material that surrounds the cells expand, such as in the case of bone growth.

6. A patient who is face down on the examining room table would be in the prone position.

    Rationale: Being face down in a reclining position is referred to as being in the prone position.

7. When the body is standing upright with palms forward, this is the anatomical position.

   Rationale: The anatomical position is when the patient is in the forward facing position, with the head level, and eyes facing forward. The patient's feet are flat on the floor and the palms are turned forward.

8. Write the correct term or terms that denote relationships, compare positions, or denote movement.
   a. Toward the back of the body Posterior, caudal, or dorsal
   b. Toward the front of the body Anterior or ventral
   c. Farther from the middle Lateral
   d. Toward the middle Medial
   e. Toward the top of the body Superior, cranial, or cephalic
   f. Toward the lower part of the body Inferior
   g. Farthest from the point of origin Distal
   h. Nearest to the point of origin Proximal
   i. Farthest from the center Exterior
   j. Nearest to the center Interior
   k. Closest to the surface Superficial
   l. Conveying toward the center Afferent
   m. Conveying away from the center Efferent
   n. The movement causing decreased angle of a joint Flexion
   o. The movement causing straightening of a joint Extension
   p. Movement away from the median plane Abduction
   q. Movement toward the median plane Adduction
   r. Movement of lower arm that rotates the palm and forearm anteriorly Supination
   s. Movement of the lower arm that rotates the palm and forearm posteriorly Pronation
   t. Movement of the foot at the ankle away from the medial plane Eversion
   u. Movement of the foot at the ankle toward the medial plane Inversion

9. The left arm and left leg would be ipsilateral to one another.
   a. True
   b. False

   Rationale: This statement is true, as ipsilateral means on the same side of the body as another structure.

10. Because we consciously control our own skeletal muscle tissues, this type of muscle is often referred to as voluntary muscle.

    Rationale: Skeletal muscle is commonly referred to as voluntary muscle because its activity, either contraction or relaxation, is under conscious control.

Integumentary System

1. A furuncle is also known as a boil and is typically found in a gland or a hair follicle.

   Rationale: Furuncles are localized skin infections that exist mainly in glands and hair follicles where a core of dead tissue is formed, which causes pain, redness, and swelling.

2. The following are all layers of the skin and subcutaneous tissue, except:

   a. Epidermis

   b. Dermis

   c. Muscle and fascia

   d. Hypodermis

   Rationale: The muscle and fascia are not layers of the skin and subcutaneous tissue. They are in layers underneath the subcutaneous tissue.

3. What is the key role of the sudoriferous glands in the body?

   a. Releasing oil onto the skins surface

   b. Releasing perspiration to cool the body

   c. Assisting in hair growth

   d. Serving as a sensory receptor

   Rationale: The sudoriferous glands are the sweat glands, whose main responsibility is to produce perspiration to cool the body.

4. Which type of response to solar radiation causes hives or wheals in response to UV radiation?

   a. Drug photoallergic response

   b. Photocontact dermatitis

   c. Drug phototoxic response

   d. Solar urticaria

   Rationale: Solar urticaria is a condition classified as hives or wheals caused specifically by exposure to the sun or UV radiation.

5. Lichenification is a thickening and hardening of the epidermis of the skin.

   Rationale: Lichenification is a symptom of many of the skin disorders examined in this chapter.

6. The most common form of psoriasis is:

   a. Psoriasis vulgaris

   b. Palmoplantar psoriasis

   c. Pustular psoriasis

   d. Guttate psoriasis

   Rationale: Psoriasis vulgaris is the most common form of psoriasis, affecting 80 to 90 percent of patients with a psoriasis diagnosis.

7. Acne vulgaris affects adolescents, not adult patients.

   a. True

   b. False

   Rationale: Many adult patients deal with this common form of acne, beginning in their adolescent years or as adults.

8. Treatment for all types of alopecia is cosmetic in nature.

   a. True

   b. False

   Rationale: Although treatment for androgenic alopecia is typically cosmetic in nature, treatment for other types of medical hair loss, such as alopecia areata or anagen effluvium, may not be considered cosmetic.

9. Which stage of pressure ulcer involves a full-thickness skin loss extending through the subcutaneous tissue but not to the muscle and bone?

   a. First stage

   b. Second stage

   c. Third stage

   d. Fourth stage

   Rationale: A pressure ulcer with a full-thickness skin loss extending through the subcutaneous tissue but not to the muscle and bone is a Stage 3 pressure ulcer.

10. What is another name for a "pins and needles" feeling in the skin?

    a. Anesthesia

    b. Paraesthesia

    c. Hyperesthesia

    d. Skin disturbance

    Rationale: Paraesthesia is a tingling or prickling feeling in the affected area, often referred to as pins and needles.

Skeletal Systems and Articulations

1. The mandible is the only bone in the face that moves.

    a. True

    b. False

    Rationale: The face consists of 13 stationary bones and one that is mobile. The mandible (jawbone) is the only facial bone that moves, and it is also the largest and strongest bone of the face.

2. The bony spine is also called the vertebral column, named after the 24 individual bones that it comprises.

    Rationale: The vertebral column is the support for the head and trunk of the body, as well as protection for the spinal cord. It is composed of 26 individual bones. Of these bones, 24 are vertebrae that are separated by cartilage called intervertebral discs.

3. There are how many vertebrae in each section of spine?

    a. 7 cervical

    b. 12 thoracic

    c. 5 lumbar

    Rationale: The vertebrae can be divided into three groups: 7 cervical (C1-C7; C1 is also known as atlas, C2 as axis), 12 thoracic (T1-T12), 5 lumbar (L1-L5).

4. The clavicle and scapula form the shoulder girdle.

    Rationale: The shoulder girdle consists of two bones on each side, the clavicle, or collar bone, and the scapula, or shoulder blade. The clavicle is found on the anterior side of the shoulder and the scapula on the posterior.

5. What is the lowest portion of the coxal bones called? ischium

    Rationale: This area is identified in the illustration of the pelvis.

6. The acetabulum is where the head of the femur sits to form the hip joint.

    Rationale: Where the three parts of the pelvic bone fuse together is referred to as the acetabulum. It is a deep-seated pocket that accepts the rounded upper epiphysis of the thigh bone, or femoral head, to form the hip joint.

7. Both the thumb and big toe have more phalanges than the other toes.

    a. True

    b. False

    Rationale: There are three phalanges in all fingers, except thumbs, which have only two. Similar to the fingers, all of the toes have three phalanges—proximal, middle, and distal—with the exception of the great toe, or hallux.

8. The two sections of the skeleton are axial and appendicular.

    Rationale: The 206 bones that make up the adult skeleton can be divided into two classifications: the axial skeleton and appendicular skeleton.

9. A ligament attaches bone to muscle.

    a. True

    b. False

    Rationale: Ligament is fibrous tissue binding joints together that connects bone to bone or bone to cartilage.

10. True or false. The shoulder is a pivot joint.

    a. True

    b. False

    Rationale: The shoulder (humeral head and glenoid depression of the scapula) and hip joints (femoral head and acetabulum of a coxa bone) are ball-and-socket articulations. The articulation between the C1 and C2 vertebrae that allows the head to move back and forth is a pivot joint.

11. There are two types of etiology of fractures: traumatic and **pathological**.

    Rationale: In ICD-9-CM, the selection of the appropriate fracture code depends on which bone was fractured and whether the fracture was pathological or traumatic.

12. A **malunion** of a fracture is when it has healed or is healing in an incorrect position.

    Rationale: A malunion is a fractured bone that has healed or is healing in an incorrect position.

13. A **nonunion** of a fracture is when it has failed to heal.

    Rationale: A nonunion is a fractured bone that has failed to heal.

14. A type IIIA open fracture requires skin grafting.

    a. True

    b. False

    Rationale: In a type IIIA fracture there is enough local soft tissue to cover the wound and bone without the need for skin grafting.

15. A peripheral meniscus tear affects the outer **third** of the meniscus.

    Rationale: Peripheral tears are located in the peripheral or outer third of the meniscus. This area is very susceptible to healing as it has access to a rich blood supply.

16. When a joint becomes inflamed as a reaction to another disease, it is referred to as **reactive** arthropathy.

    Rationale: Occasionally the joint is impacted by an infection elsewhere. Inflammation of the joint as a reaction to another disease is referred to as reactive arthropathy.

17. When osteoarthritis is due to the aging process, it is considered secondary.

    a. True

    b. False

18. **Rationale:** As the human body ages, the cartilage of the joints begins to degenerate and lose its elasticity from wear and tear and the natural aging process. This degeneration is referred to as primary osteoarthritis.

19. Spondylosis is degenerative osteoarthritis of the spine.

    Rationale: When degenerative osteoarthritis occurs in the spine, it is called spondylosis.

20. Spinal stenosis is a narrowing of the vertebral foramen, or space that the spinal nerves occupy.

    Rationale: Stenosis is the narrowing of a foramen of the spine, putting pressure on the nerves and causing pain, numbness, and weakness of limbs.

21. The three types of spinal curvature abnormalities are:

    a. Scoliosis

    b. Lordosis

    c. Kyphosis

    Rationale: Sometimes the normal curvatures in the spine become deformed. There are three types of these deformities: scoliosis, a lateral curvature of the spine; kyphosis, an abnormal posterior convex curvature of the spine; and lordosis, an exaggerated inward curvature of the lower back.

Muscular System

1. The three types of muscle are cardiac, smooth, and skeletal.

   Rationale: There are three types of muscle tissue: cardiac, smooth, and skeletal (or striated). Each type shares one or more of four functional characteristics.

2. Cardiac muscle is found only in the heart.

   Rationale: Cardiac muscle forms the heart walls and performs the contractions that push blood through the vessels of the body.

3. Smooth muscle is located lining the inside of hollow organs.

   Rationale: Smooth muscle is involuntary in its movements but is not striated, hence the name "smooth" muscle. This type of muscle lines the hollow organs of the body and contracts to force fluids and other bodily substances through the proper channels. It is found in organs such as the gastrointestinal tract, the uterus, urinary bladder, and blood vessels.

4. The basic components of muscle are:

   • Muscle tissue

   • Nerves

   • Blood vessels

   • Connective tissue

   Rationale: All skeletal muscles are composed of muscle tissue, nerves, blood vessels, and substantial amounts of connective tissue.

5. A tendon connects a muscle to bone.

   Rationale: In some cases, the fascia extends past the muscle it surrounds, forming a cordlike structure that attaches to the periosteum of a bone. This cord is referred to as a tendon.

6. An aponeurosis connects muscle to muscle.

   Rationale: In other cases, the fascia extends past its muscle to form broad, thick sheets of connective tissue that connect the muscle to an adjacent muscle, called aponeurosis.

7. Bursae are located where muscles and tendons make contact with the bone.

   Rationale: In certain instances, mainly where muscles and tendons make contact with bone, there are fluid-filled sacs called bursae, which reduce friction between the muscle or tendon and the bone it moves across.

8. The four distinctions that determine a muscle's movement are:

   • Origin

   • Insertion

   • Shape

   • Coordination with other muscles

   Rationale: Muscles provide various movements based not only their origins, insertions, and shape but also on coordination with other muscles.

9. Abduction is moving away from midline, and adduction is moving toward midline.

   Rationale: Abduction means moving away from midline (reaching out with the arm), whereas adduction means moving closer to midline (pulling the arm close to the body).

10. Skeletal muscles are usually named for one or more of the following characteristics:

    • Size

    • Shape

    • Action

    • Location

    • Attachments

    Rationale: It is important to point out that the names of skeletal muscles are based on their basic characteristics: size, shape, action, location, and/or attachments. Understanding the meaning of a muscle's name gives a clue to that muscle's specific attributes.

11. The muscles in the head are responsible only for facial expression.

    a. True

    b. False

    Rationale: The muscles in the head are responsible for three main functions: facial expression, mastication, and movement of the eyes.

12. The diaphragm is the dome-shaped muscle dividing the abdominal and thoracic cavities and aids in respiration.

    Rationale: The diaphragm is a dome-shaped divider between the thoracic and abdominal cavities. This muscle flattens when it contracts, making more space available to the lungs during inhalation.

13. The trapezius is found in both the neck and thoracic regions.

    Rationale: Most superior in the back of the neck and connecting to the tops of the shoulders, forming the "crook" of the neck, is the trapezius muscle. This muscle stabilizes and controls movements of the shoulder. Although its superior location is the neck, it extends into the posterior thorax musculature.

14. The intrinsic muscles of the hand move the fingers.

   Rationale: The muscles in the forearm tend to control the less delicate hand movements, but the intrinsic muscles in the hands perform the precise and fluid movements of the fingers.

15. A sprain is an injury to a ligament whereas a strain is an injury of muscle or tendon.

   Rationale: A sprain occurs when there is a stretch or tear of a ligament, the tissue that connects bone to bone. A strain is an injury to a muscle or tendon, usually due to overexertion, twisting, or pulling.

16. A rotator cuff tear usually involves the supraspinatus muscle.

   Rationale: A rotator cuff tear is a very common injury, sometimes classified as a sprain. It occurs in the shoulder region and usually involves the supraspinatus muscle but can occur in the other muscles or tendons in the shoulder.

17. Tendinitis and tenosynovitis are synonymous.

   a. True

   b. False

   Rationale: Tendinitis is slightly different from tenosynovitis, in that it affects only the tendon without swelling of the tendon sheath.

18. Calcification can occur without ossification.

   a. True

   b. False

   Rationale: The process of calcification occurs during the ossification process, but they are not synonymous. Calcification can occur without ossification being present.

19. A cramp is a more severe form of a spasm.

   Rationale: Both cramps and spasms are a contraction of a muscle; the difference is the duration and whether or not there is associated pain. A spasm is a brief contraction followed by little or no pain, whereas a cramp is more severe in that it is prolonged and painful.

20. An abnormal gait may be a symptom of neurological or muscular disease.

   Rationale: An abnormal gait can indicate a neurological or muscle disorder, so it is imperative to know the different ways this movement can be altered.

Nervous System

1. The central nervous system includes the brain and the spinal cord. The peripheral nervous system includes the sense organs and the nerves linking the organs, muscles, and glands to the central nervous system.

    Rationale: The nervous system is a complex network of specialized organs, tissues, and cells that coordinate the body's actions and functions. It consists of two main subdivisions: the central nervous system and the peripheral nervous system.

2. The following are all elements of the central nervous system *except*:
    a.   Brain
    b.   Spinal cord
    c.   Connective tissues associated to the brain and spinal cord
    d.   Sensory organs

    Rationale: The brain, spinal cord, and associated connective tissues are all elements of the central nervous system.

3. In the central nervous system, the brain and spinal cord receive, integrate, and interpret information, whereas in the peripheral nervous system, the cranial and spinal nerves facilitate communication between the CNS and the rest of the body.

    Rationale: CNS: The brain and spinal cord function as central processing units to receive, integrate, and interpret information, as well as to formulate a response to stimuli. PNS: Consists of cranial nerves and spinal nerves, which serve as communication lines between the CNS and the rest of the body.

4. The PNS may be subdivided into the autonomic and the somatic nervous system.

    Rationale: The autonomic nervous system facilitates automatic bodily processes. The somatic (or bodily) nervous system regulates voluntary control over skeletal muscles in response to stimuli.

5. The nervous system works closely with other anatomic systems within the body to maintain homeostatic function.

    Rationale: As an example of how the nervous system works with other body systems, it sends and receives information from the endocrine system to produce and inhibit secretion of hormones to perform a variety of bodily functions, including metabolism.

6. The myelin (e.g., myelin sheath) is a fatty-appearing insulating membrane that covers and protects nerve axons while serving as a conducting mechanism for transmission of electrical signals between nerve cells. An example of a demyelinating disease is multiple sclerosis.

    Rationale: In effect, disorders of the myelin sheath can be loosely equated to problems with electrical wire insulation. These disruptions cause multiple deleterious nervous system effects. For example, multiple sclerosis is a painful demyelinating disease that adversely affects muscle control.

7. Diplacusis is commonly known as being "tone deaf."

   a. True

   b. False

   Rationale: Diplacusis describes a cochlear dysfunction in which the patient hears a single auditory stimulus as two sounds. This condition may be colloquially described as being "tone deaf."

8. Disorders specified as "extrapyramidal" refer to the conditions affecting the areas of the brain that coordinate muscle movement.

   Rationale: Extrapyramidal disorders are so named for the complex pathways and feedback loops that lie outside the tracts of the motor cortex that extend through the pyramid-shaped regions of the medulla. Certain pyramidal pathways innervate motor neurons of the brainstem or spinal cord, whereas the extrapyramidal tracts conduct and modulate motor activity indirectly, transmitting nerve impulses to the spinal cord from the pons and medulla of the brain using motor neurons of the basal ganglia, cerebellum, and thalamus.

9. Transient ischemic attack (TIA) and related syndromes, classified to the circulatory system in ICD-9-CM, have been reclassified to the nervous system in ICD-10-CM.

   Rationale: TIA and related syndromes include basilar and carotid artery syndromes and transient global amnesia. These conditions, although vascular in origin, manifest neurological symptoms and sequelae due to the anatomy involved.

10. High intraocular pressure may be an indication of what disease?

    a. Hypotension

    b. Glaucoma

    c. Oscillopsia

    d. Madarosis

    Rationale: In glaucoma, pseudoexfoliation of the lens capsule is characterized by small, grayish particles deposited on the pupillary margin of the iris, anterior chamber, and lens. This occurs when cells within the eye release dandruff-like flakes. The outer layers of the lens slough off and block normal flow of the aqueous humor. Material deposited on the front surface of the lens in the eye may be partially rubbed off by the pupil moving over the lens. This exfoliation process may occlude the outflow track (trabecular meshwork) and cause intraocular pressure to rise.

11. Codes for ophthalmic manifestations of diabetes mellitus in ICD-9-CM depend on etiology manifestations, whereas in ICD-10-CM, they depend on combination codes.

    Rationale: ICD-10-CM effectively employs combination codes that replace etiology-manifestation coding for diabetic ophthalmic disease. The ICD-10-CM chapter 4 endocrine disease codes (E00–E88) include the causal disease (diabetes mellitus), type of disease, specific ophthalmic manifestation, and associated conditions or complications. An excludes note at the beginning of the chapter informs the coder that those conditions due to endocrine, nutritional, and metabolic diseases (E00–E88), such as diabetes mellitus, are more appropriately classified elsewhere.

12. ICD-10-CM codes have been restructured and refined to accurately reflect disease processes by reflecting advancing medical technologies and study of the patient populations. For example, in the eye and adnexa section, the term senile, which has connotations of dementia, has been replaced with the term age-related. In the ear and mastoid process chapter, central auditory processing disorder, which was classified as a developmental delay in ICD-9-CM, is reclassified as a disorder of the sense organs in ICD-10-CM.

    Rationale: ICD-10-CM code descriptions have been updated to reflect current clinical terminology and to better represent conditions as they are understood by advancing medical technologies and through study of patient populations. For example, chapter 7, "Diseases of the Eye and Adnexa," replaces the term "senile" with "age-related," where appropriate. The term "senile" has been confused with an age-related dementia, cognitive decline, or other degenerative mental health condition beyond that associated with the normal aging process. Instead, the term "age-related" associates a stated condition only with the natural aging process without implying a change in mental or cognitive status. Chapter 8, "Diseases of the Ear and Mastoid Process," includes central auditory processing disorder (ICD-9-CM 315.32), which was formerly classified as a developmental delay in chapter 5, "Mental Health Disorders." ICD-10-CM reclassified the condition to category H93 as a disorder of the sense organs. This reclassification more appropriately identifies the under-lying physiological causal factors associated with the disorder's manifestations.

13. The entire ear works as a sensory system by which sound waves are collected, amplified, and conducted to the brain for processing of the nervous impulses and to elicit a response. The three parts of the ear (the outer, middle, and inner ear) work together to achieve this goal.

    Rationale: The canals of the outer ear lead to the eardrum (middle ear). The eardrum (tympanic membrane) is attached to the ossicles, which amplify and conduct sound to the structures of the inner ear. The cochlea of the inner ear contains hair cells that vibrate when the eardrum and ossicles conduct a sound to them. The movement of these tiny hair cells transmits electrical impulses down the auditory nerve to the brain, which processes the stimuli as sound and facilitates responsive mechanisms.

14. The following are all types of cataracts *except*:

    a. Descemet's

    b. Nuclear

    c. Posterior subcapsular

    d. Cuneiform

    Rationale: Nuclear, posterior subcapsular, and cuneiform are all types of cataracts. Descemet's is actually a membrane found within the eye itself. It is the collagenous inner layer of the corneal endothelium.

15. The left side of the brain controls the motor function on the left side of the body and vice versa.

    a. True

    b. False

    Rationale: The left side of the body is controlled by the right side of the brain and vice versa.

Endocrine System

1. Where are the parathyroid glands located?
   a. Brain
   b. In the neck behind the thyroid
   c. On top of each kidney
   d. Abdomen

   Rationale: The parathyroid is located behind the thyroid gland at the front of the neck. There are four glands: a superior pair and an inferior pair.

2. The thymus gland plays a role in which of the following?
   a. Digestion
   b. Immune defenses
   c. Insulin production
   d. Sexual and reproductive function

   Rationale: Hormones produced within the thymus are known collectively as thymosins. These play a key role in the development and maintenance of immune defenses by controlling white blood cell maturation.

3. A goiter is an enlargement of what gland?
   a. Pituitary
   b. Parathyroid
   c. Thymus
   d. Thyroid

   Rationale: A goiter is described as an abnormal enlargement of the thyroid gland, commonly caused by a deficiency of dietary iodine.

4. Low blood sugar is called:
   a. Hyperglycemia
   b. Hypoglycemia
   c. Hyperparathyroidism
   d. Thyroiditis

   Rationale: Hypoglycemia is an abnormally low blood glucose level. Excessive insulin produced by the pancreas is sometimes associated with tumors or an overdose of insulin to treat diabetes.

5. What causes Cushing's disease?
   a. High blood pressure
   b. Obesity
   c. Benign tumor/hyperplasia
   d. Malignant tumor

   Rationale: Cushing's disease is specific to one cause of Cushing's syndrome, a benign tumor or hyperplasia in the pituitary gland that produces large amounts of adrenocorticotropic hormone (ACTH), which subsequently elevates cortisol.

6. Hypoparathyroidism is due to an abnormally low amount of what hormone?

    a. Follicle stimulating hormone (FSH)

    b. Parathyroid hormone (PTH)

    c. Growth hormone (GH)

    d. Thyrotropin (TSH)

    Rationale: Hypoparathyroidism is a condition in which one or more of the parathyroid glands secrete an abnormally low amount of the parathyroid hormone (PTH).

7. What part of the eye does a cataract affect?

    a. Retina

    b. Lens

    c. Choroid

    d. Sclera

    Rationale: A cataract is a clouding or opacity of the lens that prevents clear images from forming on the retina, causing vision impairment or blindness.

8. What distinguishes Type 1 diabetes from Type II?

    a. Insulin injections are always required

    b. Age of patient

    c. Glucose blood level

    d. Hypoglycemia

    Rationale: The primary factor that distinguishes Type I diabetes from Type II diabetes is the absence of naturally occurring insulin within the body. Type I diabetics require insulin injections to survive. Type II diabetics may improve their health with insulin injections, and may even come to require insulin, but the administration of insulin has no bearing on code selection for Type II diabetes, nor does the age of onset.

9. What two types of glandular tissue is the endocrine system composed of?

    a. Epithelial

    b. Connective

    c. Muscle

    d. Exocrine and endocrine

    Rationale: The endocrine system is composed of hormone-secreting cells and two different types of glandular tissue: exocrine and endocrine.

10. What is the main cause of thiamine deficiency?

    a. Malabsorption

    b. Alcoholism

    c. Diabetes

    d. Hypothyroidism

    Rationale: Alcoholism is the main cause of thiamine (vitamin B1) deficiency in the United States.

Cardiovascular System

1. In addition to supplying oxygen and nutrients to the body and carrying away carbon dioxide and other waste products, the cardiovascular system is integral to:

    a. Stabilizing body temperature

    b. Maintaining pH balance

    c. Transporting hormones

    d. All of the above

    Rationale: The primary functions of the cardiovascular system are to transport oxygen, nutrients, and hormones to the cells of the body, as well as to remove waste products, including carbon dioxide and heat. The cardiovascular system is also instrumental in regulating the body's temperature, maintaining pH balance, and regulating the cells' water content. Protective white blood cells, antibodies, complement proteins, and clotting factors circulate in the cardiovascular system and are carried to the site of an injury to protect the body when needed.

2. The tricuspid valve is found:

    a. Between the atria of the heart

    b. Between the right atrium and the right ventricle

    c. Between the ventricles of the heart

    d. Between the left atrium and the left ventricle

    Rationale: Collectively, the bicuspid and the tricuspid valves are referred to as the atrioventricular (AV) valves. The tricuspid valve is found between the right atrium and the right ventricle, and the mitral valve is between the left atrium and the left ventricle.

3. The process whereby carbon dioxide is passed from the blood to the alveoli in the lungs to be exhaled and oxygen from the air is passed from the lungs into the blood is known as:

    a. Alveolar capillary exchange

    b. Homeostasis

    c. Reoxygenation

    d. Collateral circulation

    Rationale: The layers of cells that line the alveoli and the surrounding capillaries are very thin and in close proximity to each other. It is here that carbon dioxide is passed from the blood to the alveoli to be exhaled and oxygen from the air is passed from the lungs into the blood, a process known as alveolar capillary exchange.

4. Blood in the right ventricle is:

    a. Picked up by the pulmonary circulation to be reoxygenated via the pulmonary trunk

    b. Pumped into the systemic circulation

    c. Pumped to the aorta

    d. Collected in the vena cava

    Rationale: Blood that is deficient in oxygen and laden with carbon dioxide returns to the right atrium of the heart through the superior vena cava and the inferior vena cava. The blood then goes to the right ventricle, where it is picked up by the pulmonary circulation to be reoxygenated. Blood leaves the right ventricle via the pulmonary trunk, which splits into the right and left pulmonary arteries. These branches further divide, becoming successively smaller until they become pulmonary capillaries surrounding the alveoli in the lungs.

5. The microscopic arterioles function to control blood flow into the capillary networks. Changes at this level also affect blood pressure in the following way(s):

    a. Arteriole vasodilatation decreases blood pressure

    b. Arteriole vasoconstriction increases blood pressure

    c. A and B

    d. None of the above

    Rationale: Muscular (distributing) arteries are mid-size arteries that are branches of the elastic arteries. Varying in size from the pencil-sized axillary and femoral arteries to the small, string-size arteries that carry blood to organs, the thick walls of these arteries are able to regulate blood flow with vasoconstriction and vasodilatation. Some examples of muscular arteries include the brachial and radial arteries of the arm. Branching into increasingly smaller arteries, the muscular arteries eventually branch out into the microscopic arterioles that function to control blood flow into the capillary networks. Changes at this level can impact blood pressure, with arteriole vasodilatation decreasing blood pressure and arteriole vasoconstriction increasing blood pressure.

6. Blood is supplied to the brain by the:

    a. Subclavian artery

    b. Brachiocephalic branch

    c. Ascending aorta

    d. Carotid and vertebral arteries

    Rationale: The carotid and vertebral arteries supply oxygenated blood to the brain. The carotid arteries are easily palpated under the jaw: one on the left and one on the right. At the top of the neck, the carotids bifurcate into the external and internal carotid arteries. The external carotid arteries provide blood and nutrients to the face and scalp, while the internal carotid arteries supply the anterior three-fifths of the cerebrum, with the exception of parts of the temporal and occipital lobes. The vertebral arteries course along the spinal column, joining together to create the single basilar artery (vertebrobasilar arteries) near the brain stem at the skull base. These arteries nourish the posterior two-fifths of the cerebrum, part of the cerebellum, and the brain stem.

7. Rheumatic heart disease primarily affects which area(s) of the heart:

    a. Endocardium

    b. Coronary ostia

    c. Pulmonary vein

    d. Valves

    Rationale: Acute rheumatic fever, a complication of strep pharyngitis in children, results in a variety of cardiac conditions in more than a third of patients affected. Depending on the extent of heart inflammation involved, patients with the acute form of the disease may develop heart failure, pericarditis, myocarditis, and endocarditis, which is manifested as insufficiency of the mitral (65 to 70 percent of cases) and aortic valves (25 percent of cases). Chronic disease may result in arrhythmias, ventricular dysfunction, and dilation of the atria. In adults, it is the most common cause of mitral valve stenosis and the leading cause for valvular replacement surgery. Although the mitral valve is most commonly affected, the aortic and tricuspid valves may also be involved.

8. Arteriosclerosis, also referred to as "hardening of the arteries," occurs when the arteries become narrowed due to atherosclerosis, and then become hardened by fibrous tissue and calcification. This condition can affect:

    a. Heart only

    b. Brain only

    c. Extremities only

    d. Every system in the body

    Rationale: As arteriosclerosis continues, it results in a decrease in blood and oxygen supply to the affected organ. Eventually, the plaque may cause severe or complete obstruction of the artery, causing tissue necrosis. Although this process is often associated with the heart, it may occur in any of the organs, including the brain, kidneys, intestines, eyes, and limbs.

9. Other names for unstable angina include all of the following with the exception of:

    a. Acute coronary insufficiency

    b. Prinzmetal's variant angina

    c. Preinfarction angina

    d. Intermediate syndrome

    Rationale: Other names for unstable angina include acute coronary insufficiency, preinfarction angina, and intermediate syndrome. Prinzmetal's (variant) angina is a rare form caused by vasospasm.

10. Once plaque begins to build up in an artery of the leg, the following changes take place:

    a. The flow of blood and oxygen is reduced

    b. The walls of the artery become stiff

    c. Arterial walls become unable to dilate

    d. All of the above

Rationale: The primary cause of arterial disease of the lower extremities is atherosclerosis. Once the plaque begins to build up in the artery, not only is blood flow reduced, but the arterial walls become stiffer and unable to dilate. This means the leg muscles don't receive adequate blood and oxygen when demand is increased, such as by walking and exercising.

11. Which of the following statements is false concerning aortic dissection?

    a. A dissecting aneurysm occurs when there is deterioration of the middle layer of the artery

    b. Hypertension increases and extends the damage to the damaged aorta

    c. Arteriosclerosis is not related to aortic dissection

    d. Surgery may or may not be required

    Rationale: A dissecting aneurysm occurs when the middle arterial layer (media) deteriorates (medial necrosis). Hypertension and arteriosclerosis play a role in this process, causing further damage until a rupture occurs in the innermost arterial layer, which allows blood to fill the wall of the aorta, causing separation of the layers. When the rupture extends through the outermost wall, fatal hemorrhage occurs. There are two types of aortic dissections. Type A dissection may be treated medically for a period of time with interventional catheterization or using open surgical techniques. Type B is treated medically with regular monitoring and medications that include antihypertensive and cholesterol lowering agents.

12. The single greatest risk factor for superficial venous thrombosis and DVT is:

    a. A past medical history of these conditions

    b. Varicose veins

    c. Stroke

    d. Pregnancy

    Rationale: Although the greatest single risk factor for superficial venous thrombosis and DVT is a past medical history, other risk factors include:

    *   Aging
    *   Abdominal cancer
    *   Blood coagulation disorders
    *   Extended bed rest or sitting (e.g., such as on an airplane)
    *   Heart failure
    *   Intravenous (IV) catheter usage/use of irritating medications in the IV
    *   Oral contraceptives
    *   Pregnancy
    *   Stroke
    *   Trauma
    *   Varicose veins

13. The difference between the two pressures, the systolic and the diastolic, is referred to as:

    a. Perfusion gradient

    b. Pulse pressure

    c. Ventricular differential

    d. Stroke volume

    Rationale: Blood pressure measures the force exerted against the arterial walls produced by the left ventricle during contraction (systole), and pressure that remains in the arteries when the ventricle relaxes (diastole). Blood pressure readings are measured in millimeters of mercury (mmHg) and expressed as two numbers (e.g., 120/80). Either one or both of these numbers may be too high (hypertension). The difference between the two pressures, the systolic and the diastolic, is referred to as the pulse pressure.

14. Examining the dilated retina is integral to assessing damage sustained due to hypertension because it:

    a. Allows visualization of the inner arterial and venous systems (e.g., arteriole narrowing and vessel sclerosis)

    b. Indicates systemic disease prior to the onset of symptoms

    c. Can indicate malignant and accelerating hypertension

    d. All of the above

    Rationale: Examining the dilated retina is integral to assessing damage sustained due to hypertension. Examining the retinal microvascular allows a view of the inner arterial and venous systems and detects the onset of systemic diseases before symptoms becoming evident. Manifestations of arteriosclerosis include narrowing of the arterioles and sclerosis of the vessels. Cotton wool spots and flame-shaped hemorrhages are often found in hypertensive retinopathy. Edema of the disc indicates malignant hypertension. In many instances, the retinal examination provides the first clue the patient has hypertension. A diagnosis of malignant hypertension includes the presence of papilledema, with swelling of the optic disc in the eye, caused by an increase in intracranial pressure. On the other hand, accelerated hypertension is a recent major increase over the patient's baseline blood pressure, not associated with target organ damage. Fundoscopic examination often reveals flame-shaped hemorrhages or soft exudates, but without papilledema.

15. The precerebral arteries are designated as the:

    a. Left anterior descending, circumflex, and marginal branch

    b. Carotid, subclavian, and cerebral

    c. Basilar, carotid, and vertebral arteries

    d. Vertebral, mesenteric, anterior communicating

    Rationale: The precerebral arteries are designated as the basilar, carotid, and vertebral arteries. The internal-carotid and vertebral arteries converge at the circle of Willis. It is from the circle of Willis that other arteries—the anterior cerebral artery (ACA), the middle cerebral artery (MCA), and the posterior cerebral artery (PCA)—arise and travel to all parts of the brain. The mesenteric artery is in the abdomen, and the left anterior descending, circumflex, and marginal branch are all coronary arteries.

Blood and Blood-Forming Organs

1. What are the three main functions of blood?

    a. Transportation

    b. Regulation

    c. Protection

    Rationale: Blood serves many purposes that can be divided into three main functions: transportation, regulation, protection.

2. What are the formed elements found in blood?

    a. Red blood cells

    b. White blood cells

    c. Platelets

    Rationale: There are formed elements, consisting of red blood cells, white blood cells, and platelets, and plasma, in which the formed elements "float."

3. The plasma is the liquid that suspends the formed elements.

    Rationale: There are formed elements, consisting of red blood cells, white blood cells, and platelets, and plasma, in which the formed elements "float."

4. Erythrocytes are also known as red blood cells.

    Rationale: Red blood cells, or erythrocytes, make up more than 99 percent of the formed elements.

5. The red blood cells' main function is to carry oxygen to cells and transport some carbon dioxide away.

    Rationale: Red blood cells travel throughout the body delivering oxygen and removing some of the carbon dioxide the cells release.

6. Hemoglobin is the protein responsible for the red color of blood.

    Rationale: The protein molecules, known as *hemoglobin*, are responsible for the blood's color. When the RBCs are carrying oxygen, the blood appears bright red; when the hemoglobin is de-oxygenated, the blood appears blue when viewed through blood vessel walls.

7. What are the four blood types?

    a. A

    b. B

    c. AB

    d. O

    Rationale: The blood type group is determined by identifying up to two antigens on the surface of an erythrocyte. These antigens are known as antigen A and antigen B. The absence or presence of these determine the four blood types:

    - **A:** Antigen A is present.

    - **B:** Antigen B is present.

    - **AB:** Both antigens are present.

    - **O:** Neither antigen is present.

8. Rh-negative means there are negative antigens present on the surface of the red blood cell.

   a. True

   b. False

   Rationale: Also attached to erythrocytes, there are many types of Rh antigens and if any of these are present, the blood is considered Rh-positive. If none are present, Rh-negative.

9. The main function of leukocytes is to fight infection.

   Rationale: Unlike the red blood cells, there is more than one type of white blood cell, but they all share the same basic function, to fight infection.

10. Name the three types of granulocytes.

    a. Neutrophil

    b. Eosinophils

    c. Basophils

    Rationale: There are three types of granulocytes: neutrophils, eosinophils, and basophils.

11. Most lymphocytes are stored in the body's lymphoid tissue.

    Rationale: These types of cells can live for years in the body's lymphoid tissue (e.g., lymph nodes, spleen, etc.), hence the name lymphocyte.

12. Thrombocytes are also called platelets.

    Rationale: Platelets, also known as thrombocytes, are different from the other formed elements found in the blood in that they are not cells in the strict sense, since they lack a nucleus.

13. Plasma helps maintain the Ph of the blood.

    a. True

    b. False

    Rationale: The constant adjusting of the different components of the plasma is what maintains an acceptable pH of blood.

14. Name the three steps in hemostasis.

    a. Vessel spasm

    b. Platelet plug

    c. Coagulation

    Rationale: First, the vessel induces a local spasm of its smooth-muscle lining, constricting the flow of blood to the area to allow more time for the other two responses to occur. At this point, platelets flood the area and form a platelet plug, temporarily sealing it. To form the plug, the normally smooth platelet cells begin to swell and grow spike-like processes in order to stick to other platelets and the exposed collagen fibers of the endothelial lining of the vessel. The last step, referred to as coagulation, takes more than 30 substances, called factors, to complete.

15. Three examples of foods containing vitamin B12 are meat, poultry, and dairy.

    Rationale: Dietary B12 deficiency occurs most commonly in chronic alcoholics and elderly on a "tea and toast" diet; occasionally, this does impact people with strict vegan diets as the majority of dietary B12 comes from the ingestion of meat, poultry, and dairy products.

16. Sickle cell anemia occurs only in patients who also have thalassemia.

    a. True

    b. False

    Rationale: Sickle cell can occur with or without thalassemia, depending on the patient's genetics.

17. Other than acute and chronic, what are the two main types of leukemia?

    a. Lymphocytic

    b. Myeloid

    Rationale: Most leukemias can be classified as myeloid or lymphoid, depending on the malfunctioning stem cell producing the abnormal cells. Lymphocytic leukemia evolves from the lymphoid stem cells and myeloid leukemia the myeloid cells. These can be further divided into acute and chronic types—acute developing suddenly and chronic developing over a period of time.

18. The three phases of leukemia are active, in remission, and in relapse.

    Rationale: An important factor in choosing a code for any type of leukemia in either classification system is whether the cancer is active, in remission, or in relapse. The disease is considered active when it is first discovered and is current and causing signs and symptoms. Once treatment is rendered, usually in the form of chemotherapy or induction therapy, the abnormal blood cells disappear from the blood and the disease disappears. When this occurs, the patient is considered in remission. Relapse occurs when the disease returns after the patient has achieved remission. A patient can relapse multiple times.

Lymphatic System

1. What lymphatic structure is bean-shaped and encapsulated?

   a. Lymphatic nodules

   b. Spleen

   c. Adenoids

   d. Lymph nodes

   Rationale: Lymph nodes are encapsulated, unlike lymphatic nodules. In addition, lymph nodes are bean-shaped, and lymphatic nodules do not have a singular shape.

2. What is the name of the fluid that flows through the lymphatic system?

   a. Interstitial fluid

   b. Lymph

   c. B-cells

   d. Microphages

   Rationale: Interstitial fluid enters the lymphatic vessel and becomes lymph. Lymph is the name for the fluid that flows through the lymph vessels and nodes.

3. What is the main purpose of the lymphatic system?

   a. Move fluid though the blood vessels

   b. Provide immunity to foreign substances

   c. Aid in development of leukocytes

   d. Provide nourishment to the spleen

   Rationale: The main purpose of the lymphatic system is to provide immunity to foreign substances. Although interstitial fluid enters the lymphatic system, it flows through the lymphatic vessels, not blood vessels. The lymphatic system includes the spleen, whose main purpose is to aid in immunity.

4. Where is interstitial fluid found?

   a. In the tissues at the cell level

   b. In the lymphatic trunk

   c. In the thymus vessels

   d. In lymph nodules

   Rationale: Interstitial fluid is found within the tissues at the cell level, and the lymphatic capillaries collect interstitial fluid from the tissues via a one-way structure.

5. What tissues do not contain lymphatic vessels?

    a. Cardiac

    b. Avascular

    c. Thymus

    d. Gastrointestinal

    Rationale: Avascular tissues do not have lymphatic vessels. These include cartilage, epidermis, and corneal tissue.

6. What role does the thymus play in immune response?

    a. T-cells mature within the thymus

    b. B-cells mature within the thymus

    c. Provides nutrients for the lymph nodes

    d. Both a and b

    Rationale: B-cells are not located in the thymus. T-cells mature in the thymus and learn to identify foreign matter before moving as mature T-cells into the lymph nodes, spleen, and lymphatic tissue.

7. Lymph nodes are found along the lymphatic vessels and may be solitary or in groups.

    a. True

    b. False

    Rationale: Lymph nodes are located along the lymphatic vessels and although they may be solitary, they are often grouped together or fairly close together.

8. What are the main categories of lymphatic cancer?

    a. Hodgkin's lymphoma and all other lymphomas

    b. Non-Hodgkin's lymphoma and Hodgkin's lymphoma

    c. Hodgkin's lymphoma and sarcoidosis

    d. All lymphomas are terminal

    Rationale: Lymphatic cancer is categorized as Hodgkin's lymphoma and all other lymphomas. Reticulosarcoma, lymphosarcoma, Burkitt's tumor, marginal zone lymphoma, mantle cell, large cell lymphoma, primary central nervous system, anaplastic large cell, and other variants of lymphoma are all included in the other lymphomas category.

9. What is the primary function of microphages?

    a. Ingest and destroy foreign matter

    b. Destroy immune cells

    c. Ingest and destroy dead tissue and cells

    d. Both a and c

    Rationale: Microphages are small phagocytes that ingest foreign matter and other small things like dead tissue and cells.

10. What organ contains red and white pulp?

    a. Adenoids

    b. Thymus

    c. Spleen

    d. Peyer's patches

    Rationale: The spleen contains red and white pulp. The red pulp consists of splenic cords or tissue that contains microphages, lymphocytes, red blood cells, plasma cells, and granulocytes. The white pulp contains lymphatic tissue with lymphocytes and microphages.

11. What is hyposplenism?

    a. A reduction in the size of the spleen

    b. A reduction in spleen function

    c. An increase in spleen function

    d. An increase in the size of the spleen

    Rationale: "Hypo" is the root word meaning low or deficient. In this case, hyposplenism describes a reduction in spleen function.

12. Localized enlarged lymph nodes typically involve 1 area(s) of the body, whereas generalized enlarged lymph nodes typically involve 2 or more area(s) of the body.

    Rationale: Although not official guidelines, these are the common guidelines followed when assigning localized versus generalized lymphadenopathy codes.

13. What additional information do coders need to report infectious mononucleosis in ICD-10-CM?

    a. Type of virus, such as gammaherpesviral mononucleosis or cytomegaloviral mononucleosis

    b. Whether the patient incurred complications

    c. Both a and b

    d. None of the above

    Rationale: In ICD-10-CM, the type of virus and whether the patient incurred complications are both important factors when coding infectious mononucleosis.

14. Match the types of follicular lymphoma grades with the types of cells involved:

    a. Grade I   <u>d</u>   Centrocytes are still present

    b. Grade II   <u>a</u>   < 5 centroblasts per high power field

    c. Grade III   <u>c</u>   > 15 centroblasts per high power field

    d. Grade IIIa   <u>e</u>   Follicles consist almost entirely of centroblasts

    e. Grade IIIb   <u>b</u>   6–15 centroblasts per high power field

    Rationale: Although there is some controversy over the grading system, the World Health Organization recommends the following:

    • Grade I: < 5 centroblasts per high power field

    • Grade II: 6–15 centroblasts per high power field

    • Grade III: > 15 centroblasts per high power field

    – grade IIIa: centrocytes are still present

    – grade IIIb: follicles consist almost entirely of centroblasts

15. Immune reconstitution syndrome is limited to HIV-positive patients.

    a. True

    b. False

    Rationale: Immune reconstitution syndrome can affect any patient who has been immunocompromised.

Respiratory System

1. What is the function of cilia?

   a. They prompt the sneezing reaction

   b. They have no known function

   c. They trap particles entering with air and prevent them from entering further into the respiratory system

   d. They are the first step in the body's immune response system

   Rationale: Within the nose there are hairs, or cilia, that catch germs and other particles inhaled with air. However, cilia do not catch all germs, which is why infections can occur within the bronchial tubes and lungs.

2. Which structure is included in the upper respiratory tract?

   a. Diaphragm

   b. Alveoli

   c. Pharynx

   d. Lung

   Rationale: The upper respiratory tract contains the nose, pharynx, and larynx. The lower respiratory tract contains the trachea, bronchial tree, and the lungs.

3. What is the primary function that occurs within the lungs?

   a. Oxygen and carbon dioxide exchange

   b. Fluid waste expulsion

   c. Involuntary muscle contraction

   d. Absorption of dust particles

   Rationale: The air moves into the lungs and bronchial tubes, reaching the alveoli, which transport the oxygen to the capillaries where hemoglobin helps it flow into the bloodstream. As the oxygen is absorbed, the carbon dioxide is also extracted from the capillaries into the alveoli to be exhaled as a waste gas. Gas exchange that takes place within the lungs is referred to as external respiration, and exchange taking place within body tissues is referred to as internal respiration.

4. The trachea is commonly referred to as:

   a. Larynx

   b. Pharynx

   c. Esophagus

   d. Windpipe

   Rationale: The trachea, or windpipe, begins at the larynx and splits into two bronchi branches within the chest: the left and right primary bronchi. The trachea is 12 centimeters in length and 2½ centimeters wide and is made up of C-shaped rings of cartilage within the smooth muscle.

5. How many bronchial tubes branch off into the lungs?

    a. One

    b. Two

    c. Three

    d. Four

    Rationale: The bronchial tubes are part of the respiratory structure connecting the lungs to the trachea, allowing for air exchange within the lungs. The trachea, or windpipe, begins at the larynx and splits into two bronchi branches within the chest: the left and right primary bronchi. The right bronchus enters the right lung and is shorter and wider than the left. The left bronchus enters the left lung. Once the bronchi enter the lungs, they split into secondary bronchi, one for each lobe within the lung.

6. Where is the carina located?

    a. In the lungs

    b. In the sinuses

    c. In the diaphragm

    d. In the trachea

    Rationale: The carina is the area where the division in the trachea leads to the right and left bronchi and is made up of the last of the tracheal cartilage. The membrane in this area is the most sensitive to foreign matter and primarily responsible for the reflex to expel any irritants.

7. How many lobes are in the left lung?

    a. Two

    b. Three

    c. One

    d. Five

    Rationale: The left lung contains two lobes while the right lung contains three. This is due to the placement of the heart within the thoracic cavity, leaving the left lung somewhat smaller than the right lung. The right lung is thicker and wider than the left lung, but it is shorter than the left since the diaphragm is slightly higher on the right side due to the position of the liver.

8. What is aspergillosis?

    a. A virus

    b. An injury

    c. A genetic disorder

    d. A fungal infection

    Rationale: Aspergillosis is a fungal infection that typically does not affect people with a normal immune system. The fungus grows in stored grain, compost, and other vegetation during the decay process. This condition presents as pneumonia or a fungal growth where there was a previous lung disorder such as tuberculosis or a lung abscess.

9. What physiological changes occur in emphysema?

    a. Deterioration of the bronchioles

    b. A pH imbalance

    c. Fluid accumulation within the lungs

    d. None of the above

    Rationale: Emphysema is considered a factor in chronic obstructive pulmonary disease (COPD). This condition restricts the air flow during exhalation because of gradual deterioration of the bronchioles. This air restriction causes difficulty in breathing. As this condition progresses, the spherical air sacs within the lungs become irregular and contain holes, reducing not only the number of air sacs but also the amount of oxygen that can circulate into the blood from the lungs. As the air sacs deteriorate, the openings collapse, trapping air within the lungs.

10. What structures are responsible for speech?

    a. Vocal cords

    b. Pharynx

    c. .Sinuses

    d. All of the above

    Rationale: Ligaments within the vocal cords stretch into the airway, which constricts the glottis. When air hits this area, vibrations produce sound. To create understandable speech, the pharynx, mouth, nasal cavity, and sinuses provide a type of echo chamber.

11. Which body part houses the adenoids?

    a. Sinuses

    b. Nasopharynx

    c. Oropharynx

    d. Mouth

    Rationale: The back wall of the nasopharynx is where the adenoids are positioned. The oropharynx is the middle portion of the pharynx at the back of the mouth, starting at the soft palate and running to the hyoid bone. The palatine and lingual tonsils are within the oropharynx.

12. What is the common name of the disease caused by the *Bordetella pertussis* bacteria?

    a. Strep throat

    b. Asthma

    c. Ascariasis

    d. Whooping cough

    Rationale: Whooping cough is a common symptom/condition associated with pneumonia called pertussis, named after the bacterium *Bordetella pertussis* that is the cause. Before widespread vaccination for these bacteria began in the 1940s, whooping cough killed 5,000 to 10,000 people in the United States every year. With vaccination, that number has dropped to fewer than 30 per year. Parapertussis is similar to whooping cough in etiology and symptoms and can occur at any age, although it typically affects children ages 3 to 5 years. Parapertussis occurs less frequently than pertussis and has a shorter duration as well. Vaccination against whooping cough does not provide immunity to parapertussis, and most people recover completely. Complications due to this infection are extremely rare.

13. What is the cure for pneumoconiosis?

    a. Removal of irritant causing the symptoms

    b. Antibiotics

    c. There is no cure

    d. Rest and plenty of fluids

    Rationale: Pneumoconiosis is due to the inhalation of dust particles typically associated with occupations that require regular exposure to mineral dusts. This condition is a form of interstitial lung disease that contributes to the inflammation of the air sacs, causing the lung tissue to harden. There is no cure for this disease, and treatment focuses on managing the patient's symptoms.

14. What is one of the major complications of a pulmonary contusion?

    a. There are none, a contusion is a superficial injury

    b. Fluid accumulation within the alveoli

    c. High mortality rate

    d. A life-long, chronic lung condition

    Rationale: A contusion is a superficial injury, often a bruise, resulting from trauma without a break in the skin. However, even this kind of injury can have serious complications when the contusion affects the respiratory system, particularly the lungs. A pulmonary contusion affects the lung tissue itself, leading to fluid and blood accumulation within the alveoli of the lung. About 20 percent of blunt chest injury cases also report pulmonary contusions. In some cases, crackling noises can be heard in the chest through a stethoscope. If the contusion is left undiagnosed, complications such as atelectasis, pneumonia, and respiratory failure may occur. Once diagnosed, most lung contusions resolve in less than a week with fluid restriction and careful observation. Larger contusions may require more extensive treatment like oxygen or mechanical ventilation.

15. How can a physician differentiate a pleural friction rub from a pericardial rub?

    a. By a chest x-ray

    b. Grating sounds within the chest

    c. Absence of irregular sounds when the patient holds his or her breath

    d. Indicated by whether or not patient has chest pain

    Rationale: Pleural friction rub causes low, grating sounds heard when pleural surfaces rub against each other. This may be confused with a pericardial rub, so cessation of the sound when the patient holds his or her breath would indicate pleural friction rub. When the lungs are affected by SLE, symptoms include chest pain when breathing deeply, coughing up blood, and shortness of breath. A physician may hear a pleural friction rub when the patient is examined, and a chest x-ray may show pleuritis or pleurisy.

Digestive System

1. The digestive system consists *only* of the mouth, pharynx, esophagus, small intestine, large intestine, and anus.

   a. True

   b. False

   Rationale: The digestive system consists of an alimentary canal and several accessory organs.

2. What are some examples of the digestive system accessory organs?

   a. Pancreas, liver, gallbladder

   b. Spleen, tonsils, lymph nodes

   c. Esophagus, stomach, large intestine

   d. All of the above

   Rationale: The accessory organs of the digestive system include teeth, tongue, salivary glands, liver, gallbladder, and pancreas.

3. What are the wave-like movements of a tubular structure, where alternate contraction and relaxation occurs and the contents of the tube are propelled forward, an example of?

   a. Rhythm method

   b. Peristalsis

   c. Wave current

   d. Body wave locomotion

   Rationale: Peristalsis is the movement of a tubular structure, characterized by waves of alternate circular contraction and relaxation of the tube by which contents are propelled forward.

4. The secretion of pancreatic juices aid the digestive process by breaking down which substances?

   a. Carbohydrates

   b. Proteins and Fats

   c. Nucleic Acids

   d. All of the above

   Rationale: The pancreas plays an important part in digestion by secreting pancreatic juice. Pancreatic juice contains enzymes that digest carbohydrates, fats, proteins, and nucleic acids.

5. The cause of edentulism is no longer significant when selecting the appropriate code in ICD-10-CM.

   a. True

   b. False

   Rationale: Coders still need to identify the cause of edentulism when selecting codes in ICD-10-CM.

6. What additional details need to be documented to accurately code sialoadenitis?

    a. The presence of any obstructions

    b. Any additional complications

    c. Whether the disease is acute, chronic, or recurrent

    d. None of the above

    Rationale: To code this disease accurately in ICD-10-CM, coders need to know if the disease is acute, acute recurrent, chronic, or unspecified.

7. What condition is now included in codes for alcoholic hepatitis and cirrhosis of the liver?

    a. Abscess

    b. AIDS

    c. Ascites

    d. Aggression

    Rationale: In ICD-10-CM, coding for alcoholic hepatitis and cirrhosis has been further specified as occurring with or without ascites.

8. Peliosis hepatitis is one of the several conditions that were included in the code for unspecified hepatitis in ICD-9-CM, but will now have its own code in ICD-10-CM.

    a. True

    b. False

    Rationale: Conditions such as toxic liver disease, nonalcoholic steatohepatitis, and peliosis hepatitis have been expanded in ICD-10-CM to have their own code.

9. What are some of the causal conditions of acute/chronic pancreatitis that are now important to know when coding pancreatitis?

    a. Drug/alcohol-induced pancreatitis

    b. Iron deficiency pancreatitis

    c. Dysplastic pancreatitis

    d. None of the above

    Rationale: Some of the causal conditions of pancreatitis that are included in the codes for the disease in ICD-10-CM are cytolomegaloviral pancreatitis, idiopathic pancreatitis, biliary pancreatitis, alcohol-induced pancreatitis, and drug-induced pancreatitis.

10. What is the major physiological difference between coding for Barrett's esophagus in ICD-9-CM as opposed to ICD-10-CM?

    a. Coders need to determine if dysplasia is present and identify the grade

    b. Coders need to identify the root cause of the condition

    c. Coders need to identify if esophagitis is present

    d. All of the above

    Rationale: In addition to coding the Barrett's esophagus, coders now have to look for details on the presence of dysplasia and understand how the grades of dysplasia will be documented.

11. What clinical concept from ICD-9-CM will no longer be required in ICD-10-CM for proper code selection of the various types of gastric ulcers?

    a. With or without hemorrhage

    b. With or without obstruction

    c. With or without perforation

    d. All of the above

    Rationale: Coders no longer need to identify whether an obstruction is present. The only two complications of ulcers included in the code descriptions for ICD-10-CM are hemorrhage and perforation.

12. What new clinical concepts must be considered when coding in ICD-10-CM for diverticular disease?

    a. With or without abscess/perforation

    b. With or without hemorrhage

    c. With or without obstruction

    d. All of the above

    Rationale: When coding for diverticular disease in ICD-10-CM, coders need also to look for documentation on whether there is a perforation or abscess. In ICD-9-CM, the only distinguishing factor is whether a hemorrhage is present.

13. What complications of Crohn's disease are identified by the sixth character of the codes?

    a. Rectal bleeding

    b. Intestinal obstruction

    c. Fistula or abscess

    d. All of the above

    Rationale: Coding for Crohn's disease and its complications in ICD-10-CM depends on selecting the appropriate fifth and sixth characters. The fifth character 0 (zero) indicates that there are no complications. The fifth character 1 indicates that there are complications—coders need to identify the complications such as rectal bleeding, intestinal obstructions, fistulas, or abscess.

14. The ICD-9-CM code category regional enteritis has been renamed Crohn's disease in ICD-10-CM.

    a. True

    b. False

    Rationale: ICD-9-CM category 555 Regional enteritis currently maps to ICD-10-CM category K50 Crohn's disease.

15. Why is it important that coders pay close attention to the specific location of the stomal malfunction/complication in ICD-10-CM?

    a. Complications occur only in certain parts of the intestine

    b. The specific part of the intestine determines which codes to use

    c. Colostomy and enterostomy complications are no longer included in the same code category

    d. Both B and C

    Rationale: In ICD-9-CM, colostomy and enterostomy complications are grouped together under category 569.6. In ICD-10-CM, these have been split into two separate categories. Coders need to pay close attention to the specific part of the intestine experiencing the complication to determine if it is a colostomy or enterostomy complication.

16. What is an inflammation of the meninges due to *Salmonella typhi* or associated with typhoid fever?

    a. Typhoid pneumonia

    b. Typhoid arthritis

    c. Typhoid osteomyelitis

    d. Typhoid meningitis

    Rationale: Meningitis is an inflammation of the meninges. Inflammation documented as being due to *Salmonella typhi* or with typhoid fever is considered typhoid meningitis.

17. Intestinal trichomoniasis is classified as a protozoal intestinal disease in ICD-10-CM.

    a. True

    b. False

    Rationale: In ICD-10-CM, the condition intestinal trichomoniasis is classified as a protozoal intestinal disease along with other protozoal intestinal diseases like microsporidiosis, sarcocystosis, and sarcosporidiosis.

Urinary System

1. Name the six organs of the urinary system.

   a. Two kidneys, two ureters, one bladder, and one urethra

   b. Two kidneys, two ureters, and two sphincter muscles

   c. Two kidneys, two sphincter muscles, and two urethras

   d. Two kidneys, two ureters, and two urethras

   Rationale: The urinary system is a collection of various organs, tubes, muscles, and nerves whose function is to create, store, and transport urine out of the body. It comprises two kidneys, two ureters, the bladder, two sphincter muscles, and the urethra.

2. What is the primary function of the urinary system?

   a. Create, store, and transport urine

   b. Promote absorption ofnutrients

   c. Regulate blood volume and pH

   d. Excrete hormones

   Rationale: The urinary system, in conjunction with the lungs, skin, and intestines, excretes waste and keeps chemicals and water in the body in balance. Specifically, the urinary system removes urea from the blood. Urea is generated when foods containing proteins (meat, poultry, some vegetables) break down in the body.

3. Approximately how many nephrons does each kidney have?

   a. 100,000

   b. 500,000

   c. 1,000,000

   d. More than 1,000,000

   Rationale: Blood comes into the kidneys by way of arteries that branch within the kidneys into small clusters of looping blood vessels. These clusters are called glomeruli, the tiny units in the kidney where blood is cleaned. Approximately 1 million glomeruli (filters) are in each kidney.

4. What is the functional unit of the kidney?

   a. Medulla

   b. Calices

   c. Nephron

   d. Glomerulus

   Rationale: Every glomerulus and tubule unit combined is called a nephron, or the functional unit of the kidneys.

5. The kidneys:

    a. Help regulate blood volume

    b. Help control blood pressure

    c. Help control pH

    d. All of the above

    Rationale: The kidneys perform other necessary functions, including regulating blood ionic composition, blood pH, blood pressure, and blood glucose level, and aiding in the production of three important hormones (erythropoietin [EPO], renin, and calcitriol).

6. What organ in the urinary system is the reservoir for urine?

    a. Kidneys

    b. Bladder

    c. Renal pelvis

    d. Ureters

    Rationale: The urinary bladder is a triangular or pear-shaped, expandable hollow organ located in the pelvic area, held in place by ligaments that bind to the pelvic bones. It is the organ in the urinary system that stores urine and allows urination to be infrequent and voluntary. The urinary bladder muscles relax in order to allow urine to enter from the ureters and contract to excrete urine from the body by way of the urethra. Layers of muscle tissue stretch to house urine with a capacity of 400 to 600 mL being considered normal.

7. What drains urine from the kidneys to the ureters?

    a. Sphincter muscles

    b. Nephrons

    c. Urethra

    d. Renal pelvis

    Rationale: Once the urine is formed, it passes through the nephrons and down the renal tubules of the kidney and is subsequently funneled from the renal pelvis, the area at the center of the kidney, into the ureters, which then transport the urine to the bladder.

8. The ureters are tube-shaped structures about _____ to_____ long and connect the kidneys to the bladder.

    a. 24–30 inches

    b. 10–20 inches

    c. 15–24 inches

    d. 8–10 inches

    Rationale: The ureters are tube-shaped structures approximately 8 to 10 inches long that connect the kidney to the urinary bladder.

9. What is the capacity of an adult bladder?

    a. 400–500 mL

    b. 100–300 mL

    c. 700–900 mL

    d. Greater than 1,000 mL

    Rationale: In the average healthy adult, approximately two cups, or 400 to 500 mL, of urine can be stored in the bladder for approximately two to five hours.

10. All of the following belong in the urinary system, except:

    a. Bladder

    b. Prostate

    c. Ureters

    d. Urethra

    Rationale: The urinary system comprises two kidneys, two ureters, the bladder, two sphincter muscles, and the urethra.

Male Reproductive System

1. Which organs make up the external male reproductive system?

   a. Penis, prostate, and scrotum

   b. Penis, scrotum, and testicles

   c. Penis, testicles, and vas deferens

   d. Penis, seminal vesicles, and scrotum

   Rationale: Three primary organs make up the external male reproductive system: the penis, scrotum, and testicles (testes).

2. Which is not considered an internal accessory organ of the male reproductive system?

   a. Bulbourethral gland

   b. Ejaculatory duct

   c. Epididymis

   d. Testicle

   Rationale: The male reproductive system consists of internal organs, also referred to as accessory organs, that include the epididymis, vas deferens, ejaculatory ducts, urethra, seminal vesicles, prostate gland, and the bulbourethral glands.

3. What are the three hormones primarily involved in the regulation of the male reproductive system?

   a. FSH, LH, and testosterone

   b. FSH, TSH, and LH

   c. TSH, LH, and testosterone

   d. ADH, LH, and testosterone

   Rationale: Hormones primarily involved in the regulation of the male reproductive system include follicle-stimulating hormone (FSH), luteinizing hormone (LH), and testosterone.

4. How many ejaculatory ducts are in the male reproductive system?

   a. Four

   b. Three

   c. Two

   d. One

   Rationale: There are two ejaculatory ducts, approximately 2 cm in length, formed by the fusing of the vas deferens and the seminal vesicles. The ducts begin at the base of the prostate, running both forward and downward between the middle and lateral lobes, as well as along the sides of the prostatic utricle and ending just within the utricle margins, diminishing in size as they do so.

5. What is phimosis?

    a. Abnormal enlargement of the scrotal veins

    b. Constriction or tightening of the prepuce or foreskin

    c. Urological emergency requiring immediate treatment

    d. Condition that describes a total absence of sperm in the ejaculate fluid

    Rationale: Phimosis is a constriction, or tightening, of the prepuce (foreskin). In this condition, the foreskin contracts and is not able to be retracted or pulled back behind the glans or tip of the penis.

6. What organ in the male reproductive system controls the temperature of the testes to ensure normal sperm development?

    a. Epididymis

    b. Vas deferens

    c. Scrotum

    d. Bulbourethral gland

    Rationale: The main function of the scrotum is to control the temperature of the testes to that of slightly lower-than-normal body temperature in order to ensure healthy sperm development. The scrotum wall contains special muscles that contract and relax, thereby allowing the testicles to move closer to the body as necessary for warmth or further away in order to cool the temperature back down.

7. What organ has the task of ejaculating semen upon orgasm?

    a. Ejaculatory duct

    b. Prostate

    c. Seminal vesicle

    d. Urethra

    Rationale: As discussed in the urinary chapter, the tube that carries urine from the bladder is called the urethra. In males, the urethra has the additional responsibility of ejaculating semen upon orgasm. During intercourse, the penis is erect and the flow of urine is blocked from the urethra, thereby permitting only the release of semen upon orgasm.

8. Which organ is described as small, pea-sized, and yellow in color?

    a. Bulbourethral gland

    b. Seminal vesicle

    c. Vas deferens

    d. Epididymis

    Rationale: Bulbourethral glands, also known as Cowper's glands, are small, pea-sized, yellowish colored, lobular-like bodies located behind and to the sides of the urethra, below the prostate gland.

9. What condition describes a burning or aching type of pain coming from the area of the prostate?

    a. Prostatosis syndrome

    b. Proctalgia

    c. Oligospermia

    d. Prostatodynia syndrome

    Rationale: Prostatodynia syndrome describes a deep burning or aching type of pain that appears to originate from the prostate.

10. Which organ makes testosterone and generates sperm?

    a. Testes

    b. Prostate

    c. Scrotum

    d. Vas deferens

    Rationale: The last of the external male sex organs are the testicles (testes), which make the primary male sex hormone, testosterone, and generate sperm. Most men have two testes. The testicles are oval in shape and approximately the size of large olives, protected at either end by the spermatic cord.

Female Reproductive System

1. Which organs make up the external female reproductive system?

    a. Labia majora, labia minora, vagina, and clitoris

    b. Labia majora, labia minor, clitoris, and Bartholin's glands

    c. Bartholin's glands, clitoris, vagina, and uterus

    d. Vagina, clitoris, ovaries, and labia majora

    Rationale: The female reproductive system comprises external and internal structures. External structures include the labia majora, labia minora, Bartholin's glands, and the clitoris. These organs allow sperm to enter the body, as well as to safeguard the internal genital organs from infection.

2. Which is not an internal organ of the female reproductive system?

    a. Vagina

    b. Ovaries

    c. Fallopian tubes

    d. Bartholin's glands

    Rationale: The internal female reproductive organs include the vagina, uterus, ovaries, and fallopian tubes.

3. What are the four hormones involved in the regulation of the female reproductive system?

    a. FSH, LH, estrogen, and progesterone

    b. FSH, TSH, LH, and estrogen

    c. TSH, LH, estrogen, and progesterone

    d. TSH, LDH, testosterone, and progesterone

    Rationale: During the follicular phase, two of the four major hormones involved in the menstrual cycle are released, follicle stimulating hormone (FSH) and luteinizing hormone (LH). These two hormones activate the production of estrogen, a third hormone involved in the menstrual cycle. In the third phase of the cycle, after release of the egg, the corpus luteum emits the hormones estrogen and progesterone. As the fourth hormone in the menstrual cycle, progesterone prepares the uterus for the possibility of receiving a fertilized egg to implant. Progesterone and estrogen stimulate the endometrium (lining of the uterus) to thicken, filling it with fluids and nutrients necessary to nourish the fetus.

4. How many lobes are in each female breast?

    a. 5–10

    b. 10–15

    c. 15–20

    d. Greater than 20

    Rationale: Approximately 15 to 20 lobes are in each breast, emanating from the nipple and areolar area, that appear to be arranged in a wheel-spoke pattern.

5. What is dysplasia?

    a. Twisting of ovarian artery and vein

    b. Abnormal changes in cells

    c. A gynecological emergency requiring immediate treatment

    d. Bleeding into the fallopian tubes

    Rationale: Dysplasia describes abnormal changes in the cells found on the surface of the vagina. It is categorized by three stages: mild, moderate, and severe.

6. What organ in the female reproductive system is also referred to as the birth canal?

    a. Uterus

    b. Ovary

    c. Vagina

    d. Cervix

    Rationale: The vagina, often referred to as the birth canal, is a passageway that adjoins the lower part of the uterus, called the cervix, to the outside of the body.

7. Which disorder is considered the fifth most common gynecological emergency condition?

    a. Torsion of the fallopian tube

    b. Moderate dysplasia

    c. Vulvovaginitis

    d. Torsion of the ovary

    Rationale: As the fifth most common gynecologic emergency, torsion, or twisting of the ovary, affects females of all age ranges.

8. Which organ is described as pear-shaped and hollow?

    a. Uterus

    b. Fallopian tube

    c. Vagina

    d. Bartholin's glands

    Rationale: The hollow, pear-shaped organ, which houses the fetus during development, is called the uterus. It has two parts: the cervix or lower portion, and the corpus or main body. Naturally, the corpus is designed to expand to accommodate a developing baby. The cervix contains a channel that permits sperm to enter and menstrual blood to exit when fertilization does not occur.

9. What common condition affecting the female reproductive system causes swelling, itching, and burning in the vagina, as well as an abnormal discharge from bacteria related to a variety of different kinds of germs?

    a. Dysplasia

    b. Acquired atrophy

    c. Acute salpingitis

    d. Vaginitis

    Rationale: Vaginitis is a condition that encompasses symptoms such as swelling, itching, and burning in the vagina, often accompanied by an abnormal discharge that can be caused by several different kinds of germs.

10. Name the phases of the menstrual cycle.

    a. Follicular, ovulation, and luteal

    b. Follicular, luteal, and pregnancy

    c. Ovulation, luteal, and menstruation

    d. Follicular, ovulation, and menstruation

    Rationale: The menstrual cycle is the process by which a woman's body prepares for the possibility of pregnancy. The term "menstru" means monthly; hence the word menstruation describes the monthly shedding of the uterine lining. On average, a menstrual cycle is 28 days long and takes place in three phases: follicular phase, ovulation, and the luteal phase.

Pregnancy, Childbirth, and the Puerperium

1. What does the seventh character for multiple gestations indicate?

    a. The specific fetal anomaly affecting the fetus

    b. The identity of the affected fetus

    c. The episode of care

    d. None of the above

    Rationale: A seventh-character extension for multiple gestations in categories that designate maternal care for a fetal anomaly, damage, or other problem is required in order to indicate the affected fetus.

2. What is afibrinogenemia?

    a. A type of spontaneous abortion

    b. A protein required to stop bleeding

    c. An abnormal attachment by the placenta to the uterine wall

    d. A rare, inherited blood disorder

    Rationale: Afibrinogenemia is an uncommon, inherited blood disorder that affects the blood's ability to clot by causing a serious deficiency in fibrinogen, a protein produced by the liver. This protein is required to stop bleeding by forming clots.

3. What degree of blood loss is considered a severe postpartum hemorrhage?

    a. 1,000 ml

    b. 500 ml

    c. 1,500 ml

    d. Between 500 and 1,000 ml

    Rationale: A postpartum hemorrhage is defined as a blood loss of greater than 500 ml after the birth of a baby, and a severe postpartum hemorrhage constitutes blood loss of more than 1,000 ml after delivery.

4. What is the third stage of labor?

    a. The period of time just before delivery

    b. The period of time immediately following delivery

    c. The period of time between the birth and expulsion of the placenta

    d. The period of time after expulsion of the placenta

    Rationale: The third stage of labor is the period of time between the birth of the baby and the expulsion of the placenta. It is during this time frame when the uterine muscles contract downward and the placenta begins to separate from the uterine walls.

5. What condition is defined as the premature removal of the products of conception from the uterus?

   a. Placenta increta

   b. Spontaneous abortion

   c. Placenta percreta

   d. Legally induced abortion

Rationale: A spontaneous abortion is defined as the premature expulsion or removal of the products of conception from the uterus.

6. What is disseminated intravascular coagulation (DIC)?

   a. A type of gestational diabetes

   b. A postpartum hemorrhage

   c. A serious disorder where proteins that control blood clotting become abnormally active

   d. An uncommon, inherited blood disorder that affects the blood's ability to clot by causing a serious deficiency in fibrinogen, a protein produced by the liver

Rationale: Disseminated intravascular coagulation (DIC) is a serious disorder in which the proteins that control blood clotting become abnormally active.

7. What condition is defined as the intentional expulsion of the products of conception by a medical professional?

   a. Spontaneous abortion

   b. Placenta percreta

   c. Afibrinogenemia

   d. Legally induced abortion

Rationale: A legally induced abortion is the intentional expulsion of the products of conception from the uterus performed by a medical professional within the boundaries of the law. This often occurs by the patient's choice (elective), through a court order or other mandated action (legal), or for reasons such as the mother's health or life is at risk (therapeutic).

8. What are the three subclassifications under gestational diabetes?

   a. Diet controlled, insulin controlled, and unspecified

   b. Pregnancy, childbirth, and the puerperium

   c. First, second, and third trimester

   d. Antepartum, delivered, and postpartum

Rationale: Codes classified to category O24.4 Gestational diabetes mellitus, have three subcategories: O24.41 Gestational diabetes in pregnancy, O24.42 Gestational diabetes in childbirth, and O24.43 Gestational diabetes in the puerperium. Under each subcategory, there are three subclassifications denoted by characters 0, 4, or 9, indicating whether the gestational diabetes is diet controlled, insulin controlled, or unspecified, respectively.

About The Technical Editors

Jillian Harrington, MHA, CPC, CPC-P, CPC-I, CCS-P, MHP,
Clinical/Technical Editor
Ms. Harrington has more than 19 years of experience in the health care profession. She recently served as President and CEO of ComplyCode, a health care compliance consulting firm based in Binghamton, NY. She is the former Chief Compliance Officer and Chief Privacy Official of a large academic medical center, and also has extensive background in both the professional and technical components of CPT/HCPCS and ICD-9-CM coding. She teaches CPT coding and is an approved instructor of the Professional Medical Coding Curriculum, awarded by the American Academy of Professional Coders (AAPC). She has spoken frequently on health care compliance and health information management issues at regional and national professional conferences. Ms. Harrington holds a Bachelor of Science degree in Health Care Administration from Empire State College and a Master of Science degree in Health Systems Administration from the Rochester Institute of Technology. She is a member of AAPC and a former member of its National Advisory Board, a member of the American Health Information Management Association (AHIMA) and the Health Care Compliance Association (HCCA), and is an associate of the American College of Healthcare Executives (ACHE).

Kristin Bentley, BS, CPC, *Clinical/Technical Editor*
Ms. Bentley has 10 years of experience in the health care profession. She has an extensive background in professional component coding, with expertise in radiation therapy, chemotherapy, radiology, and ambulatory surgery procedure coding. She has conducted chart-to-claim audits and physician education. Ms. Bentley has functioned as a billing specialist and has extensive denial management experience. She is an active member of the American Academy of Professional Coders.

Kelly V. Canter, BA, RHIT, CCS, *Clinical/Technical Editor*
Ms. Canter has expertise in hospital inpatient and outpatient coding and reimbursement; ambulatory surgery coding; and ICD-9-CM, CPT, and HCPCS coding. Ms. Canter's experience includes conducting coding audits and coding staff education, revenue cycle management, and concurrent review. Most recently she was responsible for auditing and compliance of a health information management services company. She is an active member of the American Health Information Management Association (AHIMA).

Beth Ford, RHIT, CCS, *Clinical/Technical Editor*
Ms. Ford has extensive background in both physician and facility ICD-9-CM and CPT/HCPCS coding. Ms. Ford has served as a coding specialist, coding manager, coding trainer/educator and coding consultant, as well as a health information management director. She is an active member of the American Health Information Management Association (AHIMA).

Deborah C. Hall, *Clinical/Technical Editor*
Ms. Hall is a new product subject matter expert for OptumInsight. Ms. Hall has more than 25 years of experience in the health care field. Her experience includes 10 years as office manager for large multi-specialty medical practices. Ms. Hall has written several multi-specialty newsletters and coding and reimbursement manuals, and served as a health care consultant. She has taught seminars on CPT/HCPCS and ICD-9-CM coding and physician fee schedules. She is an active member of the American Academy of Professional Coders.

Karen H. Kachur, RN, CPC, *Clinical/Technical Editor*

Ms. Kachur has expertise in CPT/HCPCS and ICD-9-CM coding, in addition to physician billing, compliance, and fraud and abuse. Prior to joining Ingenix, she worked for many years as a staff RN in a variety of clinical settings including medicine, surgery, intensive care, and psychiatry. In addition to her clinical background, Ms. Kachur served as assistant director of a hospital utilization management and quality assurance department and has extensive experience as a nurse reviewer for Blue Cross/Blue Shield. She is an active member of the American Academy of Professional Coders and the American College of Medical Coding Specialists.

Temeka Lewis, MBA, CCS, *Clinical/Technical Editor*

Ms. Lewis has expertise in hospital and physician coding, including ICD-9-CM, CPT, and HCPCS coding. Ms Lewis' past experience includes conducting coding audits and physician education, teaching ICD-9-CM and CPT coding, functioning as a member of a revenue cycle team, chargemaster maintenance, and writing compliance newsletters. Most recently she was responsible for coding and compliance in a specialty hospital. She is an active member of the American Health Information Management Association (AHIMA).

Nannette Orme, CCS-P, CPC, CPMA, CEMC, *Clinical/Technical Editor*

Ms. Orme has more than 15 years of experience in the health care profession. She has extensive background in CPT/HCPCS and ICD-9-CM coding. Her prior experience includes physician clinics and health care consulting. Her areas of expertise include physician audits and education, compliance and HIPAA legislation, litigation support for Medicare self-disclosure cases, hospital chargemaster maintenance, workers' compensation, and emergency department coding. Ms. Orme has presented at national professional conferences and contributed articles for several professional publications. She is a member of the American Academy of Professional Coders.

Karen M. Prescott, CMM, CPC, CPC-I, CCS-P, *Clinical/Technical Editor*

Ms. Prescott has more than 16 years of experience in the health care profession. She has an extensive background in professional component coding and billing. Her prior experience includes establishing and maintaining a coding and billing service, directing physician practice start ups, functioning as director of physician credentialing, negotiating insurance contracts, and functioning as a health care consultant. Her areas of expertise include coding and reimbursement, documentation education, compliance, practice management, and revenue cycle management. Ms. Prescott is a member of the American Academy of Professional Coders, the American Health Information Management Association (AHIMA), and the Professional Association of Health Care Office Management (PAHCOM).

Nichole VanHorn, CPC, CCS-P, *Clinical/Technical Editor*

Ms. VanHorn has more than 15 years of experience in the health care profession. Her areas of expertise include CPT and ICD-9-CM coding in multiple specialties, auditing, and education. Most recently she served as Clinical Auditor for the Children's Hospital Physicians at Blank Children's Hospital, Des Moines, Iowa where she functioned as an auditor for a multi-specialty group. Ms. VanHorn was responsible for the oversight of the physician coding and education section of the Corporate Compliance Program. She has been an active member of her local American Academy of Professional Coders chapter for several years and served as an officer.